Applied Veterinary Anatomy

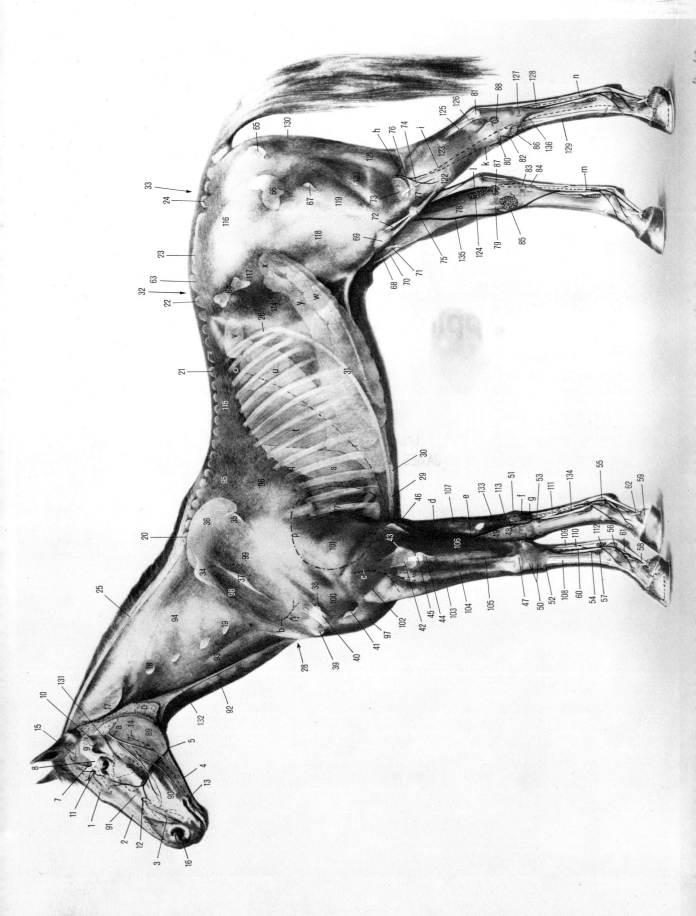

Plate I. SURFACE ANATOMY OF THE HORSE

SKELETON, JOINTS, AND LIGAMENTS

Head. 1, frontal sinus; 2, nasal bone; 3, incisive bone; 4, mandible; 5, vascular groove for facial vessels and parotid duct; 6, facial crest and maxillary sinus; 7, temporal line; 8, zygomatic proc.; 9, zygomatic arch; 10, temporomandibular joint; 11, supraorbital for. and n.; 12, infraorbital for. and n.; 13, mental for. and n.; 14, mandibular for. and inferior alveolar n. on the med. side of the mandible; 15, scutiform cartilage; 16, alar cartilage.

Neck and Trunk. 17, wing of atlas; 18, transverse proc. of C3; 19, transverse proc. of C6; 20, spine of T4; 21, spine of L1; 22, spine of L6; 23, spines of sacrum; 24, spine of Cd1; 25, lig. nuchae; 26, rib 18; 27, rib 5; 28, manubrium sterni; 29, sternum; 30, xiphoid proc.; 31, costal arch; 32, lumbosacral space; 33, space between Cd1 and Cd2.

Forelimb. 34, 35, cran. and caud. angles of scapula; 36, scapular cartilage; 37, scapular spine; 38, 39, caud. and cran. parts of the greater tubercle of humerus; 40, tendon of infraspinatus; 41, deltoid tuberosity; 42, lat. supracondyloid crest; 43, lat. epicondyle; 44, head of radius; 45, lat. collat. lig. of elbow; 46, olecranon; 47, styloid proc. of ulna; 48, styloid proc. of radius; 49, subcut. surface of radius; 50, prox. and distal rows of carpal bones; 51, accessory carpal bone; 52, metacarpal tuberosity; 53, 54, prox. and distal extremities of splint bones; 55, sesamoid bones; 56, prox. collat. tubercle of P I; 57, pouch of fetlock joint capsule; 58, prox. collat. tubercle of P II; 59, cartilage of hoof; 60, interosseus; 61, oblique sesamoid lig.; 62, lig. from P I to cartilage of hoof.

Hind Limb. 63, tuber sacrale; 64, tuber coxae; 65, tuber ischiadicum; 66, greater trochanter; 67, third trochanter; 68, med. ridge of femoral trochlea; 69, patella; 70, intermediate; 71, med.; 72, lat. patellar ligaments; 73, lat. epicondyle of femur; 74, lat. condyle of tibia and head of fibula; 75, tibial tuberosity; 76, lat. collat. lig. of stifle; 77, extensor groove of tibia; 78, subcut. surface of tibia; 79, 80, med. and lat. malleoli; 81, tuber calcanei; 82, lat. ridge of trochlea of talus, 83, second tarsal bone; 84, splint bone; 85, med. dorsal; 86, lat. dorsal; 87, med. plantar; 88, lat. plantar pouches of the tarsocrural joint capsule.

MUSCLES, TENDONS, AND TENDON SHEATHS

89, masseter; 90, buccinator; 91, levator labii; 92, sternocephalicus; 93, brachiocephalicus; 94, splenius; 95, trapezius thoracis; 96, latissimus dorsi; 97, supf. pectoral and biceps brachii; 98, supraspinatus; 99, infraspinatus; 100, deltoideus; 101, triceps; 102, lower border of lat. head of triceps (line crosses brachialis); 103, ext. carpi radialis; 104, common dig. ext.; 105, lat. dig. ext.; 106, ulnaris lateralis; 107, flexor carpi ulnaris; 108, common and lat. dig. ext. tendons; 109, supf. dig. flexor tendon; 110, deep dig. flexor tendon; 111, deep flexor accessory lig.; 112, prox. pouch of dig. sheath; 113, prox. pouch of the carpal sheath of flexor tendons; 114, flank; 115, longissimus thoracis; 116, glutei; 117, tensor fasciae latae; 118, quadriceps femoris, 119, 120, 121, cran. middle, and caud. parts of biceps femoris; 122, long dig. ext.; 123, deep dig. flexor; between 122, and 123, lat. dig. ext.; 124, deep flexor sheath; 125, gastrocnemius tendon; 126, supf. dig. flexor tendon; 127, 128, supf. and deep flexor tendons; 129, common tendon of long and lat. ext.; 130, semitendinosus.

BLOOD VESSELS

131, transverse facial a.; 132, external jugular v.; 133, cephalic v.; 134, med. palmar a.; 135, med. saphenous v.; 136, dorsal metatarsal a.

NERVES

a, facial; b, suprascapular; c, radial; d, ulnar; e, median; f, lat. palmar; g, med. palmar; h, common peroneal; i, deep peroneal; k, supf. peroneal; l, tibial; m, med. plantar; n, lat. plantar.

INTERNAL ORGANS

o, parotid gland; p, heart; q, dome of diaphragm; r, basal border of lung; s, left lobe of liver; t, stomach; u, spleen; v, left kidney; w, left ventral colon; x, pelvic flexure; y, left dorsal colon.

(From E. Seiferle, Angewandte Anatomie am Lebenden. Schweizer Arch. Tierhlk. 94 (1952):280–286.)

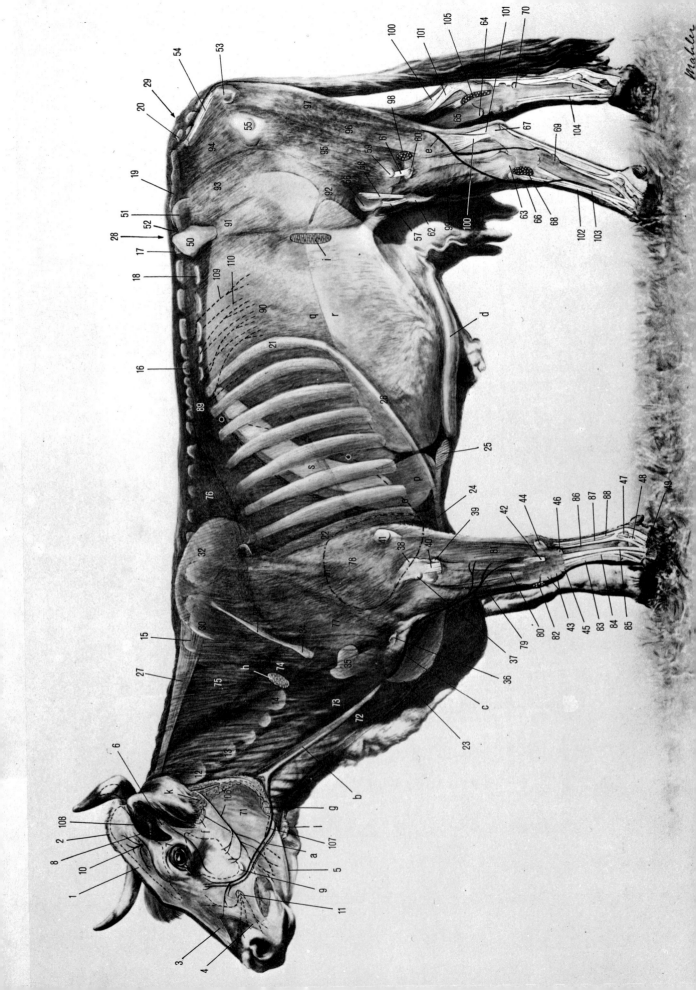

Plate II. SURFACE ANATOMY OF THE COW

SKELETON, JOINTS, AND LIGAMENTS

Head: 1, outline of frontal sinuses; 2, intercornual protuberance; 3, nasal bone; 4, incisive bone; 5, mandible; 6, zygomatic arch; 7, zygomatic proc.; 8, temporal line; 6, 7, and 8 bound the temporal fossa; 9, facial tuberosity and outline of maxillary sinus; 10, supraorbital for. and frontal v. (see Fig. 5–3), 11, infraorbital for. and n.

Neck and Trunk. 12, wing of atlas; 13, transverse proc. of C3; 14, transverse proc. of C6; 15, spine of T1, covered by expansion of lig. nuchae; 16, spine of L1; 17, spine of L6; 18, transverse proc. of L5; 19, crest of sacrum; 20, spine of Cd1; 21, rib 13; 22, rib 6; 23, manubrium sterni; 24, sternum; 25, xiphoid proc.; 26, costal arch; 27, lig. nuchae; 28, lumbosacral space; 29, point for epidural anesthesia.

Forelimb. 30, 31, cran. and caud. angles of scapula; 32, scapular cartilage; 33, scapular spine; 34, acromion; 35, greater tubercle of humerus; 36, deltoid tuberosity; 37, cran. part of lat. epicondyle; 38, caud. part of lat. epicondyle; 39, head of radius; 40, lat. collat. lig. of elbow; 41, olecranon; 42, styloid proc. of ulna; 43, prox. and distal rows of carpal bones; 44, accessory carpal bone; 45, metacarpal tuberosity; 46, lat. prominence of metacarpal bone; 47, sesamoid bone; 48, prox. collat. tubercle of P I; 49, prox. collat. tubercle of P II.

Hind Limb. 50, tuber coxae; 51, tuber sacrale; 52, iliac crest; 53, tuber ischiadicum; 54, sacrotuberous lig.; 55, greater trochanter; 56, patella; 57, 58, intermediate and lat. patellar lig.; 59, lat. epicondyle of femur; 60, lat. condyle of tibia; 61, lat. collat. lig. of stifle; 62, tibial tuberosity; 63, malleolar bone; 64, med. malleolus; 65, subcut. surface of tibia; 66, med. ridge of distal trochlea of talus; 67, tuber calcanei; 68, lat. pouch of the tarsocrural joint sac; 69, 70, lat. and med. prominences of metatarsal bone.

MUSCLES, TENDONS, TENDON SHEATHS, AND BURSAE

71, masseter; 72, sternocephalicus; 73, brachiocephalicus; 74, omotransversarius; 75, trapezius cervicis; 76, trapezius thoracis; 77, deltoideus; 78, triceps; 79, ext. carpi radialis; 80, common dig. ext.; 81, ulnaris lateralis; 82, subcut. carpal bursa; 83, med. dig. ext. tendon; 84, common dig. ext. tendon; 85, lat. ext. tendon; 86, interosseus; 87, 88, deep and supf. dig. flexor tendons; 89, longissimus thoracis; 90, flank; 91, tensor fasciae latae; 92, quadriceps femoris; 93, gluteus medius; 94, vertebral head of biceps femoris; 95, 96, cran. and caud. parts of biceps; 97, semitendinosus; 98, femorotibial joint sac; 99, flexors of hock and extensors of digits; 100, gastrocnemius tendon; 101, supf. flexor tendon; 102, long dig. ext. tendon; 103, lat. dig. ext. tendon; 104, med. dig. ext. tendon; 105, deep dig. flexor sheath.

NERVES

106, dorsal buccal; 107, ventral buccal; 108, cornual; 109, 110, dorsal and ventral branches of L2 (closer to the tip of the fourth transverse process).

BLOOD VESSELS AND LYMPH NODES

a, facial vessels; b, external jugular v.; c, cephalic v.; d, subcut. abdominal (milk) v.; e, lat. saphenous v.; f, parotid ln.; g, mandibular ln.; h, supf. cervical ln.; i, subiliac ln.

INTERNAL ORGANS

k, parotid gland; l, mandibular gland; m, heart; n, dome of the diaphragm; o, basal border of lung; p, reticulum; q, r, dorsal and ventral sacs of rumen; s, spleen.

(From E. Seiferle, Angewandte Anatomie am Lebenden. Schweizer Arch. Tierhlk. 94 (1952): 280–286)

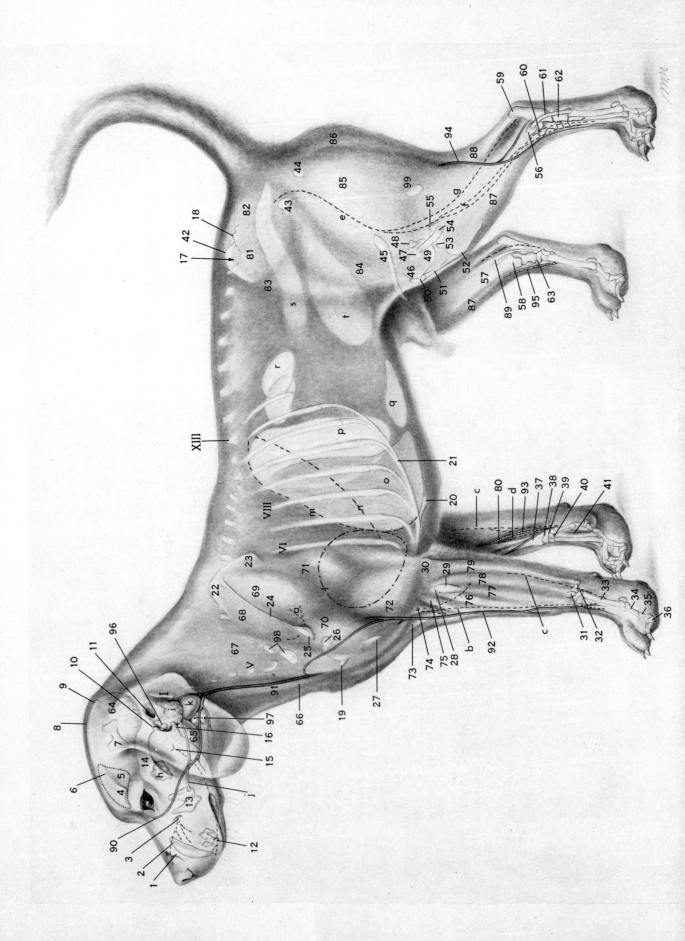

Plate III. SURFACE ANATOMY OF THE DOG

SKELETON, JOINTS, AND LIGAMENTS

Head. 1, incisive bone; 2, root of canine tooth; 3, infraorbital for. and n.; 4, zygomatic proc.; 5, frontal sinus; 6, temporal line; 7, scutiform cartilage; 8, external sagittal crest; 9, external occipital protuberance; 10, temporomandibular joint; 11, external acoustic meatus; 12, mental for. and n. on the mandible ventral to premolars 1 and 2; 13, premolar 4; 14, zygomatic arch; 15, mandibular for. and inferior alveolar n. on the med. side of ramus of mandible; 16, angular proc. of mandible.

Neck and Trunk. I, wing of atlas; V, transverse proc. of C5; VI, rib 6; VIII, rib 8; XIII, spine of T13; 17, lumbosacral space; 18, crest of sacrum; 19, manubrium sterni; 20, xiphoid proc.; 21, costal arch.

Forelimb. 22, cran. angle of scapula; 23, caud. angle of scapula; 24, spine of scapula; 25, acromion; 26, greater tubercle of humerus; 27, deltoid tuberosity; 28, lat. epicondyle of humerus; 29, lat. collat. lig. of elbow; 30, olecranon; 31, styloid proc. of ulna; 32, accessory carpal bone; 33, 5th metacarpal bone; 34, P I; 35, P II; 36, P III; 37, subcut. surface of radius; 38, radiocarpal joint; 39, midcarpal joint; 40, carpometacarpal joint; 41, 2nd metacarpal bone.

Hind Limb. 42, cran. dorsal iliac spine; 43, trochanter major; 44, tuber ischiadicum; 45, os penis; 46, femoral trochlea; 47, epicondyle of femur; 48, sesamoid bone of gastrocnemius; 49, lat. condyle of femur; 50, patella; 51, patellar lig.; 52, tibial tuberosity; 53, lat. condyle of tibia; 54, lat. collat. lig. of stifle; 55, head of fibula; 56, lat. malleolus; 57, subcut. surface of tibia; 58, med. malleolus; 59, tuber calcanei; 60, trochlea tali; 61, lat. collat. lig.; 62, 4th tarsal bone; 63, central tarsal bone.

MUSCLES AND TENDONS

64, temporalis; 65, masseter; 66, sternocephalicus; 67, brachiocephalicus; 68, supraspinatus; 69, infraspinatus; 70, deltoideus; 71, triceps, long head; 72, triceps, lat. head; 73, biceps brachii; 74, brachialis; 75, ext. carpi radialis; 76, ext. dig. communis; 77, ext. dig. lat.; 78, ulnaris lat.; 79, flexor carpi ulnaris; 80, flexor carpi radialis; 81, gluteus med.; 82, gluteus supf.; 83, sartorius; 84, quadriceps femoris; 85, biceps femoris; 86, semitendinosus; 87, tibialis cranialis; 88, gastrocnemius; 89, deep flexor tendon.

BLOOD VESSELS AND LYMPH NODES

90, v. angularis oculi; 91, external jugular v.; 92, cephalic v.; 93, median a.; 94, lat. saphenous v.; 95, a. dorsalis pedis; 96, parotid ln.; 97, mandibular ln.; 98, supf. cervical ln.; 99, popliteal ln.

NERVES

a, suprascapular; b, supf. branch of radial; c, ulnar; d, median; e, sciatic; f, peroneal; g, tibial.

INTERNAL ORGANS

h, zygomatic gland; i, parotid gland; j, parotid duct; k, mandibular gland; l, heart (radiograph); m, diaphragm (radiograph); n, basal border of lung (percussion); o, liver (percussion); p, stomach (radiograph), 24-hour fast, barium meal); q, spleen (radiographic section of ventral end); r, left kidney (radiograph); s, descending colon (radiograph); t, bladder (radiograph).

Applied Veterinary Anatomy

Alexander de Lahunta, D.V.M., Ph.D.

Professor of Anatomy
Chairman, Department of Clinical Sciences
New York State College of Veterinary Medicine
Cornell University, Ithaca, New York

Robert E. Habel, D.V.M., M.Sc., M.V.D.

Professor of Veterinary Anatomy, Emeritus
New York State College of Veterinary Medicine
Cornell University, Ithaca, New York

W. B. Saunders Company

A Division of Harcourt Brace & Company

Philadelphia   London   Toronto
Montreal   Sydney   Tokyo

W.B. SAUNDERS COMPANY
A Division of
Harcourt Brace & Company

The Curtis Center
Independence Square West
Philadelphia, PA 19106

Listed here is the latest translated edition of this book together with
the language of the translation and the publisher.

Spanish *(1st Edition)*—Nueva Editorial Interamericana S.A. Mexico D.F., Mexico

Library of Congress Cataloging in Publication Data

De Lahunta, Alexander, 1932–
    Applied veterinary anatomy.

    Includes index.
    1. Veterinary anatomy.   I. Habel, Robert Earl,
1918–   II. Title.
SF761.D42   1986   636.089'1   85–8379
ISBN 0-7216-1431-0

Designer: Bill Donnelly
Production Manager: Laura Tarves
Manuscript Editor: Susan Colaiezzi-Short
Illustration Coordinator: Walt Verbitski
Page Layout Artist: Patti Maddaloni

Applied Veterinary Anatomy   ISBN 0-7216-1431-0

Last digit is the print number: 9   8   7   6   5   4

PREFACE

This book is a revision and expansion of a laboratory guide published first in 1948 and last as the fifth edition in 1965. The material added in 1973 in the first edition of this title consisted of many illustrations and the information formerly given in lectures. It is intended for a two-semester course in the third year of the veterinary curriculum, but may also be useful to the practitioner. The purpose of the course is to develop the ability to reason from an anatomical basis in the solution of clinical problems and to give actual practice in the recognition of the anatomical features that form the groundwork of surgical, diagnostic, medical, obstetrical, and post-mortem procedures.

The application of anatomy to the practice of veterinary medicine is completely dependent upon a thorough understanding of the fundamentals of anatomy, beginning with the development, and including the microscopic and neuroanatomy as well as the gross anatomy of domestic animals. This book leans heavily upon the standard textbooks and dissection guides used in our system of instruction: H.E. Evans and G.C. Christensen: *Miller's Anatomy of the Dog,* 2nd ed., Philadelphia: Saunders, 1979; H.E. Evans and A. de Lahunta: *Miller's Guide to the Dissection of the Dog,* 2nd ed., Philadelphia: Saunders, 1980; R. Getty: *Sisson and Grossman's the Anatomy of the Domestic Animals,* 5th ed., Philadelphia: Saunders, 1975; A. Schummer, R. Nickel, and W.O. Sack: *The Viscera of Domestic Mammals,* 2nd ed., New York: Springer, 1979; A. Schummer, H. Wilkens, B. Vollmerhaus, and K.H. Habermehl: *The Circulatory System, the Skin, and the Cutaneous Organs of the Domestic Mammals,* New York: Springer, 1981; W.O. Sack and R.E. Habel: *Rooney's Guide to the Dissection of the Horse,* revised reprint, Ithaca, N.Y.: Veterinary Textbooks, 1982; R.E. Habel: *Guide to the Dissection of Domestic Ruminants,* 3rd ed., Ithaca, N.Y.: R.E. Habel, 1977; and A. de Lahunta: *Veterinary Neuroanatomy and Clinical Neurology,* 2nd ed., Philadelphia: Saunders, 1983.

The material for the course was assembled by searching the clinical literature in a continuous reviewing process for applications of anatomy. The resulting notes were organized by regions and verified by reference to the anatomical literature, dissections, radiographs, and the living animals.

The course has always been taught in accordance with the autotutorial principles of active learning. Each chapter or topographic region may be regarded as a ''minicourse'' and need not be taken in the sequence of the book, but may be correlated with surgical exercises or instruction in physical diagnosis.

We are indebted to the late Professor Eugen Seiferle of the University of Zurich for permission to use the plates showing the surface anatomy of the horse and cow. These, together with a similar illustration of the dog, have been placed in the front of the book, and references to them have been inserted throughout the text. We wish to acknowledge the important contribution of the artists, Pat Barrow Wallace, Marion E. Newson, Lewis L. Sadler, W.P. Hamilton, IV, and Michael A. Simmons. Dr. H.P.A. de Boom taught the course in 1975–76 and compiled a valuable detailed critique, which was carefully considered in the revision of 1978. We also wish to thank the staffs of the clinics and the departments of physiology and pathology for their help in providing live animals for the class work and dissection material for the demonstrations. We shall be grateful for further criticism and suggestions.

ALEXANDER DE LAHUNTA

ROBERT E. HABEL

CONTENTS

INTRODUCTION

The nomenclature used in this laboratory guide consists of English translations of the terms in *Nomina Anatomica Veterinaria* (N.A.V.), 3rd ed., 1983. A few general principles of the nomenclature will be explained here, and the details will be incorporated in appropriate lessons. The World Association of Veterinary Anatomists has adopted the principle that the nomenclature should be applicable to all animals and their embryos and that homologous parts should have the same name in all species. This means that all terms of position and direction must refer to parts of the animal's body itself and not to the supporting surface or to the direction in which the animal faces (Fig. 1). For example, cranial and caudal are preferred to anterior and posterior for reference to the trunk because anterior means ventral in the standing man and cranial in the standing dog. A more extreme example of the confusion introduced into comparative anatomy by the use of standard positions is in the nomenclature of the forepaw and hand. In the human standard anatomical position, the palm is turned forward. In the canine standing position, the palm is turned backward. Therefore the anterior surface of the human hand is the opposite of that of the paw. The veterinary anatomist uses the terms dorsal and palmar, which do not change in meaning, regardless of species or position. The following terms refer to position and direction (Fig. 1).

Median. Refers to the median plane, which divides the body, including the head and tail, into right and left halves. The term has been also applied to a plane dividing a limb longitudinally into halves, as in naming the median artery, vein, and nerve.

Sagittal. A plane parallel to the median plane.

Transverse. Refers to a plane perpendicular to the long axis of the body or part.

Medial. The direction toward the median plane; of two structures, the one closer to the median plane.

Lateral. The direction away from the median plane; of two structures, the one farther from the median plane.

Intermediate. Designates the position between a medial and a lateral structure; for example, in the cow and horse there are medial, intermediate, and lateral patellar ligaments.

Cranial, Caudal. When used as terms of direction, these adjectives are employed on the neck and trunk and on the limbs proximal to the carpus and tarsus. The term caudal is also used on the head.

Middle. Refers to a structure between two other structures that are cranial and caudal, dorsal and ventral, superficial and deep, external and internal, or proximal and distal.

Anterior, Posterior, Superior, Inferior. These terms cannot be generally applied in comparative medicine because they refer to a standard anatomical position that is different in man and quadrupeds. The use of these terms is limited in veterinary anatomy to certain structures on the head, where no confusion with human nomenclature can arise.

Rostral. Toward, or nearer to, the tip of the nose. This term is used only on the head, where "cranial" would be ambiguous. The antonym is "caudal."

Dorsal. Refers to the back or dorsum of the tail, trunk, neck, and the corresponding surface of the head. It also refers to the back of the hand (manus: carpus, metacarpus, and digits) and to the corresponding surface of the foot (pes: tarsus, metatarsus, and digits). A dorsal plane is one parallel to the dorsal surface of the body or part. It is perpendicular to the median and transverse

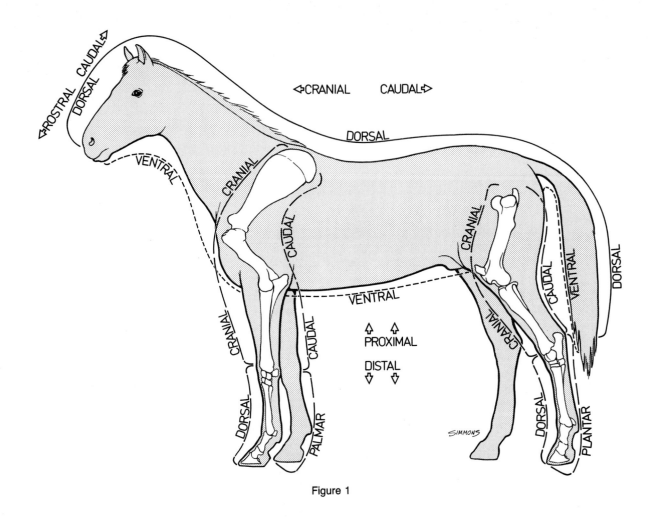

Figure 1

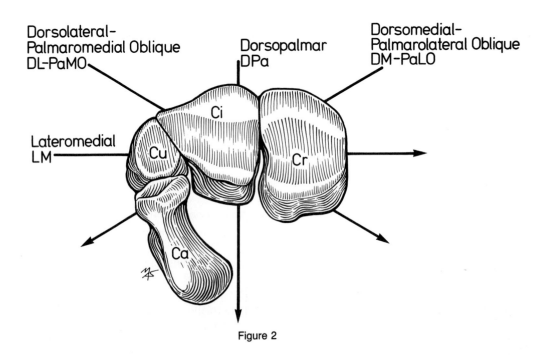

Dorsolateral-
Palmaromedial Oblique
DL-PaMO

Dorsopalmar
DPa

Dorsomedial-
Palmarolateral Oblique
DM-PaLO

Lateromedial
LM

Ci

Cu

Cr

Ca

Figure 2

planes. The term frontal, referring to the plane of the human forehead, is not applicable to quadrupeds.

Ventral. Refers to the direction toward the belly—the opposite of dorsal. It has nothing to do with the plane of support and should not be thought of as the underside. It is used on the tail, trunk, neck, and head but never on the limbs.

Internal, External. Used only in reference to the walls of hollow organs or body cavities.

Proximal. As used on the limbs, nearer to the trunk; applied to vessels and nerves, nearer to the heart or to the central nervous system.

Distal. The opposite of proximal.

Axial, Abaxial. It is convenient to use these terms on the digits of species in which the functional axis of the limb passes between the third and fourth digits, as in artiodactyls and carnivores. For example the axial palmar nerve of the third digit is the same as the lateral proper palmar nerve of the third digit, but the use of the term lateral in this situation is confusing. (See also the description of the attachments of the cruciate ligaments to the femoral condyles.)

Palmar, Plantar. Refer to the surface opposite the dorsum of the manus or pes, respectively. The term volar is no longer used because it referred either to the hollow of the hand or the hollow of the sole of the foot.

Anatomical terms for the designation of radiographic views have historically differed considerably from accepted anatomical terms. Attempts have been made to reconcile these differences and are still in progress.[2] In keeping with the goal to use only the directional terms that are accepted anatomical nomenclature published in the *Nomina Anatomica Veterinaria,* the following principles will be adhered to in this book:

1. All radiographic views are described by the direction in which the central x-ray penetrates the body part, from point of entrance to point of exit where the radiographic film is exposed (Fig. 2).

2. Combined terms will be used to accurately describe oblique designations, with a hyphen between the point of entrance and the point of exit. In some instances, the degrees of angle of obliquity will be inserted in the combined term for the point of entrance.

To conclude this general discussion of the principles of nomenclature, we wish to make it clear that terminology is not the substance of anatomy. Form, structure, relationships, and function are the significant characteristics. The name is only a short substitute for the description. The description is always an acceptable, and sometimes a preferable, substitute for the name.

In the appendix of this book there are lists of the ossification centers for the horse and the dog and cat accompanied by the approximate age at which growth plate closure is observed on radiographs.

References

1. Habel, R. E., J. Frewein, and W. O. Sack (eds.): Nomina Anatomica Veterinaria. 3rd ed., Ithaca, N.Y.: International Committee on Veterinary Gross Anatomical Nomenclature, 1983.

2. Smallwood, J. E., M. J. Shively, V. T. Rendano, and R. E. Habel: A standardized nomenclature for radiographic projections used in veterinary medicine. Vet. Radiol. 26(1985):2–9.

CHAPTER 1

TEETH

OBJECTIVES

1. To be able to identify any tooth in the mouth of a domestic animal by name, number, and dentition. It is essential to be able to tell deciduous from permanent teeth.
2. To be able to identify the three hard tissues of a tooth and to understand their arrangement in the complex crown of the tooth of a herbivore.
3. To be able to estimate within 6 months the age of a horse, ox, sheep, cat, or dog during the period of eruption of the permanent teeth.
4. To be able to estimate the age from the wear of the permanent teeth up to 17 years in the horse and 9 years in the ox.
5. To understand that eruption and wear are subject to biological variation and should never under any circumstances, and especially not in a lawsuit, be made the basis for a statement of the actual age of a particular animal. The tables contain only averages. An acceptable statement is: The teeth of this horse are like those of an average 2-year-old.
6. To know the number of roots of the premolars and molars in the dog and cat. This is useful in order to avoid unnecessary difficulty in extraction.
7. To recognize the radiographic features of the teeth in all species and to distinguish permanent and incisor teeth in young dogs and cats.

The only way to age an animal accurately is to know its date of birth. Without this knowledge, various features of the animal's growth may be used to estimate the age. The most practical on physical examination are the eruption and wear of teeth; eruption is considerably more reliable.

The estimation of the age of ungulates by the teeth is usually based on the lower incisors and canines. The eruption of the premolars and molars is a more accurate indication of age but is seldom considered. The periods of eruption given here for large animals are from *Sisson and Grossman's The Anatomy of the Domestic Animals*.[5]

After the permanent teeth are in wear, the estimation of age becomes highly speculative. The various systems that have been devised do not agree, and the actual age of the individual may not be indicated by the amount of wear of the teeth. Often the ages are rounded for easy memorization. An estimate of age should always be cautiously phrased. One should never say that the animal is X years old but that it has the teeth of an average animal of X years.

Note on the Nomenclature: Of the domestic animals, only the pig has a full dentition, which is expressed by the formula:

$$2(I\frac{3}{3}\ C\frac{1}{1}\ P\frac{4}{4}\ M\frac{3}{3}) = 44$$

In applying the dental formula to other species in which several teeth are missing, one must distinguish between molars and premolars. These are the cheek teeth, which are behind the canines. Molars are the caudal group and have no deciduous predecessors. Premolars are the cheek teeth rostral to the molars, and all except P 1 replace deciduous premolars. When the number of molars is reduced, the congenitally absent teeth are the most caudal ones. Missing premolars are the most rostral. The evolutionary instability of P 1 is shown by the following: it is not replaced, it does not appear at all in the ruminants or in the cat, and it erupts in the horse, in the upper jaw only, as the vestigial wolf tooth. Thus each cheek tooth retains its comparative anatomical designation in spite of the reduction in the number of teeth in different species. The most rostral cheek tooth in ruminants is P 2. In carnivores the reference points are the sectorial teeth, which are always P 4 above and M 1 below, regardless of the number of cheek teeth that fail to develop. Beginning at the midline, the permanent incisors are designated I 1, I 2, I 3. Deciduous incisors are Di 1, Di 2, Di 3.

Special terms of direction are used in dentistry to refer to the borders, or contact surfaces, of the teeth. On the first incisor the mesial surface is next to the median plane; on all other teeth it is directed toward the first incisor. The opposite contact surface is the distal surface.

Brachydont teeth are short or low-crowned teeth that have a distinct crown, neck, and root(s) and stop growing after eruption. These include all the teeth of the dog, cat, and pig (except the pig's canines) and the incisors and canines of ruminants. Hypsodont teeth have a large crown called the body and small late-forming root(s). These teeth continue to grow for a variable number of years after birth, which accounts for their unique pattern of wear and for the clinical problems that occur when the wear is abnormal. Hypsodont teeth include the cheek teeth of ruminants, the pig's canine tusks, and all the teeth of horses, except P 1.

1a. INCISORS, HORSE

The dental formulae are:

$$2(Di\frac{3}{3}\ Dc\frac{0}{0}\ Dp\frac{3}{3}) = 24 \qquad 2(I\frac{3}{3}\ C\frac{1}{1}\ P\frac{3-4}{3}\ M\frac{3}{3}) = 40\text{–}42$$

Estimate the ages of the specimens. The signs of age are discussed first in order of usefulness, then they are employed to describe the teeth at various ages. Reference is to lower teeth unless otherwise indicated. Changes in the upper incisors occur later, but their evaluation greatly increases the difficulty of the examination without a corresponding improvement in accuracy.[4]

The most valuable criterion for estimating age is eruption, the tooth breaking through the gum. It is necessary at this time to be able to tell deciduous from permanent teeth. Deciduous teeth are smaller, have a constricted neck, show many fine longitudinal grooves on the labial surface, and, at the time of replacement, are well worn (see Fig. 1–3). At eruption the permanent teeth are covered by yellow cement, whereas the remaining deciduous teeth are white, the cement having been

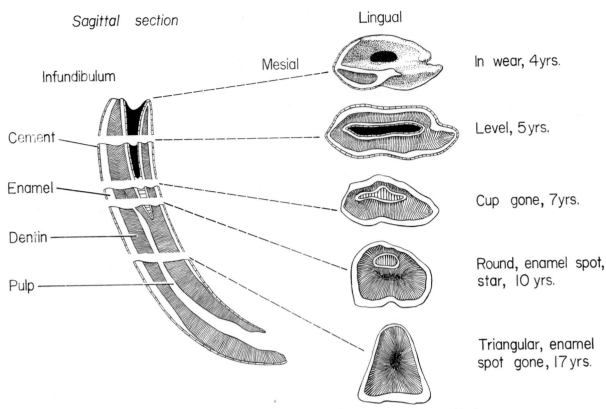

Figure 1–1. Sagittal section and occlusal surfaces of an equine second incisor.

worn off the enamel. Permanent incisors have one large central groove on the labial surface. During the period of eruption, it is only necessary to part the lips and determine which permanent incisors have erupted. The best results will be attained with minimum disturbance of the animal. After eruption, it takes about 6 months for the tooth to grow out far enough to be in wear. When the preliminary examination reveals that all of the permanent lower incisors are in wear, the mouth must be opened far enough to see the occlusal surfaces and to evaluate the degree of wear. Even then strong-arm measures such as seizure of the tongue should be avoided. The horse can usually be induced to display the worn surfaces of the lower incisors if the examiner grasps the upper lip and lower jaw and inserts a finger into the diastema.

The changes caused by wear of the occlusal surface are shown in Figure 1–1 and are brought into relation with the anatomy of the tooth. Notice that the infundibular enamel is continuous with the outer enamel when the tooth first erupts. When the crest where they meet is worn off, the dentin is exposed. The bottom of the infundibulum contains cement, so that when the infundibulum is worn down to that level it no longer has a cup to hold black decaying feed. Only the enamel spot is left. Because the pulp cavity is on the labial side of the infundibulum, the dental star formed by the closure of the pulp cavity is in the same relation to the enamel spot.

The wearing process begins on the mesiolabial side of the occlusal surface. When the entire surface is in wear, the outer and inner enamel rings are completely separated by yellow dentin, and the tooth is said to be level. Evidence derived from the eruption and leveling of the teeth should be given more weight than the signs discussed subsequently.

The disappearance of the black cavity or cup in the infundibulum is often used to estimate age. This sign is not reliable because it depends upon the depth of the enamel infundibulum and the amount of cement in the bottom, both of which are variable. The cups are supposed to disappear from lower I 1, I 2, and I 3 at 6, 7, and 8 years, but this sign should be disregarded if it is not in agreement with the leveling of the teeth. For example, if the cup is gone from I 1, but I 3 is not yet in wear, the age is probably less than 5 years—not 6 years (see Fig. 1–3). The cup often persists in I 3 in horses older than 8 years.

After the cup has disappeared, the bottom of the infundibulum remains, first as a long oval containing cement, then as a small round spot of enamel near the lingual side of the tooth. Disappearance of the enamel spot varies from 13 to 16 years (see Fig. 1–4).[12]

The dental star is the darker dentin that fills the pulp cavity as the tooth wears. It appears first as a dark yellow transverse line in the dentin on the labial side of the infundibulum of lower I 1 at 8 years. As the enamel spot recedes toward the lingual side, the dental star becomes oval and moves to the middle of the occlusal surface. It reaches this position in all the lower incisors when the animal is about 13 years old. At 15 years the dental stars are round. The star should not be confused with the enamel spot, which wears more slowly than the dentin and therefore remains elevated.

The shape of the occlusal surface changes as the tooth is worn down. It is at first oval, with the long diameter extending from side to side. Then the lingual border becomes much more strongly curved, the two diameters become equal, and the tooth is said to be round, although its actual shape is that of an equilateral triangle with round corners. The term triangular is applied to the wearing surface when the labiolingual dimension or altitude of the triangle is longer than the labial border. In the final stage, when the root is exposed in very old horses, the wearing surface is oval, with the long diameter in the labiolingual direction. The transitional forms are hard to classify, and I 3 does not follow the pattern. The following table gives the most reliable stages in this process.

	Round	**Triangular**
I 1	9 years	16 years
I 2	10 years	17 years

The so-called seven-year hook is the result of the failure of the lower I 3 to wear all of the occlusal surface of the upper I 3. An overhang is left at the back of the upper tooth. This hook is supposed to appear at 7, wear off at 9, and appear again at 11 years. The hook may or may not be present in any horse over 6 years old.[11, 12] In one study, about 60 percent of the horses in any age class from 8 to 18 years had the hook on one side or the other or on both sides.[12]

Galvayne's groove is a longitudinal mark in the labial surface of upper I 3. The cement in the groove remains as a dark line, whereas that on the rest of the tooth is worn off to expose the white enamel. The groove is located midway in the length of the tooth; it is at first concealed in the alveolus, then gradually emerges from under the gum as the tooth grows out, and finally disappears as the ungrooved proximal part of the tooth comes into view. According to Galvayne, the groove appears at the gum line at 10 years, extends halfway down the tooth at 15 years, reaches the wearing surface at 20 years, and disappears by 30 years. The groove is of little value as a single indicator of age. If it is present, the horse is probably over 10 years old. The length of the groove or the absence of it can only be used in conjunction with other signs (Fig. 1–2).

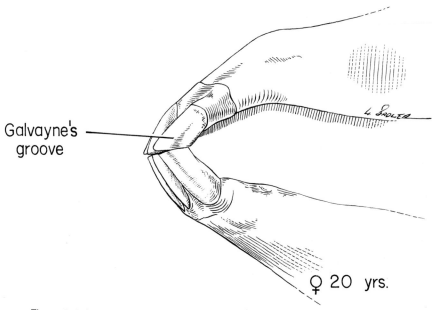

Galvayne's
groove

♀ 20 yrs.

Figure 1–2. Lateral aspect of the incisors of an aged mare.

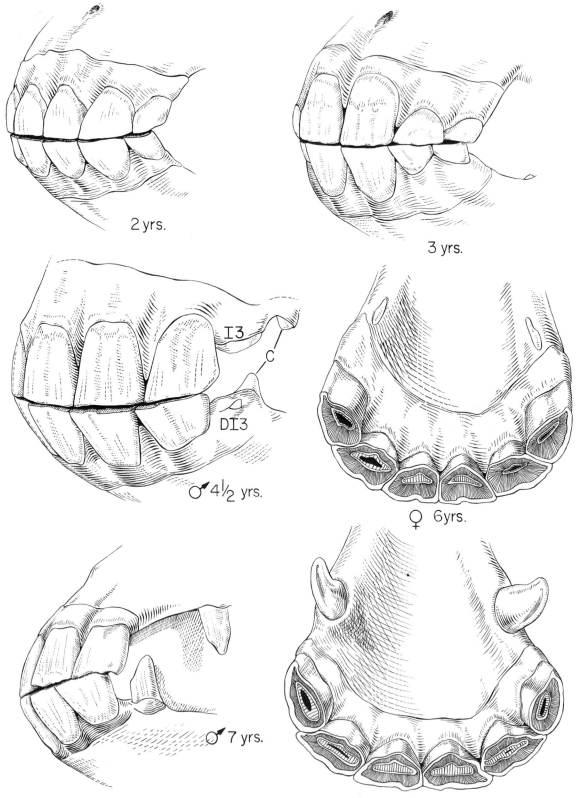

Figure 1–3. Equine incisors at various ages; two views at 7 years.

There are three other general indications of age. (1) When the teeth are viewed in profile, the angle between the upper and lower incisors becomes more acute with age. (2) When the teeth are viewed from the front, they are seen to diverge from the median plane in a young horse and to converge in an old one. (3) The arcade of the incisors when seen from the occlusal surface is a semicircle in the young horse and a straight line in the older animal.

The more useful signs are arranged chronologically in the following list:

1 week. Di 1 has erupted.

1 month. Di 2 has erupted.

8 months. Di 3 has erupted.

1 year. Di 1 and Di 2 are in wear. Upper and lower Di 3 are not in contact. There is no deciduous canine.

2 years. Di 1 and Di 2 are level, Di 3 is in wear. It is easy to confuse this stage with the adult if the general appearance of the animal and the differences between deciduous and permanent incisors are not considered.

2½ years. I 1 erupts.

3½ years. I 2 erupts.

4½ years. I 3 erupts.

5 years. I 1 and I 2 are level, labial border of I 3 is in wear. Canines erupt at 4 to 5 years, usually only in males.

6 years. Cup is gone from I 1.

7 years. All lower incisors are level. Cup is gone from I 2. Hook is in upper I 3. Cement has worn off, changing the color from yellow to bluish-white.

8 years. Dental star appears in I 1. Cup is gone from I 3.

9 years. I 1 is round.

10 years. I 2 is round. Galvayne's groove begins to emerge from the gum on upper I 3.

13 years. The enamel spot is small and round in the lower incisors. The dental stars are in the middle of the occlusal surfaces.

15 years. Dental stars are round, dark, and distinct. Galvayne's groove extends halfway down to the occlusal surface.

16 years. I 1 is triangular.

17 years. I 2 is triangular. Enamel spots are gone from lower incisors.

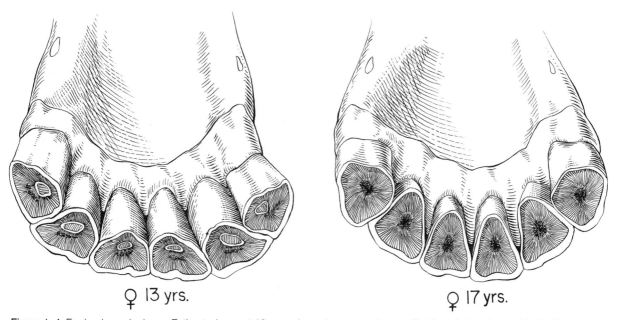

♀ 13 yrs.   ♀ 17 yrs.

Figure 1–4. Equine lower incisors. Estimated age at 13 years based on enamel spots (light) and dental stars (dark). The shapes of the occlusal surfaces do not conform to the average.

In addition to the changes in the incisors, it is important in dentistry to know that the permanent premolars erupt as follows: P 1 (wolf tooth) at 5 to 6 months, P 2 at 2½ years, P 3 at 3 years, P 4 at 4 years. The molars erupt: M 1 at 1 year, M 2 at 2 years, M 3 at 3½ to 4 years. Note that the large cheek teeth erupt at ages that correspond with their numerical designations.

The upper cheek teeth are slightly lateral to the lower cheek teeth; therefore, the labial edge of the upper cheek teeth and lingual edge of the lower cheek teeth do not wear and must be filed (floated) to prevent injury to the lip and palate. Caps are remnants of deciduous teeth that remain attached to the erupting surfaces of permanent teeth.

1b. INCISORS AND CANINES, OX

The dental formulae are:

$$2(Di\frac{0}{3} \, Dc\frac{0}{1} \, Dp\frac{3}{3}) = 20 \qquad 2(I\frac{0}{3} \, C\frac{0}{1} \, P\frac{3}{3} \, M\frac{3}{3}) = 32$$

The ruminant canine tooth has the form of an incisor.

Test the following rules for age determination on specimens of known ages. The eruptions are relatively accurate, but the wear of the occlusal surface and the exposure of the necks of the teeth are quite variable.

At birth. Most of the incisors have broken through the gum but are still largely covered by a thin, pink membrane.

2 weeks. The gum has receded to the neck of I 1.

3 to 4 weeks. The gum has receded to the necks of all the incisors and canines. Eruption of all the deciduous teeth has occurred.

1½ to 2 years. I 1 erupts.

2 to 2½ years. I 2 erupts.

3 years. I 3 erupts.

3½ to 4 years. C erupts.

5 years. All incisors and canines are in wear (Fig. 1–5).

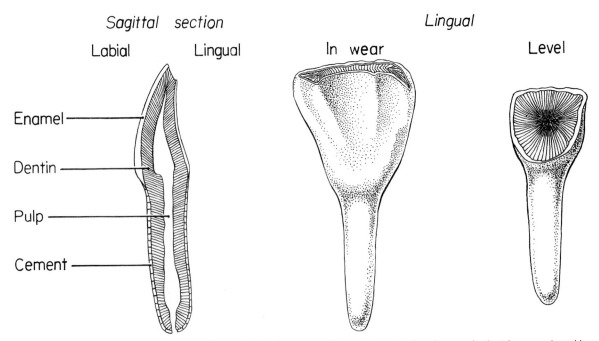

Sagittal section

Labial   Lingual   In wear   Level

Lingual

Enamel

Dentin

Pulp

Cement

Figure 1–5. Sagittal section and occlusal surfaces of a bovine second incisor showing the changes in the shape and markings of the occlusal surface with increasing age.

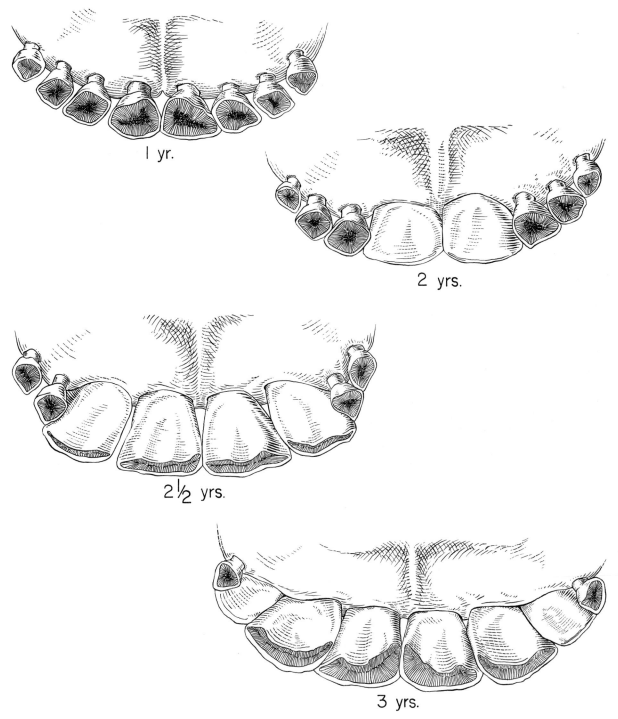

Figure 1–6. Bovine incisors and canines. Compare the level deciduous teeth at 1 year with the level permanent teeth at 9 years in Figure 1–7. The necks of permanent teeth are much larger.

The best criterion for estimating age in the next 4 years is the process of leveling of the incisors and canines. This term has a special meaning in the ox: a tooth is level when the occlusal surface shows a smooth lingual convexity (Figs. 1–5 and 1–7). The tooth becomes level because it is worn down so far that the ridges on the lingual surface have disappeared and no longer make the lingual border of the occlusal surface zigzag.

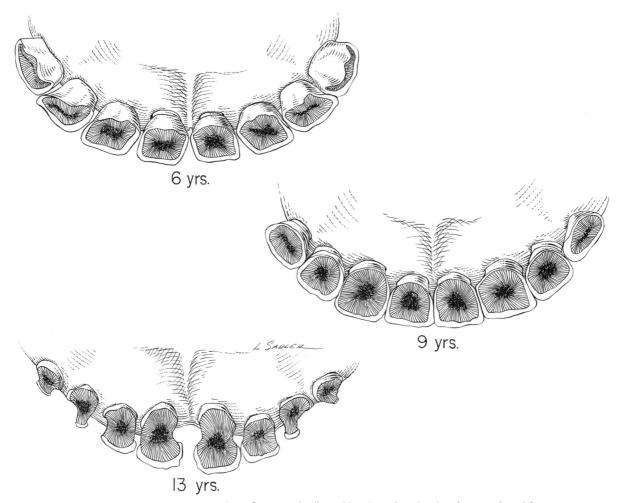

6 yrs.

9 yrs.

13 yrs.

Figure 1–7. Bovine incisors and canines. Compare the lingual borders of occlusal surfaces at 6 and 9 years.

6 years. I 1 is level, and the neck has emerged from the gum.
7 years. I 2 is level, and the neck is visible.
8 years. I 3 is level, and the neck is visible. C may be level.
9 years. C is level, and the neck is visible.
15 years. The teeth that have not fallen out are reduced to small round pegs.

1c. INCISORS AND CANINES, SHEEP AND GOAT

The dental formulae are the same as those of the ox.

1 to 1½ years. I 1 erupts.
1½ to 2 years. I 2 erupts.
2½ to 3 years. I 3 erupts.
3 to 4 years. C erupts.

1d. TEETH, PIG

The dental formulae are:

$$2(\text{Di}\frac{3}{3}\,\text{Dc}\frac{1}{1}\,\text{Dp}\frac{3}{3}) = 28 \qquad 2(\text{I}\frac{3}{3}\,\text{C}\frac{1}{1}\,\text{P}\frac{4}{4}\,\text{M}\frac{3}{3}) = 44$$

The deciduous third incisors and canines are erupted at birth, project laterally, and have sharp points; they are called needle teeth. These points are often cut off I 3 and C to prevent injury to the sow and to other piglets.

1e. TEETH, DOG

The dental formulae are:

$$2(Di\frac{3}{3} \, Dc\frac{1}{1} \, Dp\frac{3}{3}) = 28 \qquad 2(I\frac{3}{3} \, C\frac{1}{1} \, P\frac{4}{4} \, M\frac{2}{3}) = 42$$

Eruption of the deciduous teeth begins with the incisors at 4 to 5 weeks and ends with Dp 4 at 6 to 8 weeks.

The data given for wear of the teeth are accurate in about 90 percent of large dogs.[2] The wear of the teeth in small dogs and dogs with undershot or overshot jaws is often misleading. "Cusp worn off" means that the largest cusp of the incisor is worn down to the level of the small cusp or cusps. The upper I 1 and I 2 have two small cusps; lower incisors have one (Fig. 1–8).

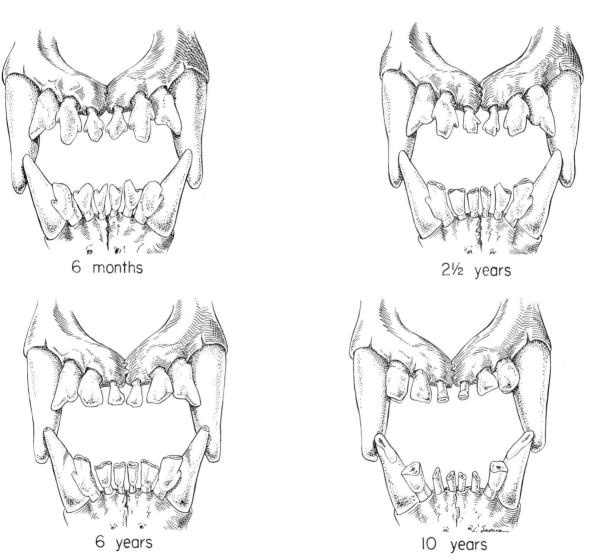

6 months 2½ years

6 years 10 years

Figure 1–8. Wear of teeth in the dog.

5 months. Permanent incisors have erupted. I 3 is not yet in wear.

6 months. Permanent canines have erupted (see Fig. 1–8).

1½ years. Cusp is worn off lower I 1.

2½ years. Cusp is worn off lower I 2.

3½ years. Cusp is worn off upper I 1.

4½ years. Cusp is worn off upper I 2.

5 years. Cusp of lower I 3 is slightly worn. The occlusal surfaces of lower I 1 and I 2 are rectangular. The canines are slightly worn.

6 years. Cusp is worn off lower I 3. Canines are worn blunt. Lower canine shows impression of upper I 3 (see Fig. 1–8).

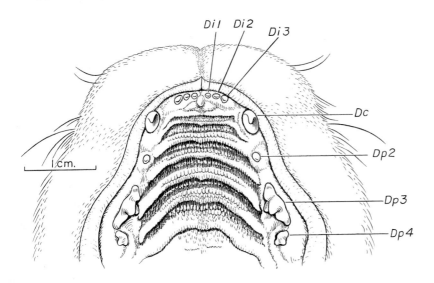

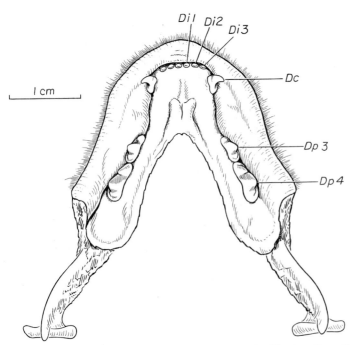

Figure 1–9. Deciduous dentition in a 2-month-old cat.

7 years. Lower I 1 is worn down to the root, so that the occlusal surface is elongated in the labiolingual direction.

8 years. Occlusal surface of the lower I 1 is beveled in front.

10 years. Lower I 2 and upper I 1 have occlusal surfaces elongated labiolingually (see Fig. 1–8).

12 years. 1 1s begin to fall out.

16 years. Incisors are gone.

20 years. Loss of canines occurs.

The cheek teeth erupt at about 6 months. In connection with tooth extraction in the dog, it is of interest that the last three upper teeth have triple roots. (P 4, M 1, M 2). All the first premolars and the last lower molars have one root. All the other cheek teeth have two roots.

1f. TEETH, CAT

The dental formulae are:

$$2(\text{Di}\frac{3}{3}\,\text{Dc}\frac{1}{1}\,\text{Dp}\frac{3}{2}) = 26 \qquad 2(\text{I}\frac{3}{3}\,\text{C}\frac{1}{1}\,\text{P}\frac{3}{2}\,\text{M}\frac{1}{1}) = 30$$

As in the dog, the sectorial teeth in the permanent dentition are the upper P 4 and lower M 1. The missing premolars are P 1 above and P 1 and P 2 below. The deciduous dentition begins to erupt at 15 to 21 days and is complete when the upper Dp 2 erupts at 2 months (Fig. 1–9). The permanent dentition is complete at 6 months (Fig. 1–10). Only upper P 4 has three roots in the permanent dentition. Note that the roots of this tooth are in the ventral wall of the orbit. An apical abscess here may rupture into the conjunctival sac and drain from the eye. In the deciduous dentition upper Dp 3 and Dp 4 have triple roots.

Cats' incisors have cusps that give them a scalloped appearance. These cusps are usually worn off by 4 years in upper I 1 and I 2. In older cats the upper canine projects farther from the gum and beyond the level of the lip, and teeth begin to fall out.

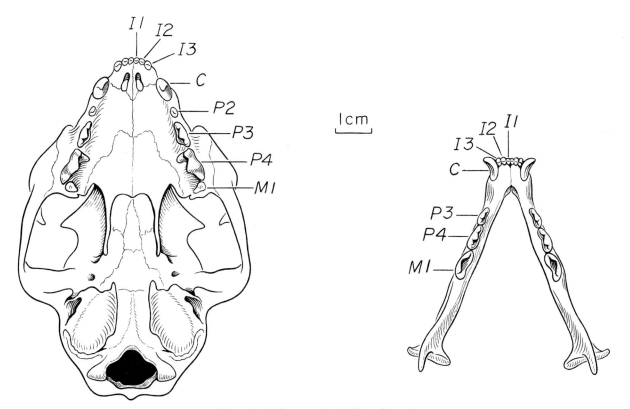

Figure 1–10. Permanent dentition of a cat.

1g. RADIOGRAPHS

Identify the radiographic features of the teeth of all the domestic animals.[10, 13] In the young dog and cat distinguish permanent from deciduous teeth. During eruption of a permanent tooth the bone covering it is resorbed as well as the root(s) of the deciduous tooth it replaces.

The lamina dura is the thin layer of dense cortical bone that lines the alveolus. It is most evident in the young dog, and it disappears in diseases associated with calcium deficiency. The periodontal ligament is in the radiolucent space between the lamina dura and the cementum of the root. It is also attached to the gingiva. Its fibers are so directed that they prevent the tooth from being driven into the alveolus by the pressure of mastication. The interalveolar margin is the free border of the interalveolar septum. In radiographs the margin appears flat between cheek teeth and sharp between incisors. Demineralization of the septum is an indication of disease or aging.

References

1. Baker, A. J.: Dental disorders in the horse. Comp. Cont. Ed. *4* (1982):507–514.
2. Boenisch, F.: Beitrag zur Altersbestimmung des Hundes nach den Schneidezähnen. Archiv für Tierheilkunde *39* (1913):289–327.
3. Brown, G. T.: Dentition as Indicative of the Age of the Animals of the Farm, 8th ed. London: John Murray, 1927.
4. Davis, R. W. (ed.): Official Guide for Determining the Age of the Horse. Golden, Colorado: American Association of Equine Practitioners, 1966.
5. Getty, R.: Sisson and Grossman's The Anatomy of the Domestic Animals, 5th ed. Philadelphia: W. B. Saunders, 1975.
6. Habermehl, K. H.: Die Altersbestimmung bei Haus- und Labortieren, 2nd ed. Berlin: Parey, 1975.
7. Huidekoper, R. S.: Age of the Domestic Animals, Philadelphia: F. A. Davis, 1891.
8. Judging the Age of Sheep by Their Teeth. Circ. 149, Mont. Agr. Exp. Sta., 1936.
9. Pope, G. W.: Determining the Age of Farm Animals by Their Teeth. USDA Farmer's Bull. 1727, 1934.
10. Quick, C. B. and V. R. Rendano: The equine teeth. Mod. Vet. Pract. *60* (1979):561–567.
11. Sassen, W.: Beitrag zur Beurteilung der Furche und des Einbisses an den Eckzähnen des Pferdes für dessen Altersbestimmung. Diss. Hannover, 1950.
12. Weekenstroo, H. J.: Onderzoekingen betreffende de veranderingen aan de tanden van het paard op verschillende leeftijden en hun waarde voor de leeftijdsbepaling. 'S-Hertogenbosch: P. Stokvis en Zoon, 1918.
13. Zontine, W. J.: Canine dental radiology: radiographic technic, development and anatomy of the teeth. J. Am. Vet. Rad. Soc. *16* (1975):75–83.

CHAPTER 2

MOUTH, PHARYNX, LARYNX, AND CRANIAL NERVES V (MAXILLARY, MANDIBULAR), IX, X, AND XI

OBJECTIVES

1. To know the sensory innervation of the teeth in all species.
2. To be able to diagnose a lesion of the maxillary nerve by sensory deficits in the areas it innervates.
3. To be able to block the maxillary nerve at the most effective site for the desired purpose.
4. To be able to diagnose a lesion of the mandibular nerve by motor paralysis and sensory deficits in the structures innervated.
5. To be able to block the mandibular nerve at the most effective site for the desired purpose.
6. To be able to palpate the infraorbital foramen in all species.
7. To understand the normal relation of the epiglottis to the soft palate in the horse and dog and to be able to diagnose malfunction caused by paresis of the pharynx (cranial nerves IX, X, XI), an elongated or displaced soft palate, epiglottic entrapment in the horse, and brachycephaly in the dog.
8. To understand the innervation and function of the larynx. To be able to diagnose laryngeal hemiplegia by endoscopy and to understand the surgical anatomy of the larynx.
9. To understand the pathogenesis of inspiratory dyspnea.
10. To be able to palpate the thyroid and cricoid cartilages in all species, the lingual process of the basihyoid in the horse, and most of the hyoid bones in the dog.
11. To be able to palpate the temporomandibular joint in all species and to know how to reduce a luxation of the mandible in the dog.
12. To understand the surgical anatomy of pharyngostomy in the dog and to be able to palpate the site of pharyngostomy.
13. To understand the surgical anatomy of tonsillectomy.
14. To be able to find the orifices of the salivary ducts.
15. To appreciate the danger of injury to the pharyngeal diverticulum in treating swine with a dose syringe.
16. To know the relationship of major vessels and nerves to the tympanic bulla to avoid them during surgical drainage.

Cranial Nerves

Chapters 2 to 6 contain many references to the cranial nerves. Cranial nerves are important in making a clinical diagnosis and in administering local anesthesia, and they should be avoided during surgery. This general review and functional classification will be followed by more detailed applied study when the appropriate region of the head is discussed.

A. Special Sensory
   I. Olfactory. Smell
   II. Optic. Vision
   VIII. Vestibulocochlear
      1. Vestibular. Equilibrium, motion of the head
      2. Cochlear. Hearing
B. Motor (except proprioceptive fibers)
   III. Oculomotor. Dorsal, ventral, and medial recti; ventral oblique; and levator palpebrae superioris
   IV. Trochlear. Dorsal oblique
   VI. Abducent. Lateral rectus and retractor bulbi
   XI. Accessory
      1. Internal branch (from cranial roots). Joins the vagus and is distributed through vagal branches to the striated muscles of the pharynx, larynx, and esophagus
      2. External branch (from spinal roots). Motor to sternocephalicus, cleidocephalicus, and trapezius
   XII. Hypoglossal. Muscles of the tongue
C. Mixed
   V. Trigeminal
      1. Ophthalmic. Somatic sensory to eyeball, upper eyelid, forehead, frontal sinus, and nasal mucosa
      2. Maxillary. Sensory to nasal mucosa, upper oral cavity, upper teeth, skin of nose, upper lip, eyelids, temporal region, and horn
      3. Mandibular
         a. Motor to muscles of mastication (branches to salivary glands for fibers derived from N. VII and IX)
         b. Sensory to lower teeth and lip, cheek, skin and mucosa of lower jaw, tongue, and part of external ear
   VII. Facial
      1. Motor to muscles of expression (cutaneous muscles of head: orbicularis oculi, muscles of nose, lips, cheek, and ear), cutaneous muscles of neck, mandibular and sublingual salivary glands (via chorda tympani and lingual nerve), and lacrimal gland (via N. V).
      2. Sense of taste to tongue via chorda tympani and lingual nerve
   IX. Glossopharyngeal
      1. Motor to pharynx, and the parotid and zygomatic glands (through N. V, mand.)
      2. Sensory to middle ear, pharynx, and taste buds in root of tongue
   X. Vagus
      1. Motor to pharynx, most of digestive tract, larynx, trachea, lungs, and heart
      2. Sensory to pharynx, larynx, trachea, esophagus, and part of external ear
      3. Afferent fibers for many visceral reflexes

Cranial Nerve V. The trigeminal nerve (cranial nerve V) consists of the ophthalmic, maxillary, and mandibular nerves. The ophthalmic nerve is sensory to the eyeball (ciliary nerves), eyelids, forehead, frontal sinus, nasal mucosa, and sometimes the horn (see Chapters 4 and 6). The maxillary nerve is sensory to almost all of the head dorsal to a line between the upper and lower lips and rostral to the orbit: nasal mucosa, hard and soft palate, upper teeth and gums, upper lip, skin of nose, eyelids, temporal region, and horn. The mandibular nerve is sensory to part of the external ear and most of the head ventral to a line between the upper and lower lips and the zygomatic arch, including: the lower teeth and lip, cheek, skin and mucosa of lower jaw, and tongue (lingual nerve). The mandibular nerve is motor to muscles of mastication. The muscles that close the jaw are the most powerful and include the pterygoids, masseter, and temporal.

A dropped jaw indicates bilateral mandibular nerve paralysis. This is most common in the dog, where it is the only clinical sign and is associated with a transient neuritis of the trigeminal nerve. Unilateral mandibular nerve paralysis is diagnosed by palpation of the denervation atrophy of the masseter and temporal muscles and analgesia of its autonomous zone (the cutaneous area supplied *only* by the mandibular nerve). Neoplasms of the trigeminal nerve or on the floor of the cranial cavity where the nerve can be compressed will cause paralysis and atrophy of these muscles and anesthesia of the face on the affected side.[39]

Inspiratory Dyspnea. The most common cause of inspiratory dyspnea is inability to abduct the vocal folds to open the glottis on inspiration. This is a sign of neuromuscular disease of the cricoarytenoideus dorsalis muscle or of its innervation by neurons in the recurrent laryngeal nerve.

The cell bodies of these neurons are in the nucleus ambiguus in the medulla. An inherited abiotrophy of these cell bodies occurs in young Bouvier des Flandres dogs causing inspiratory dyspnea, exercise intolerance, and poor growth.[49] Listeriosis in ruminants and protozoal encephalitis in horses may affect the nucleus ambiguus and produce laryngeal paralysis as part of the clinical syndrome.

The axons of these neurons leave the medulla in the cranial roots of the accessory nerve and join the vagus nerve as it leaves the skull through the jugular foramen and tympano-occipital fissure. As the vagus nerve courses caudally in the retropharyngeal area, it may be affected in horses by mycosis of the guttural pouch[7] or by abscessation of the retropharyngeal lymph nodes in horses with strangles. In cattle the vagus nerve may be affected by the cellulitis and lymph node abscessation secondary to injuries to the pharynx.[9]

The vagus nerve courses caudally in the neck, where it is subject to injury and more rarely, neoplasia. The only consistent clinical sign of a lesion in the cervical portion of one vagus nerve caudal to the pharynx is laryngeal hemiplegia.

The recurrent laryngeal nerves leave the vagi in the cranial thorax and course around the aorta or right subclavian artery into the cranial mediastinum, where they can be affected by lesions such as pleuritis or abscessed lymph nodes. Stretching of the axons in long-necked horses may be a cause of laryngeal hemiplegia.

The recurrent laryngeal nerve courses cranially adjacent to the dorsal aspect of the thyroid gland, where it can be affected by thyroid neoplasia or surgery on this gland.

The neuromuscular junctions in the cricoarytenoideus dorsalis muscle can be affected by the toxin associated with botulism or by the muscle receptor disorder of myasthenia gravis. Inspiratory dyspnea is sometimes observed in these diseases. Myositis may affect the laryngeal muscles. Inspiratory dyspnea from laryngeal paralysis has been associated with chronic hypothyroidism in some patients, who may have a neuromyopathy involving the larynx.

2a. SKULL, HORSE

The point of entry for maxillary nerve anesthesia is 2.5 cm. ventral to the lateral angle of the eye and ventral to the zygomatic arch. The needle is directed medially and slightly rostrodorsally to a depth of 6.5 to 7.5 cm. The nerve runs across the pterygopalatine fossa from the round foramen to the maxillary foramen, where it should be blocked. It runs dorsal and parallel to the maxillary artery. A maxillary nerve block will anesthetize all the upper teeth but is only necessary for the last four. To anesthetize the first two cheek teeth (P 2 and P 3) and the incisors, the much simpler infraorbital nerve block is adequate. The needle is inserted in the infraorbital foramen rostrodorsal to the end of the facial crest, and the anesthetic is injected into the canal, blocking the alveolar branches to the premolars, the branches that continue in the bone to the incisors, and the branches that emerge to supply the nose and upper lip (see Plate I).

Inferior alveolar nerve block. The mandibular foramen is on the medial side of the mandible at the apex of a right angle formed by the occlusal plane of the cheek teeth and a perpendicular drawn to the lateral angle of the eye. When the mouth is closed, the lateral border of the occlusal surface of the upper cheek teeth overhangs the lower teeth and can be palpated through the cheek from the outside. The block at the mandibular foramen anesthetizes all the teeth but is only necessary for the last four. The first two cheek teeth and the incisors can be blocked by an injection into the mental foramen halfway between the canine and the first large cheek tooth (P 2). This will block the alveolar branches to the first two cheek teeth, the branches that continue in the bone to the incisors, and the branches that emerge into the lower lip (see Plate I).

The reason for using dental blocks is that they permit very painful dental operations under narcosis rather than a surgical plane of general anesthesia, which may not be practicable or may be contraindicated.

2b. LARYNGEAL CARTILAGES AND DISSECTED LARYNX, HORSE

Articulate the laryngeal cartilages. The laryngeal prominence of the thyroid cartilage is palpable ventrally. The thyroid laminae overlap the arytenoid cartilages and the dorsal part of the cricoid cartilage. The space between the caudal thyroid notch and the arch of the cricoid is filled by the cricothyroid ligament. Study the mechanics of the arytenoid cartilages. They have a medial facet for articulation with the cricoid, a dorsolateral muscular process, and a ventromedial vocal process. The muscles that pull downward on the muscular process rotate the cartilage so that the vocal process carries the vocal fold medially, closing the intermembranous part of the glottis, while the arytenoideus transversus and the ventricularis pull the arytenoid cartilages together, closing the intercartilaginous part. The only dilator of the glottis is the cricoarytenoideus dorsalis, which originates on the cricoid lamina and pulls the muscular process of the arytenoid mediocaudally, abducting the arytenoid cartilage and the vocal fold and opening the glottis.

Study the laryngeal ventricle. It extends laterally between the ventricularis and vocalis muscles, and caudodorsally, where it is covered by the thyroid lamina.

The cranial laryngeal nerve goes directly to the larynx from the vagus. Its external branch innervates one muscle, the cricothyroideus. The internal branch enters through the thyroid foramen under the rostral horn of the thyroid cartilage and provides the sensory innervation of the mucosa. It is the sensory limb of the protective choking reflex elicited by foreign material in the larynx.

The caudal laryngeal nerve is the laryngeal end of the recurrent laryngeal nerve, which originates from the vagus in the thorax. The left recurrent laryngeal nerve loops around the aorta and ligamentum arteriosum to run back up the trachea to the larynx; the right nerve loops around the subclavian artery. The caudal laryngeal nerves innervate all the muscles of the larynx but the cricothyroideus. In horses with idiopathic laryngeal hemiplegia, the distal portion of the left nerve degenerates more than the right, resulting in a left hemiplegia.[10] The clinical effect is produced by paralysis of the only abductor of the vocal fold, the cricoarytenoideus dorsalis. Examination of a larynx from a patient with laryngeal hemiplegia shows atrophied muscles on the left side.

In the interior of the bisected larynx, note the following in rostrocaudal order: the vestibular fold, the ventricle, and the vocal fold. In a "roarer" the paralysis of the cricoarytenoideus dorsalis allows the arytenoid cartilage and vocal fold to swing into the air current on inspiration. Inflation of the ventricle contributes to the obstruction. The asymmetry of the glottis can be seen if an endoscope is passed through the ventral nasal meatus into the nasopharynx.[34] Other causes of respiratory stenosis must be eliminated. Paresis of the pharynx is seen with the endoscope as a collapse of the walls of the nasopharynx, constricting the airway above the larynx. This may occur in horses with guttural pouch mycosis and dysphagia.[7] Dorsal displacement of the soft palate is recognized by failure to see the epiglottis, which normally extends over the soft palate into the nasopharynx.[26] If their positions are reversed, the soft palate will obstruct the laryngeal opening on inspiration and interfere with expiration. Many causes have been proposed, including soft palate paresis, excessive tongue retraction, and contraction of the sternothyroid muscles. The epiglottis may be entrapped by a fold of oropharyngeal mucosa (not just the aryepiglottic folds) that is drawn caudally over the epiglottis from its lingual surface.[4, 26]

The "roaring operation" or ventriculectomy is performed through a median incision between the right and left sternohyoidei and through the cricothyroid ligament. The ventricle is everted and cut off around the margins of the orifice, leaving the cavity to close by granulation and cause the adhesion of the vocal fold and vocal process to the lateral wall of the cavity and indirectly to the thyroid lamina. A prosthetic suture may be used to replace the cricoarytenoideus dorsalis muscle.

The larynx is approached from an incision between the omohyoideus muscle ventrally and the linguofacial vein dorsally. The dorsolateral aspect of the larynx is exposed, and the prominence on the caudodorsal aspect of the cricoid cartilage is identified caudal to the cricopharyngeus muscle. The muscular process of the arytenoid is exposed through the septum between the cricopharyngeus and thyropharyngeus. The suture is placed between these two cartilaginous structures beneath the cricopharyngeus. Tension must be applied carefully to avoid excessive abduction of the vocal process. In addition, a ventriculectomy is done from the usual ventral approach.[35]

If the cricotracheal ligament is lax, it may bulge into the lumen on inspiration and cause stenosis. The cricotracheal ligament can be exposed and reefed by extending the median incision caudally through the skin and muscle.

If the soft palate is too long, a 2-cm. strip can be trimmed off the caudal free border by working through a ventral laryngotomy incision.

A ventral surgical approach through an incision in the cricothyroid ligament provides access to the laryngeal ventricle (hemiplegia), arytenoid cartilage (chondritis), soft palate (displacement), oropharyngeal mucosa (entrapment), laryngopharyngeal mucosa (follicular pharyngitis–lymphoid hyperplasia), and subepiglottic cysts.

For access to the oral cavity, oropharynx, hard and soft palate, and nasopharynx, a surgical approach is made through the intermandibular space between the tongue and mandible. This approach includes an intermandibular symphysiotomy. The soft palate is split to reach the nasopharynx.[37]

The functional anatomy of the pharynx and larynx during respiration in the horse should be understood.[6] The horse normally breathes only through its nose. During respiration the caudal end of the nasopharynx encloses the larynx, creating an airtight passageway. The palatopharyngeal arches and the free border of the soft palate form a sphincter around the rostral larynx. The free border of the soft palate is ventral to the epiglottis. The palatopharyngeal arches are ventral to the aryepiglottic folds and caudal to the corniculate cartilages of the arytenoids. Bilateral arytenoid abduction further tightens the contact with the palatopharyngeal arches. Contraction of the sternothyrohyoideus and omohyoideus will pull the larynx against these arches to tighten this seal. Functional obstruction of the nasopharynx or the "choking-up" that occurs during fast exercise is due to a dorsal displacement of the soft palate. Displacement may result from excessive contraction of these neck muscles and disengagement of the soft palate from its normal position below the epiglottis, breaking the seal and allowing the soft palate to obstruct respiration.[27] Surgical resection of the paired sternothyroideus muscles has been effective in some horses with intermittent dorsal displacement of the soft palate. Others require palatal resection. Surgery is ineffective if displacement is secondary to a short epiglottis, which may be determined by radiographs.[33]

2c. LIVE HORSE

Locate the following:

The site for a maxillary nerve block, as in 2a.

The site for an infraorbital nerve block. Palpate the levator labii superioris and displace it dorsally. The infraorbital foramen and nerve are deep to the muscle, about 6 cm. dorsal to the end of the facial crest and usually about 3 cm. rostral to the end of the crest. If the first interphalangeal joint of the index finger is placed against the end of the facial crest, the tip of the middle finger will be on the foramen.

The site for an inferior alveolar nerve block. The point of entry is medial to the caudal border of the mandible or medial to the ventral border of the mandible. Palpate through the cheek to find the lateral border of the occlusal surface of the upper cheek teeth and locate the mandibular foramen as in 2a.

The site for a mental nerve block. Palpate the mental foramen and nerve on the mandible about 3 cm. caudal to the plane of the angle of the mouth. The tendon of the depressor labii inferioris must be displaced.

Lingual process. A longitudinal bar projects rostrally from the basihyoid bone on the midline in the intermandibular space, rostral to the larynx. The junction of the right and left chains of mandibular lymph nodes is superficial here.

Laryngeal prominence (of the thyroid cartilage). Caudal to the prominence, palpate the caudal thyroid notch.

Cricoid cartilage. The ventral part of the arch forms the caudal boundary of a triangle, the other two sides of which are formed by the caudal thyroid notch. The cricothyroid ligament fills this triangle and is the site of the incision for laryngeal, palatal, and pharyngeal surgery. Palpate the cricotracheal ligament. It fills the large space that is easily felt between the cricoid and the first tracheal ring. If it is too loose, the cricotracheal ligament will be sucked up into the lumen on inspiration. This action is exaggerated if the nostrils are held closed.

M. cricoarytenoideus dorsalis. Find the dorsal or ventral border of the thyroid lamina and follow it back to the cricothyroid joint. The ventral border can be palpated as a ridge on the lateral surface of the cricoid. Just dorsal to the caudal end of the thyroid cartilage is the hard, convex muscular process of the arytenoid. The cricoarytenoideus dorsalis lies medial to the joint and terminates on the muscular process. This muscle atrophies in laryngeal paralysis, leaving a palpable hollow. The arytenoid depression maneuver is of greater significance than muscular atrophy in detecting laryngeal hemiplegia. For this maneuver, the operator stands facing the horse with its chin on his shoulder.[34] The muscular process of the arytenoid is pushed downward, forward, and inward while the larynx is supported with the other hand. The roaring sound can be produced with much less force on the affected side if laryngeal hemiplegia is present.

Palpate the temporomandibular joint, which is the most prominent lateral part of the skull on the caudal aspect of the zygomatic arch.

2d. SKULL, COW

A method for maxillary nerve anesthesia in the cow is Peterson's orbital block (see section 4f) in which a 12-cm. curved needle is passed medially in the angle between the frontal and temporal processes of the zygomatic bone. The needle crosses the rostral border of the coronoid process of the mandible to the foramen orbitorotundum. This blocks both the ophthalmic and maxillary nerves and can be used for ocular surgery. The maxillary foramen is medial to the large lacrimal bulla and is not accessible by injection.

The infraorbital foramen is 3 cm. above the gum line of the first cheek tooth and slightly rostral to it. This is a marked difference from its position in the horse (see Plate II).

The mandibular foramen is at the intersection of the plane of the occlusal surfaces of the cheek teeth and a line from the vascular groove on the ventral border of the mandible to the temporomandibular articulation.

The mental foramen is 3 to 4 cm. caudal to the canine tooth (former I 4) at the level of the caudal end of the intermandibular joint.

2e. LIVE COW

Locate the foramina described in section 2d. To find the vascular groove on the ventral border of the mandible, palpate the pulse in the facial artery. Palpate the larynx. The laryngeal prominence is near the caudal end of the thyroid cartilage in the ox, unlike that of the horse. There is no palpable caudal thyroid notch. The larynx in short-necked beef cattle can be mistaken for a foreign body in the esophagus.[12]

2f. SKULL, DOG

In luxation of the mandible the condyloid process of the mandible is displaced dorsorostrally. Malocclusion is apparent in the relation of the lower teeth to the upper teeth. Visualize the effect of placing a fulcrum between the molars and pressing the incisors together. This must be done under general anesthesia to obtain relaxation of the muscles. A dysplasia of this joint in the Basset hound may result in displacement of the coronoid process of the mandible lateral to the zygomatic arch, which fixes the jaw in an open position.[41] Fixation can be prevented by removing a ventral portion of the zygomatic arch.

Bulla Tympanica. The middle ear may be drained into the pharynx by passing a medullary pin through the ruptured eardrum and through the bulla tympanica, palpating the bulla through the

Tongue
All components of the pharynx
Larynx
Guttural pouch in the horse

Diagnosis of injury to the temporomandibular joint in dogs and cats requires ventrodorsal and lateral oblique views.[48] Appreciate the width of the condyloid process in the joint on ventrodorsal view.

The external acoustic meatus is clearly visible in the lateral view of the dog as an oval radiolucent spot rostrodorsal to the bulla tympanica. In the lateral view of the horse, the meatus is superimposed on the ventral aspect of the radiodense petrosal bone. The bulla is small in the horse. Its ventral border is at the level of the floor of the cranial cavity, the dorsal portion of the basilar part of the occipital bone. Note the very large bulla in the cat and its medial extent on ventrodorsal view. In the ventrodorsal view of the dog, the large oblique tympano-occipital fissure may be seen caudomedial to the bulla. It leads to the jugular foramen inside, and it transmits cranial nerves IX, X, and XI, the internal carotid artery, and radicles of the internal jugular and vertebral veins.

Locate the oropharynx and nasopharynx, which are separated by the thick soft palate, and the laryngopharynx over the laryngeal opening.

The best-defined features of the larynx in a lateral view are the epiglottis, the corniculate processes of the arytenoids in the horse, the lamina of the cricoid cartilage in the dog, and the radiolucent cavity. In good soft tissue exposures it is possible to see the arytenoid cartilages and the radiolucent laryngeal ventricles. In the ventrodorsal view in the dog, the thyroid laminae may be visible as two narrow sagittal lines ventral to the atlas and sometimes the axis.

The basihyoid in lateral view is seen end-on as a dense spot. From this the thyrohyoid extends caudodorsally to the rostral horn of the thyroid cartilage. The short keratohyoid extends rostrodorsally to the long epihyoid, from which the stylohyoid is linked to the radiolucent tympanohyoid. In the horse, the rudimentary epihyoid bone is united in the adult with the large long stylohyoid that extends from the keratohyoid to the temporal bone lateral to the bulla. It appears superimposed on the guttural pouch, which it invaginates, dividing it into medial and lateral compartments.

2i. LIVE DOG, CAT

Palpate the zygomatic arch and the temporomandibular articulation. In the cat, palpate for the tympanic bulla ventrally in the angle between the zygomatic arch and the wing of the atlas. Find the infraorbital foramen.

Palpate the hyoid bones and larynx and estimate the site for pharyngostomy.

2j. ANESTHETIZED DOG

Identify the following structures. The hand should be wet to avoid abrasion of the oral mucosa.

Palatoglossal arch
Tonsillar fossa and palatine tonsil
Epihyoid bone lateral to the wall of the pharynx and caudal to the tonsil. The basihyoid can be palpated from the outside. Palpate the site of pharyngostomy between the root of the tongue and the epiglottis and rostral to the epihyoid. Palpate the bulge of your fingertip on the outside of the pharynx.
Bulla tympanica, palpable in the dorsal wall of the pharynx caudal to the epihyoid and stylohyoid.
Identify each tooth and estimate the age of the animal.

Find the orifices of the principal salivary ducts. The parotid orifice is on a small papilla in the buccal mucosa opposite upper P 4. A ridge of mucosa extends caudally from the parotid papilla to the orifices of the zygomatic gland opposite upper M 1. The mandibular and sublingual ducts open on the lateral surface of the rostral end of the sublingual fold opposite P 1. The sublingual orifice is slightly caudal to the mandibular. They may have a common orifice (see section 3f).

Locate the points of insertion for maxillary, inferior alveolar, infraorbital, and mental nerve blocks as given in section 2f.

2k. LARYNX, CAT

Note the absence of ventricles and cuneiform processes. To devocalize the cat, split the thyroid cartilage, the cricothyroid ligament, and the cricoid arch on the midline and remove the vestibular and vocal folds and the intervening mucosa. Close the incision in the larynx with two sutures in the muscles.[45]

2l. DIVERTICULUM PHARYNGEUM, PIG

The diverticulum is dorsal to the esophageal orifice and may catch the stomach tube. If a dose syringe with a long metal tube is used to worm a herd of swine, many fatalities may result from rupture of the diverticula and injection of the drug into the retropharyngeal tissues. Barley awns occasionally lodge in the diverticulum, penetrate the mucosa, and cause a fatal phlegmon.[29]

Although there is no diverticulum in the ruminant, caution must be exercised in the use of a dose syringe or other rigid instrument passed into the pharynx to avoid injury and subsequent infection.

References

1. Ader, P. L. and H. A. Boothe: Ventral bulla osteotomy in the cat. J. Am. Anim. Hosp. Assoc. *15* (1979):757–762.
2. Baker, G. J.: Laryngeal hemiplegia in the horse. Comp. Cont. Ed. *5* (1983):S61–S66.
3. Böhning, R. H., et al.: Pharyngostomy for maintenance of the anorectic animal. JAVMA *156* (1970):611–615.
4. Boles, C. L., C. W. Raker, and J. D. Wheat: Epiglottic entrapment by arytenoepiglottic folds in the horse. JAVMA *172* (1978):338–342.
5. Cook, W. R.: The diagnosis of respiratory unsoundness in the horse. Vet. Rec. *77*: (1965):516–527.
6. Cook, W. R.: Clinical observations on the anatomy and physiology of the equine upper respiratory tract. Vet. Rec. *79* (1966):440–446.
7. Cook, W. R., R. S. F. Campbell, and C. Dawson: The pathology and aetiology of guttural pouch mycosis in the horse. Vet. Rec. *83* (1968):422–428.
8. Cook, W. R.: Skeletal radiology of the equine head. J. Am. Vet. Radiol. Soc. *11* (1970):35–55.
9. Davidson, H. P., W. C. Rebhun, and R. E. Habel: Pharyngeal trauma in cattle. Cornell Vet. *71* (1981):15–25.
10. Duncan, I. D., I. R. Griffiths, A. McQueen, and G. J. Baker: The pathology of equine laryngeal hemiplegia. Acta Neuropathol. *27* (1974):337–348.
11. Duncan, I. D., I. R. Griffiths, and R. E. Madrid: A light and electron microscopic study of the neuropathy of equine idiopathic laryngeal hemiplegia. Neuropathol. Appl. Neurobiol. *4* (1978):483–501.
12. Fox, F. H.: *In* W. J. Gibbons, E. J. Catcott, and J. F. Smithcors (eds.): Bovine Medicine and Surgery. Wheaton, Ill.: American Veterinary Publications, Inc. 1970.
13. Frank, E. R.: Dental anesthesia in the dog. JAVMA *73* (1928):232–233.
14. Goulden, B. E. and L. J. Anderson: Equine laryngeal hemiplegia, Part 1: Physical characteristics of affected animals. N.Z. Vet. J. *29* (1981):150–153.
15. Goulden, B. E. and L. J. Anderson: Equine laryngeal hemiplegia, Part 2: Some clinical observations. N.Z. Vet. J. *29* (1981):194–198.
16. Goulden, B. E. and L. J. Anderson: Equine laryngeal hemiplegia, Part 3: Treatment by laryngoplasty. N.Z. Vet. J. *30* (1982):1–5.
17. Gourley, I. M., H. Paul, and C. Gregory. Castellated laryngofissure and vocal fold resection for the treatment of laryngeal paralysis in the dog. JAVMA *182* (1983):1084–1086.
18. Hare, W. C. D.: Radiographic anatomy of the feline skull. JAVMA *134* (1959):349–356.
19. Harvey, C. E.: Everted laryngeal saccule surgery in brachycephalic dogs. J. Am. Anim. Hosp. Assoc. *18* (1982):545–547.
20. Harvey, C. E.: Partial laryngectomy in brachycephalic dogs. J. Am. Anim. Hosp. Assoc. *18* (1982):548–550.
21. Harvey, C. E.: Soft palate resection in brachycephalic dogs. J. Am. Anim. Hosp. Assoc. *18* (1982):538–544.
22. Harvey, C. E.: Stenotic nares surgery in brachycephalic dogs. J. Am. Anim. Hosp. Assoc. *18* (1982):535–537.
23. Harvey, C. E.: Treatment of laryngeal paralysis in dogs by partial laryngectomy. J. Am. Anim. Hosp. Assoc. *18* (1982):551–556.
24. Haynes, P. F., T. G. Snider, J. R. McClure, and J. J. McClure: Chronic chondritis of the equine arytenoid cartilage. JAVMA *177* (1980):1135–1142.
25. Haynes, P. F.: Persistent dorsal displacement of the soft palate associated with epiglottic shortening in two horses. JAVMA *179* (1981):677–681.
26. Haynes, P. F.: Dorsal displacement of the soft palate and epiglottic entrapment: diagnosis, management, and interrelationship. Comp. Cont. Ed. *5* (1983):S379–S389.
27. Heffron, C. J. and G. J. Baker: Observations on the mechanism of functional obstruction of the nasopharyngeal airway in the horse. Equine Vet. J. *11* (1979):142–147.
28. Hofmeyr, C. F. B.: Surgery of the pharynx. Vet. Clin. North Am. *2* (1972):3–16.
29. Jubb, K. V. F. and P. C. Kennedy: Pathology of Domestic Animals. 2nd. ed. New York: Academic Press, 1970, Vol. II p. 6.
30. Koch, D. B. and L. P. Tate, Jr.: Pharyngeal cysts in horses. JAVMA *173* (1978):860–862.
31. Lantz, G. C.: Pharyngostomy tube installation for the administration of nutritional and fluid requirements. Comp. Cont. Ed. *3* (1982):135–142.
32. Leonard, H. C.: Collapse of the larynx and adjacent structures in the dog. JAVMA *137* (1960):360–363.
33. Linford, R. L., T. R. O'Brien, J. D. Wheat, et al.: Radiographic assessment of epiglottic length and pharyngeal and laryngeal diameters in the Thoroughbred. Am. J. Vet. Res. *44* (1983):1660–1666.
34. Marks, D., M. P. Mackay-Smith, L. S. Cushing, et al.: Etiology and diagnosis of laryngeal hemiplegia in horses. JAVMA *157* (1970):429–436.
35. Marks, D., M. P. MacKay-Smith, L. S. Cushing, et al.: Use of a prosthetic device for surgical correction of

laryngeal hemiplegia in horses. JAVMA *157* (1970):157–163.

36. Mayer, K., J. V. Lacroix, and H. P. Hoskins (eds.): Canine Surgery. 4th ed. Evanston, Ill.: Am. Vet. Public., 1957.

37. Nelson, A. W., B. M. Curley, and R. A. Kainer: Mandibular symphysiotomy to provide adequate exposure for intraoral surgery in the horse. JAVMA *159* (1971):1025–1031.

38. Ott, R. L.: *In* Archibald, J. (ed.): Canine Surgery. Wheaton, Ill.: Am. Vet. Public., 1965.

39. Palmer, A. C.: Clinical signs associated with intracranial tumors in dogs. Res. Vet. Sci. *2* (1961):526–339.

40. Raphel, C. F.: Endoscopic findings in the upper respiratory tract of 479 horses. JAVMA *181* (1982):470–473.

41. Robbins, G. and J. Grandage: Temporomandibular joint dysplasia and open-mouth jaw locking in the dog. JAVMA *171* (1977):1072–1076.

42. Rosin, E. and G. F. Hanlon: Canine cricopharyngeal achalasia. JAVMA *160* (1972):1496–1499.

43. Rosin, E. and K. Greenwood: Bilateral arytenoid cartilage lateralization for laryngeal paralysis in the dog. JAVMA *180* (1982):515–518.

44. Schreiber, J.: Die Leitungsanästhesie der Kopfnerven beim Rind. Wiener tierärztl. Msch. *42* (1955):129–153.

45. Sis, R. F., J. T. Yoder, and C. J. Starch: Devocalization of cats by median laryngotomy and dissection of the vocal folds. Vet. Med. (Small Anim. Clin.) *62* (1967):975–980.

46. Sokolovsky, V.: Cricopharyngeal achalasia in a dog. JAVMA *150*(1967):281–284.

47. Stick, J. A. and C. Boles: Subepiglottic cyst in three foals. JAVMA *177*(1980):62–64.

48. Ticer, J. W. and C. P. Spencer: Injury of the feline temporomandibular joint: radiographic signs. J. Am. Vet. Radiol. Soc. *19*(1978):146–156.

49. Venker-Van Haagen, A. J., W. Hartman and S. A. Goedegebuure: Spontaneous laryngeal paralysis in young Bouviers. J. Am. Anim. Hosp. Assoc. *14*(1978):714–720.

50. Westhues, M. and R. Fritsch: Die Narkose der Tiere. Band I: Lokalanästhesie. Berlin: Parey, 1960.

51. Whalen, L. R. and R. L. Kitchell: Electrophysiologic studies of the cutaneous nerves of the head of the dog. Am. J. Vet. Res. *44*(1983):615–627.

52. Wykes, P. M.: Canine laryngeal diseases. Part I. Anatomy and disease syndromes. Comp. Cont. Ed. *5*(1983):8–13.

53. Wykes, P. M.: Canine laryngeal diseases. Part II. Diagnosis and treatment. Comp. Cont. Ed. *5*(1983):105–110.

54. Yoder, J. T. and C. J. Starch: Devocalization of dogs by laryngofissure and dissection of the thyroarytenoid folds. JAVMA *145*(1964):325–330.

CHAPTER 3

SALIVARY GLANDS AND LYMPH NODES OF HEAD AND CRANIAL NERVES VII, VIII, IX, AND XII

OBJECTIVES

1. To be able to recognize the clinical signs of a lesion of the facial nerve or its branches and to relate these signs to the location of the lesion.
2. To be able to diagnose a lesion of the vestibular apparatus.
3. To be able to diagnose hypoglossal nerve paralysis.
4. To be able to palpate the parotid and mandibular salivary glands and differentiate the mandibular salivary glands from lymph nodes.
5. To be able to trace the ducts of the salivary glands and palpate the parotid duct in the cheek of the dog.
6. To be able to differentiate canine ranula, salivary mucocele, and branchial cyst.
7. To be able to extirpate the mandibular and monostomatic sublingual salivary glands in the dog.
8. To be able to palpate the mandibular, retropharyngeal, cervical, and parotid lymph nodes where possible in different species and to be able to find these nodes at autopsy and in meat inspection. Where would you examine a cow for lymphosarcoma involving lymph nodes in the head?
9. To know the surgical landmarks for access to the diseased guttural pouch and retropharyngeal lymph nodes via Viborg's triangle.
10. To be able to palpate the pulse in the facial artery.
11. To be able to reflect the masseter muscle for tooth expulsion, sparing the buccal and masseteric veins in the horse.
12. To know the anatomical aspects of the surgery to transplant the parotid duct to the conjunctival sac.

Cranial Nerves. The facial, vestibulocochlear, glossopharyngeal, and hypoglossal nerves will be discussed in this chapter. The other cranial nerves have either been dealt with in Chapter 2, or will be considered in Chapter 4.

The facial nerve (VII) is primarily a motor nerve to the superficial muscles of the head, often called the muscles of expression. Although some of these muscles are active in eating, they should not be confused with the muscles of mastication, which are innervated by the mandibular nerve. Another diagnostic distinction that must be kept clear is that the sensory nerve to the skin covering the muscles of expression is the trigeminal—not the facial.

The extent of facial paralysis is important in the prognosis. A common site of injury in the horse is at the caudal border of the mandible, where the dorsal and ventral buccal branches cross the masseter ventral to the temporomandibular joint. It is common for a halter buckle to bruise the nerves if the animal is carelessly cast. An injury at this point will paralyze the lips, nostrils, and cheek and will cause hypalgesia of the field of the branches of the auriculotemporal nerve (V) that course with the transverse facial artery and the buccal branches of the facial nerve. (In ruminants and carnivores, the ventral buccal branch runs along the ventral border of the masseter so a superficial injury is less likely to involve both branches.) In the horse and small ruminants but not in the ox and dog, the tonus of the muscles on the opposite, normal side will pull the nose and lips in that direction. The paralysis of the lateral nasal muscle, which dilates the nostril, may be the earliest sign in the race horse, as maximum speed cannot be attained without dilation of the nostrils. Another sign is the accumulation of decaying feed in the oral vestibule, which is caused by paralysis of the buccinator muscle. This muscle normally presses the feed back between the dental arcades into the oral cavity proper, working in opposition to the tongue during mastication. The accumulation of feed in the mouth has been interpreted as an inability to swallow and has led to a false diagnosis of rabies. In the dog, a common sign is drooling from the corner of the mouth because of paralysis of the orbicularis oris. If the signs are limited to the mouth and nose, the prognosis is good because the lesion is peripheral and probably traumatic (see Plates I and II).

In the ox and dog, the palpebral branches of the auriculopalpebral nerve are more vulnerable to injury because they cross the zygomatic arch where it is prominent. Cattle that resist restraint in a stanchion and forcefully pull their heads back may injure one or both nerves at this point, causing an inability to close the eyelids. The lower lid may droop and permit tears to cross the face. Traumatic keratitis is always a danger following eyelid paralysis. In the horse, the auriculopalpebral nerve leaves the facial nerve caudal to the temporomandibular joint and passes dorsally caudal to the mandible, where it is protected. The palpebral branch passes forward over the highest point of the zygomatic arch, where it is palpable, and crosses the supraorbital foramen to the orbicularis oculi. It is not likely to be injured along with the buccal branches. For ocular examination, the eyelids can be immobilized by blocking the palpebral branch where it can be palpated on the zygomatic arch.

In the horse and ox, ptosis accompanies paralysis of branches of the auriculopalpebral nerve, because in the ox the frontalis muscle is a strong levator of the upper lid and in the horse the small levator anguli oculi medialis has a similar action. This ptosis should not be confused with that accompanying oculomotor nerve paralysis, sympathetic nerve paralysis, or a sunken eyeball due to atrophy of the temporal and pterygoid muscles. In small animals, the size of the palpebral fissure is unchanged or slightly wider in facial paralysis.

In any species, paralysis of the ear along with the eyelids, lips, and nose indicates a complete facial nerve paralysis and a lesion in its course from the medulla to the stylomastoid foramen. The ear muscles are supplied by auricular branches of the auriculopalpebral nerve and the caudal auricular nerve. The latter leaves the facial nerve as it emerges from this foramen. The paralyzed ear will droop in the horse, ox, sheep, and some breeds of dogs. In cats and some dogs, the immobile ear will be held erect by its cartilage.

Unless there are other clinical signs of a lesion in the medulla, the lesion is in the facial nerve. A common site of involvement is in its course through the facial canal of the temporal bone, where it is exposed to inflammation in the middle ear.[3, 9, 15] This same otitis media often affects the vestibulocochlear nerve in the inner ear, simultaneously causing signs of vestibular disturbance on the same side as the facial paralysis. In the dog and cat, the postganglionic sympathetic axons that course through the middle ear may be affected by the otitis and cause Horner's syndrome. Complete unilateral idiopathic facial paralysis occurs in the dog. Some biopsy specimens have revealed degenerative lesions, and chronic hypothyroidism has been implicated in some patients. A few dogs recover spontaneously.

Listeriosis is an inflammation of the brain stem of ruminants. Involvement of the facial nucleus or the nerve in its course through the medulla is a common cause of facial paresis or paralysis in these species. These animals are usually depressed and have an ataxic and paretic gait and other clinical signs indicating a lesion in the pons and medulla.

Remember the location of the stylomastoid foramen caudal to the external acoustic meatus when doing aural surgery in the dog. The facial nerve courses rostrally from this foramen adjacent to the ventral wall of the external ear canal where the canal changes from a vertical to a horizontal position.

Hemifacial spasm is seen in dogs as an idiopathic disease or associated with otitis media.[2, 16] The nose and philtrum are pulled toward the affected side, the lips are taut and retracted, the palpebral fissure is narrowed, and the ear is elevated. A deviated philtrum in the dog is usually a sign of hemifacial spasm. In facial paralysis in the dog the philtrum is rarely pulled toward the normal side as it is in horses and small ruminants. Hemifacial spasm is thought to be a continual activity of facial neurons; it is less likely to be a contracture of denervated muscles, because the muscles relax in patients that have been examined under anesthesia.

A lesion in the vestibular receptor or vestibular part of the eighth cranial nerve in the inner ear causes a loss of balance and an inability to orient the head with the limbs, trunk, and eyes. This is referred to as peripheral vestibular disease. Characteristically, there is a head tilt with the lower ear toward the affected side and a tendency to fall toward that side or stumble, lean, or drift that way. Occasionally, the patient will fall and roll forcefully toward the affected side, but this usually occurs only in the first few hours after an acute peripheral lesion. Strength is normal, as are the postural reactions. An abnormal horizontal or rotatory nystagmus may be present, with the quick phase always directed toward the normal side. This may be continual (spontaneous) for the first 3 or 4 days after an acute lesion or may be observed only when the head is held in extension or flexion to one or both sides (positional). Peripheral vestibular disease most commonly occurs secondary to otitis media and interna. A transient idiopathic disorder is observed in cats during the summer months in the northeast[2] and in older dogs at any time of year.[20] Similar signs may occur when lesions affect the vestibular nuclei in the medulla or vestibular components of the cerebellum, but the other signs of medullary or cerebellar disease will locate the lesion centrally.[2]

Disease of the cochlear part of the eighth cranial nerve results in deafness. Unilateral deafness is difficult to detect on clinical examination.

The glossopharyngeal nerve (IX) is both motor and sensory to the pharynx. The pharyngeal branch joins those of the vagus and accessory nerves, and the signs of pharyngeal paralysis are common to these three nerves.

The hypoglossal nerve (XII) supplies the muscles of the tongue. Paralysis results in a weak tongue that is best detected by the lack of resistance to pulling it out of the mouth, the inability to retract it, and decreased movement associated with dysphagia. Atrophy may also be observed. The most reliable sign of unilateral paralysis is atrophy of one-half of the tongue.

3a. DISSECTION, HEAD, HORSE

Facial nerve. Trace the dorsal and ventral buccal branches to the facial muscles. Note the origin of the caudal auricular nerve. Trace the auriculopalpebral nerve dorsally in the groove between the ear and the zygomatic process, where it gives off its rostral auricular branches. It then turns forward over the most dorsal part of the zygomatic arch and runs across the supraorbital foramen to the muscles of the eyelids.

Mandibular lymph nodes. A chain of nodes about 10 to 12 cm. long in the intermandibular region, lateral to the omohyoid muscles. The right and left groups of nodes meet ventral to the lingual process and the body of the hyoid bone, which is the point of termination of the muscles. The nodes diverge caudally. They are superficial and easily palpated.

Facial artery. Turns around the ventral border of the mandible at the rostral border of the masseter. The facial vein and parotid duct are caudal to the artery at the turn (see Plate I).

Reflection of the masseter for repulsion of the last lower molar. Two large veins must be avoided: the buccal vein at the rostral end of the incision and the large ventral masseteric vein, which is more caudal within the masseter muscle.

Retropharyngeal lymph nodes. This group of nodes lies medial to the mandibular salivary gland and the digastricus muscle. The lateral retropharyngeal lymph nodes lie near the wing of the atlas, on the internal carotid artery and the caudodorsal surface of the guttural pouch. The medial retropharyngeal lymph nodes are larger and more numerous. They lie on the dorsolateral surface of the pharynx, ventral to the guttural pouch and medial to the external carotid and linguofacial arteries (Fig. 6–1, 24).

Cranial deep cervical lymph nodes. On the common carotid artery near the thyroid gland and under the cervical angle of the parotid gland.

Viborg's triangle is one means of access to the frequently abscessed retropharyngeal nodes. The triangle is formed by the angle of the mandible, the linguofacial vein, and the tendon of the sternocephalicus.

Parotid lymph nodes have been described on the deep surface of the rostral dorsal part of the parotid salivary gland.

3b. LIVE HORSE

Identify the following structures:

Facial artery, facial vein, and parotid duct where they pass around the ramus of the mandible. Be sure that you can count the pulse.

Basihyoid bone and the lingual process.

Termination of the sternohyoid and omohyoid muscles on the basihyoid and lingual process.

Mandibular lymph nodes in the intermandibular region lateral to the omohyoid muscles.

Mandibular and parotid salivary glands. Outline their positions; they cannot be palpated, except the cervical angle of the parotid (see Plate I).

Viborg's triangle: Angle of the mandible
                                 Linguofacial vein (distend the jugular)
                                 Tendon of the sternocephalicus (extend the head)

The retropharyngeal lymph nodes are not normally palpable but are incised from Viborg's triangle when they are abscessed. Palpate the retropharyngeal region through the triangle.

3c. DISSECTION, HEAD, COW

Mandibular lymph node. Between the mandibular attachment of the sternocephalicus and the mandibular salivary gland, medial to the facial vein.

Facial artery. Medial and deep to the vein at the lymph node, in front of the vein at the turn around the ventral border of the mandible.

Parotid lymph node. Ventral and slightly rostral to the temporomandibular articulation. It is partially covered by the parotid salivary gland. Note the proximity of the dorsal buccal branch of the facial nerve.

Lateral retropharyngeal (atlantal) lymph node. Dorsal to the common carotid artery, medial to the caudodorsal border of the mandibular salivary gland, and cranioventral to the wing of the atlas.

Medial retropharyngeal lymph node. On the median cut surface of the head, between the caudodorsal wall of the pharynx and the longus capitis muscle. Swelling of these nodes causes dyspnea and dysphagia. The palatine tonsil is also exposed. It may be mistaken for the lymph node at autopsy if the topographical relations are destroyed.

3d. LIVE COW

Take the pulse from the facial artery in the groove at the rostral border of the masseter muscle (see Plate II).

Distend the linguofacial vein by compression of the jugular vein.

Identify the mandibular attachment of the sternocephalicus. (Extend the head.)

Palpate the mandibular salivary gland. The palpable part is discoid and pendant near the midline in the caudal intermandibular region (see Plate II). The ventral ends of the right and left glands are usually adjacent here. Do not confuse these glands with lymph nodes.

Mandibular lymph node. Lateral to the mandibular salivary gland, small, firm, and covered by the sternocephalicus. It is best palpated by grasping the mandible and the sternocephalicus with the thumb on the lateral surface and the fingertips medial to the mandible. Roll the sternocephalicus mediolaterally under the fingertips to feel the node against the mandible (see Plate II).

Parotid lymph node. It is large and movable at the rostral border of the parotid salivary gland ventral to the temporomandibular joint (see Plate II).

Lateral retropharyngeal (atlantal) lymph node. This is difficult to palpate if normal. Extend the head and examine the fossa between the mandible and the wing of the atlas.

Medial retropharyngeal lymph node. Must be palpated through the mouth and the dorsal wall of the pharynx in the normal state. This is not recommended in rabies territory.

Hyoid apparatus. Palpate the angle of the stylohyoid in the dorsal part of the triangle formed by the mandible and the atlas. The medial retropharyngeal node would be palpable here if enlarged.

3e. DISSECTION, HEAD, PIG

Mandibular lymph nodes. Ventromedial to the angle of the mandible near the ventral part of the rostral border of the mandibular salivary gland.

Parotid, lateral retropharyngeal, and ventral superficial cervical lymph nodes. They form a chain that begins at the rostral border of the large parotid salivary gland near the temporomandibular joint and extends caudoventrally deep to the caudal border of the gland to the external jugular vein.

Medial retropharyngeal lymph nodes. On the dorsal wall of the pharynx, dorsal to the external carotid artery, and caudoventral to the paracondylar process. They are ventral to the longus capitis muscle.

Dorsal superficial cervical (prescapular) lymph node. If the head is cut off with a long jowl attached, the node will be found with the head. Normally it is at the cranial border of the subclavius muscle, under cover of the trapezius and omotransversarius.

3f. SIALOGRAMS, DOG

Sialography is the radiographic visualization of a salivary gland with a radiopaque material. For the monostomatic sublingual and the mandibular salivary glands, the ducts are cannulated with small needles (24 gauge) at their openings on the sublingual caruncle.[4-6] The ducts course caudally beside the tongue. The oval mandibular gland is caudal to the mandible. The caudal part of the elongate monostomatic sublingual gland is applied to the cranial curvature of the mandibular gland. The rostral part is medial to the ramus of the mandible.

3g. DISSECTION, HEAD, DOG

Cervical cysts in the dog are usually salivary mucoceles that result from a rupture in the monostomatic sublingual duct or gland.[5, 10] The saliva collects in a connective tissue space, which expands caudally along the ventral surface of the neck. The wall of the mucocele is neither epithelial nor secretory. The mucocele will not recur if the affected salivary gland is removed. Branchial cysts are rare vestiges of the embryonic pharyngeal pouches or branchial grooves.[22] They are usually dorsolateral in position. The lining of a cyst is pseudostratified secretory epithelium and must be entirely removed. Branchial cysts may be identified by biopsy. A ranula is a swelling under the tongue; usually it is a salivary mucocele caused by a defect in the duct of the monostomatic sublingual gland or by an abnormal solitary lobule of the polystomatic sublingual gland.

Cervical salivary mucoceles can be diagnosed by sialography, which will identify the abnormal salivary gland. Radiopaque material will leak from the duct or gland into the mucocele. The treatment is to remove the mandibular and monostomatic sublingual glands on the side of the abnormal gland.[13] During surgery when the mucocele is dissected free, the side of its origin may be apparent. Occasionally the salivary gland defect is bilateral.

There are two sublingual glands on each side. The polystomatic sublingual gland consists of many small lobules under the oral mucosa, each with a minor sublingual duct opening into the mouth. This gland is rarely involved in a mucocele and is not removed in the operation under discussion. The monostomatic sublingual gland has two parts, both drained by the major sublingual duct. The caudal part is closely applied to the mandibular gland and enclosed in a common capsule with it. The rostral part lies along the major sublingual and mandibular ducts medial to the mandible.

The mandibular gland is removed with the monostomatic sublingual gland because of the difficulty of isolating the latter without damaging the mandibular duct. The glands are located together caudal to the mandible in the fork made by the maxillary and linguofacial branches of the external jugular vein. After the glands are mobilized and their blood supply ligated, the ducts are traced rostrally, then medially between the digastricus and the mandible.[7] The ducts are ligated rostral to the glands, and the glands are removed. Greater access to the rostral part of the ducts can be achieved by passing the glands medially between the digastricus and mandible and incising the caudal part of the mylohyoideus.

Zygomatic salivary mucoceles cause either exophthalmos or enophthalmos. Abscesses are more common and cause exophthalmos. These are very painful. Appreciate why attempting to open the jaw exacerbates this pain!

Examine the parotid duct. It can be transplanted under the skin to the dorsolateral fornix of the conjunctiva for the treatment of keratoconjunctivitis sicca.[1, 12] A dark-colored nylon filament is passed through the parotid orifice into the duct to facilitate dissection. Beware of two right angle turns in the terminal part of the duct.[23] The incision is made along the course of the duct, which can sometimes be located by palpating the groove in the masseter, in which it lies. The duct runs between the middle and ventral thirds of the muscle. After section and retraction of the cutaneous muscle, the dorsal and ventral buccal branches of the facial nerve are identified, with the duct between them. To dissect the duct to the parotid papilla it is necessary to follow it deep to the facial artery and vein and the communication between the dorsal and ventral buccal branches of the facial nerve. The parotid papilla with duct attached is cut out of the oral mucosa and sutured into a stab wound in the conjunctiva.

Mandibular lymph nodes. There are two or three mandibular lymph nodes, which are located between the angle of the jaw and the mandibular salivary gland on both sides of the facial vein (see Plate III).

Medial retropharyngeal lymph node. This node is located dorsal to the caudal part of the pharynx, medial to the sternomastoideus and mandibular salivary gland, ventral to the longus capitis, and caudal to the digastricus. It is closely related to the end of the common carotid artery.

Lateral retropharyngeal lymph node. This node is present in only one-third of dogs. It lies between the dorsal border of the mandibular salivary gland and the atlas.

Parotid lymph node. The parotid lymph node is between the dorsal part of the caudal border of the masseter and the rostral border of the parotid salivary gland. It is small, but palpable (see Plate III).

Lymph nodes are occasionally found associated with the facial vessels on the rostral border of the masseter muscle ventral to the zygomatic bone.[17, 21]

3h. LIVE DOG

Estimate the position of the parotid salivary gland from specimen 3g. It is not readily palpable (see Plate III). Palpate the duct, the facial vessels, and the dorsal buccal branches of the facial nerve in the cheek.[14]

Palpate the parotid lymph node at the rostral border of the parotid gland by drawing the fingertip forward in the notch between the ear and the angular process of the mandible.

Palpate the mandibular salivary gland in the fork between the maxillary and linguofacial veins. The external jugular vein should be distended (see Plate III).

Differentiate the mandibular lymph nodes from the salivary gland. They are small, two to three in number, and rostral to the mandibular gland. They can be picked up in a fold of skin, whereas the mandibular gland is tightly covered by fascia.

References

1. Baker, G. J. and C. Formston: An evaluation of transplantation of the parotid duct in the treatment of keratoconjunctivitis sicca in the dog. J. Small Anim. Pract. *9* (1968):261–268.

2. de Lahunta, A.: Veterinary Neuroanatomy and Clinical Neurology, 2nd ed. Philadelphia: W. B. Saunders, 1983.

3. Firth, E. C.: Vestibular disease and its relationship to facial paralysis in the horse: a clinical study of 7 cases. Aust. Vet. J. *53* (1977):560–565.

4. Glen, J. B.: Salivary cysts in the dog. Identification of sublingual duct defects by sialography. Vet. Rec. *78* (1966):488–492.

5. Glen, J. B.: Canine salivary mucoceles. Results of sialographic examination and surgical treatment of fifty cases. J. Small Anim. Pract. *13* (1972):515–526.

6. Harvey, C. E.: Sialography in the dog. J. Am. Vet. Radiol. Soc. *10* (1969):18–27.

7. Hoffer, R. E. and H. E. Jensen: Stereoscopic Atlas of Small Animal Surgery. St. Louis: C. V. Mosby, 1973, pp. 181–186.

8. Hulland, T. J. and J. Archibald: Salivary mucoceles in dogs. Can. Vet. J. *5* (1964):109–117.

9. Jensen, R., L. R. Maki, L. H. Lauerman, et al.: Cause and pathogenesis of middle ear infection in young feedlot cattle. JAVMA *182* (1983):967–972.

10. Karbe, E. and S. W. Nielsen: Canine ranulas, salivary mucoceles and branchial cysts. J. Small Anim. Pract. *7* (1966):625–630.

11. Knecht, C. D.: Diseases of the salivary glands in the dog. Comp. Cont. Ed. *2* (1980):932–936.

12. Lavignette, A. M.: Keratoconjunctivitis sicca in a dog treated by transposition of the parotid salivary duct. JAVMA *148* (1966):778–786.

13. Leonard, E. P.: Fundamentals of Small Animal Surgery. Philadelphia: W. B. Saunders, 1968. pp. 178–180.

14. McCarthy, P. H.: The anatomy of the parotid duct (ductus parotideus) of the Greyhound as appreciated by the sense of touch. Anat. Histol. Embryol. *7* (1978):311–319.

15. Power, H. T., B. J. Watrous, and A. de Lahunta: Facial and vestibulocochlear nerve disease in six horses. JAVMA *183* (1983):1076–1080.

16. Roberts, S. R. and S. J. Vainisi: Hemifacial spasm in dogs. JAVMA *150* (1967):381–385.

17. Rumph, P. F., P. D. Garrett, and B. W. Gray: Facial lymph nodes in dogs. JAVMA *176* (1980):342–344.

18. Saar, L. I. and R. Getty: The interrelationship of the lymph vessel connections of the lymph nodes of the head, neck, and shoulder regions of swine. Am. J. Vet. Res. *25* (1964):618–636.

19. Schmidt, G. M. and C. W. Betts: Zygomatic salivary mucoceles in the dog. JAVMA *172* (1978):940–942.

20. Schunk, K. L. and D. R. Averill, Jr. Peripheral vestibular syndrome in the dog: a review of 83 cases. JAVMA *182* (1983):1354–1357.

21. Shelton, M. E. and W. B. Forsythe: Buccal lymph node in the dog. Am. J. Vet. Res. *40* (1979):1638–1639.

22. Smith, D. F. and D. E. Gunson: Branchial cyst in a heifer. JAVMA *171* (1977):64–66.

23. Testoni, F. J., C. L. Lohse and R. J. Hyde: Anatomy and cannulation of the parotid duct in the dog. JAVMA *170* (1977):831–833.

CHAPTER 4

EYE, NASAL CAVITY, AND CRANIAL NERVES II, III, IV, V (OPHTHALMIC), AND VI

OBJECTIVES

1. To understand the anatomy of the eyeball and the relationship among its three coats.
2. To understand the iridocorneal angle and its relation to the drainage of aqueous humor and to intrabulbar pressure.
3. To be able to find the optic disc and to recognize the normal pattern of the retinal vessels in each species.
4. To know the normal size and shape of the tapetum lucidum in connection with the diagnosis of retinopathies.
5. To understand the disposition of the conjunctiva, the third eyelid, and the gland of the third eyelid in connection with normal function, inflammation, displacements, and bovine carcinoma of the eye.
6. To be able to interpret the pupillary reflex and its abnormalities in neuroanatomical terms.
7. To be able to interpret the failure of the wink reflex and to be able to paralyze the m. orbicularis oculi for examination of the eye.
8. To be able to anesthetize the orbit of the ox for enucleation.
9. To be able to diagnose nervous and muscular disorders by abnormal movements of the eyeball. This requires a knowledge of the origins and terminations of the muscles and their innervation.
10. To be able to find the terminations of the extrinsic muscles on the eyeball in surgery.
11. To be able to maintain hemostasis in enucleation of the eye.
12. To understand the lacrimal system in order to avoid the nasolacrimal duct in surgery, to be able to flush the duct from either end, and to remove the lacrimal gland in enucleation.
13. To be able to trephine the dorsal nasal meatus without involving the frontal sinus in the horse.
14. To be able to pass a stomach tube through the ventral nasal meatus.
15. To be able to do a retrobulbar injection in the dog.
16. To be able to inject radiopaque dye into the ophthalmic plexus and cavernous sinus.
17. To know the anatomy of the orbit to explain exophthalmos and enophthalmos.
18. To be able to recognize the radiographic features of the orbit and to be able to distinguish the orbit from the cribriform plate of the ethmoid bone.

The periorbita serves as periosteum for the bony orbit and as a thick membrane ventrolaterally, where the bony orbit is incomplete in animals. It is conical with its apex at the optic canal and orbital fissure and its base at the rim of the orbit, where it gives off the orbital septum into the eyelids. It surrounds all of the structures in the orbit including the extrabulbar muscles, vessels, and nerves and most of the globe, and it gives attachment to the fascial sheaths of these structures. Retrobulbar injections are made inside the periorbita for anesthesia of the globe and eyelids and for treatment of inflammatory diseases of the optic nerve and globe. The dura is continuous through the optic canal with the periorbita and with the external sheath around the optic nerve. The dura attaches to the sclera and to a fascial socket on the outside of the sclera, the bulbar sheath. Between the optic canal and the eyeball, the leptomeninges and the subarachnoid space continue along the optic nerve, the pia mater forming its internal sheath. This continuity of meninges and cerebrospinal fluid from the cranial cavity along the optic nerve permits disease processes to extend in either direction and may alter the cerebrospinal fluid contents in patients with optic neuritis.

The eyelids receive sensory innervation from branches of the ophthalmic and maxillary nerves within the periorbita. The ophthalmic nerve branches are the infratrochlear ventromedially, the frontal dorsomedially, and in ungulates, the lacrimal dorsolaterally. The maxillary nerve branches are the zygomaticotemporal dorsolaterally in the dog and the zygomaticofacial ventrolaterally. These nerves can be blocked by a retrobulbar injection of anesthetic into the periorbita, by a line block in the eyelids proximal to the area that requires anesthesia, or by an injection along the margin of the orbit at each quadrant where the nerve emerges.[21] In the horse, the frontal nerve emerges as the supraorbital nerve through the supraorbital foramen, where it can be blocked. There is considerable overlap of the cutaneous areas supplied by these nerves, which explains why individual nerve blocks are often not effective. For clinical diagnosis in the dog, the only autonomous zone for the ophthalmic nerve is a small area of the upper eyelid at the medial angle and for the maxillary nerve, a small area of the lower eyelid at the lateral angle.[39]

4a. DISSECTION, EYE, HORSE

The terms anterior and posterior are employed for the eyeball and inner ear in the N.A.V. because there is no conflict here with their meaning in human anatomy.

Orient the eye by means of the third eyelid and examine the gland of the third eyelid on the deep end of the cartilage. Arrange the muscles of the eyeball so that their origins, terminations, and actions can be studied. All of the muscles except the ventral oblique originate at the apex of the orbit. The retractor bulbi pulls the eyeball straight back in a protective reflex mediated by the ophthalmic and abducent nerves when pressure is applied to the anterior surface of the globe. The recti incline the optic axis dorsoventrally, mediolaterally, or, by contraction of two adjacent muscles, obliquely. The lateral rectus is innervated by the abducent nerve; the other three recti are innervated by the oculomotor nerve. The thin flat muscle on the dorsal surface of the dorsal rectus is the levator palpebrae superioris, which is also innervated by the third nerve.

The dorsal oblique muscle takes the same direction as the straight muscles until it reaches the trochlea, where it turns laterally, then passes deep to the tendon of termination of the dorsal rectus, and is inserted on the sclera. It is innervated by the trochlear nerve and rotates the globe around an anteroposterior axis that differs from the optic axis. The degree of deviation of the axis of rotation from the optic axis varies with the species, but the dorsal part of the globe is rotated medially. The ventral oblique originates from the medial wall of the orbit, passes ventral to the ventral rectus, and terminates on the sclera under the tendon of the lateral rectus. It is innervated by the oculomotor nerve and has a rotatory action opposite to that of the dorsal oblique. The dorsal oblique produces intorsion of the eyeball and the ventral oblique causes extorsion.

The external ophthalmic artery is a short trunk from the maxillary in the apex of the orbit. It gives off a long branch that runs forward on the optic nerve and supplies the ciliary arteries that pierce the sclera around the optic nerve. The external ophthalmic also gives rise to muscular branches that, in addition to supplying the muscles, give off small anterior ciliary arteries in front of the equator. Other branches are the supraorbital, lacrimal, and the large external ethmoidal.

4b. ANTERIOR HEMISPHERE, HORSE

The cornea joins the anterior sclera at the limbus where the bulbar conjunctiva is attached, and it may be pigmented. Knowledge of the structure of the cornea is clinically important in the understanding of the many diseases that affect it. The cornea consists of five layers: (1) stratified squamous anterior epithelium, (2) anterior limiting membrane of fine collagen fibrils (extremely thin in domestic animals),[25, 34] (3) thick proper substance of highly organized collagen layers, (4) posterior limiting basement membrane, and (5) posterior epithelium. There are no blood vessels in the normal cornea; it is nourished by loops of conjunctival vessels at the limbus, by tears, and by aqueous humor. The posterior and anterior epithelia maintain transparency by controlling hydration of the cornea. Corneal ulcers that extend through the proper substance allow the posterior limiting membrane and epithelium to protrude on the surface.

The vascular coat or uvea consists of the choroid, ciliary body, and iris and is attached to the inside of the sclera. The lens is suspended from the ciliary body by the noncellular zonular fibers that extend from between the ciliary processes. These radial processes can be seen on the inside of the ciliary body. Their epithelium functions in producing the aqueous humor, which enters the posterior chamber between the iris and lens. The nervous layer of the retina is continuous with this epithelium at the posterior border of the ciliary body, the ora serrata. The nervous layer appears white in preserved specimens. The ciliary muscle consists mostly of fibers that run meridionally from their origin on the inside of the sclera into the ciliary body.

Projecting from the upper pupillary border of the iris are the normal, black, iridic granules. Much smaller granules project from the lower margin. They are vascular extensions of the stroma of the iris, covered by the pigmented posterior epithelium of the iris.

At the ciliary border of the iris, the trabeculae that attach it to the inside of the corneal limbus are visible grossly. The aggregate of these trabeculae forms a radial structure, the pectinate ligament of the iridocorneal angle. Between the trabeculae and behind them are the spaces of the iridocorneal angle, in the depths of which is the trabecular meshwork composed of collagenous strands (ungulates) or fenestrated lamellae (carnivores) and covered by simple squamous epithelium.[19] The trabecular meshwork is clinically important in drainage of the aqueous humor into the venous plexus of the sclera. The aqueous humor passes through the meshwork to the small vessels of the plexus. The aqueous humor is produced by the ciliary processes and passes from the posterior chamber through the pupil to the anterior chamber. The rate of production and the rate of drainage determine the intrabulbar pressure. Congenital or acquired lesions of the trabecular meshwork cause increased pressure (glaucoma).[18] A small amount of aqueous humor passes through the ciliary body to the suprachoroidal space and sclera for absorption into vessels there (uveoscleral flow).[12]

In life, the nervous layer of the retina is transparent. Light rays must traverse its entire thickness to stimulate impulses in the layer of rods and cones adjacent to the pigmented epithelium of the retina. The fundus is the inside of the posterior portion of the eyeball that is examined with an ophthalmoscope. The relatively triangular shiny area of a combination of yellow, green, and orange colors is the tapetum lucidum. This is a layer in the inner portion of the choroid that is visible because the pigment layer of the retina that covers it lacks pigment in this region. The remainder of the visible fundus is called the nontapetal area and is dark brown from the pigment in the pigment layer of the retina and the underlying choroid. In the normal animal, these regions are visible by looking through the normally transparent nervous layer of the retina. Lesions of the retina that cause opacities will interfere with this normal appearance.

4c. POSTERIOR HEMISPHERE, HORSE

The optic disc is ventral and lateral to the posterior pole of the bulb, and this must be kept in mind in using the ophthalmoscope. The disc is below the distinct horizontal lower border of the tapetum lucidum in the horse. In the various domestic animals there is considerable variation in the position of the optic disc relative to the tapetum lucidum and in the arrangement of blood vessels at the disc (Fig. 4–1). There are no large vessels at the optic disc in the horse. Numerous small vessels extend

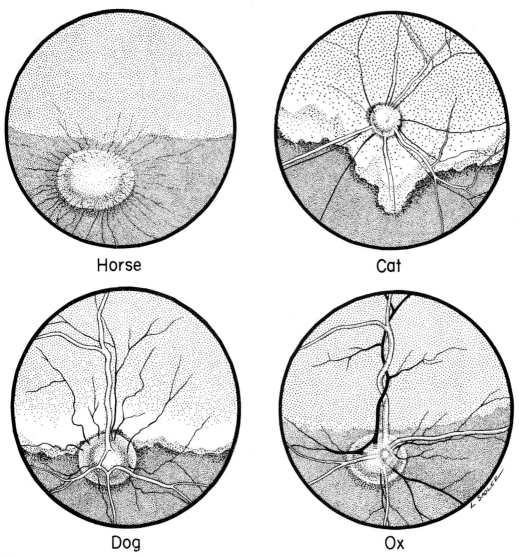

Figure 4–1. Ophthalmoscopic views of the fundus of the right eye in four species, the arteries are black; the veins are white. The position of the optic disc on the ventral border of the tapetum lucidum shown for the dog is that of middle-sized breeds. In large dogs the disc is entirely surrounded by the tapetum lucidum as in the cat. In small dogs it is ventral to the tapetum lucidum as in the ungulates.

peripherally from the entire margin of the disc. The numerous dark spots seen in the area of the tapetum lucidum are penetrating choroidal blood vessels seen on end-view.

In preserved specimens the nervous layer of the retina separates from the pigment layer of the retina, which is attached to the inside of the choroid. The nervous layer remains attached at the disc posteriorly and at the ciliary body anteriorly. This is the same site of detachment that may occur with disease conditions, and it was the lumen of the optic cup or neural canal in the embryo.

4d. TRANSVERSE AND SAGITTAL SECTIONS, NASAL CAVITY, HORSE

Identify the following structures:

The nasolacrimal duct. The duct courses dorsal to a line drawn from the medial angle of the eye to the infraorbital foramen.

Infraorbital canal. The infraorbital canal is located on the top of a septum that traverses the maxillary sinus and contains the roots of the cheek teeth.

Major palatine artery and the venous plexus of the hard palate. These vessels are the source of profuse hemorrhage in tooth extraction.

Dorsal and ventral conchae.

The four nasal meatuses on each side: dorsal, middle, ventral, and common.

The rostral extent of the frontal sinus. This is best seen on the caudal aspect of a transverse section in front of the orbit. The cavity here is actually the sinus of the dorsal concha, but because it is continuous with the sinus in the frontal bone, the two sinuses are considered one for practical purposes—the clinical frontal sinus. Note the septum separating the frontal sinus from the rostral part of the conchal cavity. Trephine caudal to this point for the frontal sinus, rostral to it for the dorsal nasal meatus. (see Section 5d).

4e. LIVE HORSE

Evert an eyelid and look for the tarsal glands. These are seen as a palisade of yellowish lines under the conjunctiva. They are about 5 mm. long and 1 mm. wide and are perpendicular to the free border of the lid. Other glands that open on the free border are the ciliary glands, which are similar to sweat glands, and sebaceous glands. The ciliary and sebaceous glands are similar to the two types of skin glands associated with hair follicles wherever they occur.

Press gently on the upper lid, forcing it into the depression between the orbit and the eyeball, which should cause protrusion of the third eyelid. This is a useful procedure in physical examination.

Elicit the palpebral reflex by lightly touching the eyelids and observe the closure of the palpebral fissure. The sensory nerve is the trigeminal (maxillary and/or ophthalmic nerves) and the motor nerve is the facial nerve to the orbicularis oculi. The same response can be elicited by lightly touching the cornea. This tests the same two cranial nerves (ophthalmic nerve of the trigeminal and the facial nerve) and is unnecessary and potentially dangerous, as the cornea of the domestic animal is much less sensitive than that of the human and can be injured. The wink reaction can also be elicited by menacing the eye with the hand, but this must be done with care to ensure that the sensory stimulus is visual, through the optic nerve, and not caused by air currents stimulating the trigeminal nerve through the hairs.

The orbit can be anesthetized by inserting a 12-cm. needle caudal to the zygomatic process of the frontal bone at the level of the palpable supraorbital foramen (see Plate I). The needle is inserted medioventrally at an angle of 40° from the sagittal plane to the orbital fissure.[8] In order to operate on the eye it is also necessary to block the motor nerve to the orbicularis oculi—the auriculopalpebral. A needle is introduced into the depression between the ear and the temporomandibular joint and directed upward to a position caudal to the most dorsal part of the zygomatic arch, where a fan-shaped injection is made.[30] Alternatively, the palpebral branch can be blocked where it is palpable on the highest part of the zygomatic arch.[16]

Locate the puncta lacrimalia. These are inside the edges of the lids, 8 mm. from the medial angle. A catheter may be inserted through the punctum of the lower lid and through the nasolacrimal duct to find an imperforate nasal orifice. Locate the nasal orifice of the nasolacrimal duct. It is on the floor of the nasal cavity about 5 cm. from the lower commissure of the nostril, near the mucocutaneous junction. Estimate, on the exterior, the course of the nasolacrimal duct.

Look for vessels of the corneal limbus. There should be no vessels in the normal cornea. The cornea and aqueous humor should be clear, and the surface and borders of the iris should be visible for examination.

Shine a light in the eye and observe the expansion of the iris to narrow the pupil. The sensory pathway involves the neurons in the retina, optic nerve, optic chiasm and tracts, and pretectal nuclei in the thalamus. The preganglionic motor neuron is in the rostral midbrain and oculomotor nerve. The second motor neuron is in the ciliary ganglion and nerves, all within the periorbita adjacent to the optic nerve. Crossing of the majority of the neurons in the optic chiasm and in the pretectal area causes the impulses generated in one retina to reach the preganglionic motorneurons of both oculomotor nerves, and both pupils constrict. The direct response is observed in the eye that is stimulated and is usually stronger. The indirect or consensual response is observed in the opposite eye.

With a lesion throughout the retina or optic nerve of one eye, there will be no response in either eye to light directed into the affected eye. Both pupils respond to light directed into the normal eye. A lesion in one oculomotor nerve causes a widely dilated pupil on that side and the iris will not respond to light directed into either eye, while the opposite pupil will constrict.

Examine the fundus with an ophthalmoscope. Find the optic disc and notice the numerous fine vessels that radiate a short distance from the periphery of the optic disc. The disc is below the tapetum lucidum.[9]

Palpate the lamina of the alar cartilage projecting from the medial side of the nostril. In the dorsal commissure of the nostril is the opening of the nasal diverticulum, which should be avoided. The stomach tube should be inserted at the ventral commissure and directed into the ventral meatus.

4f. ENUCLEATION OF THE EYE, OX

A skin incision is made 5 mm. from the margins of the lids. The conjunctival sac is dissected to its bulbar attachment, so that when the sutured margins of the lids are raised, the conjunctiva forms a closed chamber between the lids and the cornea. Note its reflection around the cartilage of the third eyelid. The deep end of the cartilage may be withdrawn to see the gland of the third eyelid, which surrounds it. The lacrimal gland is in the dorsolateral quadrant of the orbit, well inside the margin, and held against the periorbita (orbital periosteum at this point) by a layer of fascia. The eyeball may be pushed aside to see the muscle attachments, which are aponeurotic. The recti and obliqui must be severed at their terminations before the eyeball can be rotated enough to reach the retractor and the optic nerve.

To anesthetize the orbit, a 12-cm. curved needle may be inserted in the angle between the frontal and temporal processes of the zygomatic bone. The needle is passed across the rostral border of the coronoid process of the mandible to reach the oculomotor, trochlear, ophthalmic, maxillary, and abducent nerves as they emerge from the foramen orbitorotundum.[24] (See the skull.) It is also advisable to prevent closure of the eyelids by blocking the palpebral branch of the auriculopalpebral nerve as it crosses the zygomatic arch. This is done by superficial infiltration along the zygomatic arch for 7 cm. caudal to the original insertion of the needle. The palpebral branch is often blocked alone to examine the eye.

Another method is to first anesthetize the eyelids with a line block near the margin of the orbit. Then press the eyeball medially and pass a 15-cm. needle caudally through the lateral conjunctival fornix medial to the rim of the orbit to the apex of the periorbita. Injection of anesthetic blocks all the nerves within the periorbita and anesthetizes the eye and paralyzes the muscles of the globe.

4g. EYE, OX

Orient the eye by means of the third eyelid and the oblique muscles. Identify the seven muscles of the eyeball. Note that the dorsal oblique crosses between the sclera and the dorsal rectus, while the ventral oblique crosses ventral to the ventral rectus. Note the gland of the third eyelid and its relationship to the fornix of the conjunctiva.

The ophthalmic rete mirabile lies between the retractor and the dorsal rectus. From the rete a branch runs forward on the optic nerve to the eyeball, where it divides into medial and lateral branches that give off the short posterior ciliary arteries and continue as the medial and lateral long posterior ciliary arteries. The latter are accompanied by veins, which emerge from the sclera (vorticose veins). The other arteries of the orbit are like those of the horse, except that the malar, in the medial angle, is much larger. (See the groove for the malar artery in the lacrimal bulla on the skull.)

4h. SECTIONS, NASAL CAVITY, OX

Follow the infraorbital canal through the sections. Trace the conchae and identify the nasal passages. Follow the nasolacrimal duct through each section. The nasal orifice is on the medioventral surface of the alar fold, a fold of mucosa attached to the tip of the ventral concha. Although it is concealed, it can be easily exposed for cannulation and irrigation by everting the lateral margin of the nostril.

4i. SAGITTAL SECTION, HEAD, OX

A stomach tube can be passed through the nose in the ox as well as through the mouth. It must go under the rostral end of the ventral concha into the ventral meatus.

4j. LIVE COW

Palpate the thick frontalis muscle extending into the upper eyelid. A large expanse of the dorsal bulbar conjunctiva can be exposed for examination by twisting the head on its long axis. Examine the fundus with the ophthalmoscope. The optic disc is round or transversely oval and is below the tapetum lucidum.[20] Note the difference from the horse in the retinal vessels: they come from the central part of the disc; in addition to several small vessels there are usually four main veins with accompanying arteries that run dorsally, ventrally, medially, and laterally to form a cross (see Fig. 4–1). At the point where the vessels emerge from the disc is a small light spot, the vestige of the hyaloid artery. This extends toward the lens through the vitreous body in an undulating course. It can be followed by changing the focus of the ophthalmoscope. It is present in most adults and all calves.

Turn the lateral margin of the nostril upward and outward and find the nasal orifice of the nasolacrimal duct on the medioventral surface of the alar fold.

4k. DISSECTION, EYE, PIG

Closely surrounding the cartilage of the third eyelid is the superficial gland of the third eyelid, which is present in most animals. The large dark gland attached loosely to the deep end of the superficial gland is the deep gland of the third eyelid described by Harder. It is not present in other domestic animals. The deep gland is surrounded by a large orbital venous sinus that can be used to obtain blood samples. In dorsal recumbency the sinus can be penetrated by passing a needle between the third eyelid and the eyeball to a depth of 2 to 4 cm.[13]

4l. DISSECTION, ORBIT, DOG

Note the depth of the orbit and the relationship of the zygomatic salivary gland ventral to the rostral part of the orbit. Inflammation of this gland may cause the eye to bulge (see Plate III). The lacrimal gland can be exposed by removal of the orbital ligament. It lies dorsolateral to the globe within the periorbita. Numerous ducts convey its secretion into the fornix of the conjunctiva from where it passes across the cornea to the lacrimal puncta at the medial angle of the eyelids.

There are three components to the tear film that covers the cornea. A thin mucoid glycoprotein layer is secreted by the conjunctival goblet cells and adheres the aqueous layer to the cornea, which is hydrophobic. The aqueous layer is the largest and is secreted by the lacrimal gland and the gland of the third eyelid. Because of the significant contribution of the latter, surgical removal should be avoided whenever possible. The third layer is a lipid secretion from the tarsal glands, which prevents flow of the aqueous layer over the eyelids.

The lateral rectus has a branch of the abducent nerve entering it. Between the dorsal and lateral recti is a part of the retractor bulbi.

The large maxillary artery and nerve are ventral at the apex of the orbit. These are outside the periorbita on the surface of the pterygoid muscles. Just after it emerges from the alar canal, the maxillary artery gives off the external ophthalmic artery, a short trunk that penetrates the periorbita and divides into muscular and ciliary branches, and several other arteries to the lacrimal gland, upper lid, meninges and, via the external ethmoidal artery, to the nasal cavity. Because the muscular branches enter the muscles at the apex of the orbit, hemorrhage is reduced in enucleation of the eye if the muscles are cut at their scleral insertions and left in place.

There are a number of sites for retrobulbar injections.[23] Most commonly the injection is made caudal to the orbital ligament at the level of the zygomatic arch. The needle is directed medially and slightly caudal and ventral. The needle can also be inserted just ventral to the zygomatic arch at the level of the lateral angle of the eye and directed dorsomedially rostral to the coronoid process of the mandible.

4m. DISSECTION, EYE, DOG

A branch of the external ophthalmic artery runs forward on the optic nerve to the eyeball and gives off two long posterior ciliary arteries. These give off short posterior ciliary arteries that enter the sclera around the optic nerve. Branches of these are seen at the periphery of the optic disc with the ophthalmoscope. After the muscle terminations are cut in enucleation, the optic nerve and the accompanying arteries should be clamped and ligated before they are severed. The large angular vein of the eye on the medial side of the orbit should be cut between two ligatures.[27]

The facial vein rostral to the orbit is continuous with the angularis oculi vein that passes caudally on the dorsolateral aspect of the nose, across the medial side of the orbit, and through the periorbita to join the ophthalmic plexus of veins. This vein has no valves, and blood can flow in either direction. An orbital venogram can be made by injection of radiopaque dye into this vein on the side of the face. This will opacify the ophthalmic venous plexus and venous sinuses on the floor

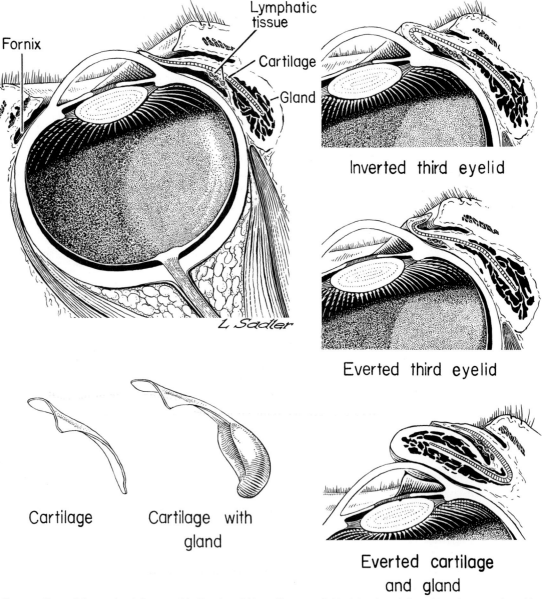

Figure 4–2. Four sections of the canine left eye cut in the dorsal plane (from medial to lateral angle) to show the normal position (upper left) and various displacements of the third eyelid and its gland. The figure in the lower left corner shows the dorsal aspect of the cartilage and gland of the third eyelid.

of the cranial cavity in radiographs. This procedure can be used to help diagnose space-occupying lesions that are retrobulbar or on the floor of the cranial cavity.

Recognize the lymphoid tissue on the bulbar side of the third eyelid. Inflammation may occur here. Recognize that the superficial gland of the third eyelid surrounds the cartilage but is thickest on the outer (medial) surface (Fig. 4–2).

4n. THIRD EYELID

This is a semilunar fold of conjunctiva supported by a plate of cartilage. The cartilage has a wide concave edge in the free border of the third eyelid and a narrower part that projects back along the medial wall of the orbit. The posterior part is covered by the superficial gland of the third eyelid. Anything that pulls or pushes the eyeball back into the periorbita will increase the pressure exerted by the intraorbital fat on the gland and cartilage, which act as a piston, pushing the third eyelid out of the fornix conjunctivae and across the cornea (See Fig. 4–2). The retractor bulbi reflex causes this passive protrusion that protects the cornea. In tetanus, the eyeball is retracted by contraction of its muscles, and the resultant third eyelid protrusion ("flashing") is a passive response.

The cat has a peculiar mechanism that actively draws the third eyelid across the cornea. A slip of striated muscle from the levator palpebrae superioris passes into the upper end of the third lid, and a slip of striated muscle from the lateral rectus passes into the lower end of the third lid.[1] Striated muscle in the lateral rectus innervated by the abducent nerve causes the active protrusion of the third eyelid independently of outward rotation or retraction of the eyeball.[28]

The third eyelid is normally held in the retracted position by the tonus of smooth muscle innervated by the sympathetic system. The smooth muscle of the orbit in domestic animals consists of a sheet in the periorbita that acts to squeeze the eyeball out of its conical sheath to make it protrude. There are also sheets that extend into the upper, lower, and third eyelids and tend to retract them. The sheets of smooth muscle attached to the three eyelids originate from the fascial sheaths of the recti.[1] Tonus of the smooth muscle of the orbit maintains the normal prominence of the globe and the width of the palpebral fissure. One sign of injury of the sympathetic nerve supply to the head is protrusion of the third lid caused by relaxation of its smooth muscle. This is usually associated with enophthalmos, narrowed palpebral fissure, vasodilation, and miosis, comprising Horner's syndrome.

Other causes of abnormal protrusion of the third eyelid include spasm of the retractor muscle caused by irritation from a corneal ulcer or foreign body, epinephrine-blocking tranquilizers, or a space-occupying lesion of the medial wall of the orbit.

The third eyelid often protrudes in chronic wasting diseases, especially in cats. This may be due to general debility, sympathetic inhibition, or vagotonus. Central stimulation of the vagus in the cat causes inhibition and relaxation of the smooth muscle of the third lid.[29]

Because the third eyelid of the dog is protruded by pressure from within the orbit, the cartilage often buckles, resulting in one of three displacements. The deep end of the cartilage with the gland often doubles forward between the third lid and the bulb and protrudes as a rounded red swelling covered by conjunctiva. A congenital defect in the cartilage may be a cause. The gland is normal, except for some congestion and edema (see Fig. 4–2); it has only been mechanically displaced. Sometimes the gland and cartilage can be replaced in the normal position, but the condition usually recurs. Another displacement is eversion of the free border of the third lid caused by buckling of the cartilage. The third variant is inversion of the free border.

These cartilaginous defects are corrected by removal of the deformed cartilage only. The gland is preserved because of its contribution to lacrimal secretion.

4o. SAGITTAL SECTION, NASAL CAVITY, DOG

Identify the dorsal and ventral conchae and the large mass of the ethmoid labyrinth. Note the narrow meatuses. On the lateral surface, note the palpebral branch of the auriculopalpebral nerve on the zygomatic arch. The palpebral branch can be blocked here to prevent closure of the eyelids.[5]

4p. LIVE DOG

Elicit the direct pupillary reflex and observe the consensual pupillary reflex in the opposite eye. This reflex will be absent with diseases of the eyeball or optic nerve that cause blindness, but it is normal with lesions of the optic radiation or visual cortex that cause blindness. The consensual pupillo-constrictor reflex affords a means of differentiating retinal or optic nerve blindness from unilateral oculomotor paralysis.

A dilated pupil occurs with:
1. Severe retinal or optic nerve lesions if bilateral (unilateral lesions may cause only slight ipsilateral dilation)
2. Oculomotor nerve lesion
3. Iris atrophy
4. Parasympatholytic drugs (used for ophthalmoscopic examinations)
5. Sympathomimetic drugs
6. Sympathetic stimulation—fear, excitement
7. Glaucoma

A constricted pupil occurs with:
1. Pain from keratitis or iritis (pain from other superficial parts of the body produces an adrenergic reaction with dilation of the pupils)
2. Iritis
3. Sympathetic paralysis
4. Sympatholytic drugs
5. Parasympathomimetic drugs
6. Upper motor neuron lesions rostral to the midbrain

Find the lacrimal puncta. The nasolacrimal system can be cannulated with a 17- to 22-ga. catheter to flush the duct, identify an obstruction, or inject radiopaque dye for dacryocystorhinography.[11, 33, 41]

Examine the fundus with the ophthalmoscope[40] (see Fig. 4–1). The tapetum lucidum is a right triangle lying on its hypotenuse, with the base lateral and the right angle dorsal. The color ranges from blue to orange. The position of the disc varies with the size of the dog: in large dogs it is within the tapetum lucidum; in small dogs it is below it. The disc in the cat is surrounded by the tapetum lucidum. Observe the pattern of the retinal vessels. There are three or four large primary veins directed dorsally, medioventrally, lateroventrally, and ventrally. The ventral one is not always present. These veins anastomose to form an incomplete ring on the optic disc about midway between the center and the periphery. The small arterioles emerge near the periphery of the disc. The cat has a smaller disc; the vessels are entirely peripheral; and the dorsal vessels are inclined medially.

References

1. Acheson, G. H.: The topographical anatomy of the smooth muscle of the cat's nictitating membrane. Anat. Rec. *71* (1938):297–311.
2. Ammann, K. and G. Pelloni: Der Bulbus oculi des Hundes (Eine topographischanatomische Darstellung). Schweiz. Arch. Tierheilkd. *113* (1971):287–290.
3. Anderson, B. G. and W. D. Anderson: Vasculature of the equine and canine iris. Am. J. Vet. Res. *38* (1977):1791–1799.
4. Anderson, B. G. and M. Wyman: Anatomy of the equine eye and orbit: histological structure and blood supply of the eyelids. J. Eq. Med. Surg. *3* (1979):4–9.
5. Bryan, G. M.: Palpebral nerve blocks in small animals. J. Am. Anim. Hosp. Assoc. *11* (1975):453–454.
6. Curtis, R.: The suspensory apparatus of the canine lens. J. Anat. *136* (1983):69–83.
7. de Lahunta, A.: Small Animal Neuroophthalmology. Vet. Clin. North Am. *3* (1973):491–501.
8. Evans, L. H.: Regional analgesia in large animals. *In* Soma, L. R. (ed.): Textbook of Veterinary Anesthesia. Baltimore: Williams & Wilkins, 1971, pp. 486–488.
9. Gelatt, K. N. and E. J. Finocchio: Variations in the normal equine eye. Vet. Med.–SAC *65* (1970):569–574.
10. Gelatt, K. N.: Surgical correction of everted nictitating membrane in the dog. Vet. Med.–SAC *67* (1972):291–292.
11. Gelatt, K.N., T. H. Cure, M. M. Guffy, et. al.: Dacryocystorhinography in the dog and cat. J. Small Anim. Pract. *13* (1972):381–397.
12. Gelatt, K. N., C. G. Gum, L. W. Williams, et. al.: Uveoscleral flow of aqueous humor in the normal dog. Am. J. Vet. Res. *40* (1979):845–848.
13. Huhn, R. G., G. D. Osweiler, and W. P. Switzer: Application of the orbital sinus bleeding technique to swine. Lab. Anim. Care *19* (1969):403–405.
14. Kornegay, J. N.: Small Animal Neuroophthalmology. Comp. Cont. Ed. *2* (1980):923–928.

15. Magrane, W. G.: Canine Ophthalmology, 2nd ed. Philadelphia: Lea & Febiger, 1971.
16. Manning, J. P. and L. E. St. Clair: Palpebral, frontal, and zygomatic nerve blocks for examination of the equine eye. Vet. Med.–SAC *71* (1976):187–189.
17. Martin, C. L.: The normal canine iridocorneal angle as viewed with the scanning electron microscope. J. Am. Anim. Hosp. Assoc. *11* (1975):180–184.
18. Martin, C. L.: Scanning electron microscopic examination of selected canine iridocorneal angle abnormalities. J. Am. Anim. Hosp. Assoc. *11* (1975):300–306.
19. Martin, C. L. and B. G. Anderson: Ocular anatomy. *In* Gelatt, K. (ed.): Veterinary Ophthalmology. Philadelphia: Lea & Febiger, 1981.
20. McCormack, J. E.: Variations of the ocular fundus of the bovine species. Scope *18* (1974):21–28.
21. Merideth, E. and E. D. Wolf: Ophthalmic Examination and Therapeutic Techniques in the Horse. Comp. Cont. Ed. *3* (1981):S426–S433.
22. Müller, A.: Das Bild des normalen Augenhintergrundes beim Rind. Berl. Münch. Tierärztl. Wochenschr. *82* (1969):181–182.
23. Munger, R. J. and H. Ackerman: Retrobulbar injections in the dog: Comparison of three techniques. J. Am. Anim. Hosp. Assoc. *14* (1978):490–498.
24. Peterson, D. R.: Nerve block of the eye and associated structures. JAVMA *118* (1951):145–148.
25. Prince, J. H., et al.: Anatomy and Histology of the Eye and Orbit in Domestic Animals. Springfield, Ill.: Charles C Thomas, 1960.
26. Rebhun, W. C.: Diseases of the bovine orbit and globe. JAVMA *175* (1979):171–175.
27. Roberts, S. R.: Eyes. *In* Archibald, J. (ed.): Canine Surgery. Wheaton, Ill.: Am. Vet. Public., 1965, pp. 190–243.
28. Rosenblueth, A. and P. Bard: The innervation and function of the nictitating membrane in the cat. Am. J. Physiol. *100* (1932):537–544.
29. Rosenblueth, A. and H. G. Schwartz: Reflex responses of the nictitating membrane. Am. J. Physiol. *112* (1935):422–429.
30. Rubin, L. F.: Auriculopalpebral nerve block as an adjunct to the diagnosis and treatment of ocular inflammation in the horse. JAVMA *144* (1964):1387–1388.
31. Rubin, L. F.: Pupillary reactions in diagnosis. Unpublished. 59th Cornell Conf. Vet., 1967.
32. Rubin, L. F.: Diseases of the eyelids and lacrimal apparatus *In* Kirk, R. W. (ed.): Veterinary Therapy III. Small Animal Practice. Philadelphia: W. B. Saunders Co., 1968, pp. 321–324.
33. Severin, G. A.: Nasolacrimal duct catheterization in the dog. J. Am. Anim. Hosp. Assoc. *8* (1972):13–16.
34. Shively, J. N. and G. P. Epling: Fine structure of the canine eye: cornea. Am. J. Vet. Res. *31* (1970):713–722.
35. Slatter, D. H. and Y. Abdelbaki: Lateral orbitotomy by zygomatic arch resection in the dog. JAVMA *175* (1979):1179–1182.
36. Slatter, D. H.: Disorders of the lacrimal system. Part 1. Deficiency of the precorneal tear film. Comp. Cont. Ed. *2* (1980):801–807.
37. Smith, J. S. and I. G. Mayhew: Horner's syndrome in large animals. Cornell Vet. *67* (1977):529–542.
38. Thompson, J. W.: The nerve supply to the nictitating membrane in the cat. J. Anat. *99* (1961):371–385.
39. Whalen, L. R. and R. L. Kitchell: Electrophysiologic studies of the cutaneous nerves of the head of the dog. Am. J. Vet. Res. *44* (1983):615–627.
40. Wyman, M. and E. F. Donovan: The ocular fundus of the normal dog. JAVMA *147* (1965):17–26.
41. Yakely, W. L.: Dacryocystorhinography in the dog. JAVMA *159* (1971):1417–1421.

CHAPTER 5

PARANASAL SINUSES

OBJECTIVES

1. To be able to outline the surgical field for trephination of the frontal sinuses in all species and to know what structures are injured when these boundaries are exceeded. To be able to palpate the supraorbital foramen in the horse and the supraorbital foramen and groove in the cow and to know what passes through the foramen in these animals.
2. To know the location of the normal opening of each sinus into the nasal cavity in each species. A few sinuses communicate with the nasal cavity indirectly through another sinus.
3. To be able to trephine the frontal sinus in the horse directly over the frontomaxillary opening for expulsion of the upper third molar or for treatment of the frontal, caudal maxillary, and sphenopalatine sinuses.
4. To be able to make an effective drainage opening from the bottom of the sinus in the usual position of the head. This is not possible for all sinuses and it is important to know which sinuses cannot be drained and must be irrigated and aspirated.
5. To be able to trephine the caudal frontal sinus of the ox close to the oblique septum that forms its rostral boundary. This is the lowest accessible part of the sinus in the normal position of the head. To be able to trephine the rostral sinuses when infection destroys the oblique septum. To be able to trephine over the postorbital and nuchal diverticula of the caudal frontal sinus of the ox and to know what signs are produced by swelling of the bony walls of these diverticula.
6. To be able to treat *Oestrus ovis* infestation of the frontal sinuses of sheep.
7. To be able to open the dorsal and common meatuses through the nasal bone for treatment of the nasal septum and conchae.
8. To be able to outline the surgical field for the maxillary sinuses in the horse and cow and to be able to avoid the nasolacrimal duct, buccal branch of the facial nerve, transverse facial vessels, and infraorbital canal in operations on the maxillary sinuses. To be able to estimate the location of the septum between the rostral and caudal maxillary sinuses in the horse. To know which roots of upper cheek teeth project into the the maxillary sinus in horses aged 6 months, 3 years, and over 5 years.
9. To be able to trephine over the apex of the root of an affected tooth. This requires a knowledge of the obliquity of the last three cheek teeth.
10. To be able to differentiate the lacrimal sinus from the lacrimal bulla in the ox. To understand the opening between the maxillary and palatine sinuses in the ox.
11. To know the location of the maxillary recess in the dog and cat and to understand the relation of the roots of the fourth premolar in the dog to the maxillary recess, and in the cat, to the orbit.
12. To know how to diagnose a frontal or maxillary sinusitis with an endoscope in the horse. Drainage occurs into the middle meatus.
13. To be able to locate on radiographs of the dog and cat: the frontal sinus, orbit, conchae of nasal cavity, ethmoid bone (cribriform plate and labyrinth), maxillary recess (dog), sphenoid sinus (cat).
14. To appreciate the vulnerability of the brain in operations to destroy the horn buds in young calves and kids. This is due to the slow postnatal development of the frontal sinuses.

The paranasal sinuses are air-filled spaces in bones that are lined with mucosa and communicate with the nasal cavity. They are small at birth and continue to enlarge as the skull grows. In the horse there are four paranasal sinuses: frontal, rostral maxillary, caudal maxillary, and sphenopalatine. A bony septum separates the two maxillary sinuses. Each maxillary sinus communicates with the middle nasal meatus by a narrow nasomaxillary opening. The caudal maxillary sinus communicates with the sphenopalatine and frontal sinuses. Therefore, for clinical purposes there are two functional sinuses: the rostral maxillary sinus and the combined caudal maxillary, sphenopalatine, and frontal sinuses. Exudate from infection of these sinuses will be seen with an endoscope in the caudal part of the middle nasal meatus.

5a. SCULPTURED SKULLS, HORSE
Lateral view (see Plate I):

The rostral and caudal maxillary sinuses are separated by an oblique septum (usually destroyed in demonstrations), which is complete in life. Its ventral end varies in position but is usually 5 cm. caudal to the end of the facial crest. The two nasomaxillary openings are narrow and confluent as they enter the middle meatus of the nasal cavity. They can be demonstrated with wires (see Fig. 5–1: *f, g*).

The infraorbital canal runs longitudinally through both maxillary sinuses, forming the dorsal border of a bony septum that contains the alveoli of the last three or four cheek teeth.

Dorsal to the infraorbital canal in the rostral maxillary sinus is the opening to the ventral conchal sinus (see Fig. 5–1:*d*).

Dorsal to the infraorbital canal in the caudal maxillary sinus is the communication with the medial part of the sinus, which opens caudally into the sphenopalatine sinus (see Fig. 5–2:*i*).

The large frontomaxillary opening is in the roof of the caudal maxillary sinus (see Fig. 5–2:*d*).

In order to remove a tooth by expulsion, it is necessary first to identify the diseased tooth and then to determine the proper point of trephination to get a punch on the root. In the young horse the roots of the first three large cheek teeth (P 2 to 4) cause palpable bulges of the maxilla and mandible (juga alveolaria). The growth of the skull causes the upper cheek teeth to move rostrally relative to the end of the facial crest for a distance of a little more than the width of P 4 between the ages of 6 months and 5 years. After 5 years the positions of the teeth are stable, except that the roots are gradually forced out by bone formation in the alveoli. This bone is then resorbed proximal to the teeth. Therefore the alveolar eminences disappear, and in the maxillary sinuses the sagittal septum under the infraorbital canal becomes thin.

Diseased teeth are more common in the older horse and landmarks are provided for the trephination points in the horse older than 5 years.[3] While the first large cheek teeth are fairly straight and perpendicular to the occlusal surface, the roots of the others are progressively more caudally inclined and curved, so that the clinical crown gives little indication of the place to put the trephine. Observe that a line drawn through the most ventral point of the orbital margin and the ventral border of the infraorbital foramen runs dorsal and parallel to the apices of the roots of the upper cheek teeth. The points of trephination are on this line. The point for P 2 is in the transverse plane of the caudal end of the nasoincisive notch. The point for P 3 is 2 cm. rostral to the infraorbital foramen; the point for P 4 is 2 cm. caudal to the foramen, and M 1 is 4 cm. caudal to it; the point for M 2 is 4 cm. rostral to the medial angle of the eye. The root of M 3 is reached by trephining the frontal sinus midway between the medial angle of the eye and the median plane. This point is dorsal to the frontomaxillary opening, and the tooth can be reached with an offset punch (see Plate I).

M 1 is the most commonly diseased tooth in the older horse. M 1 and M 2 are easily accessible through a "flap sinusotomy." The maxillary bone is cut longitudinally along the dorsal border of the facial crest from the level of the medial angle of the eye to the rostral end of the facial crest. Transverse cuts are made in the maxilla from the rostral end of the facial crest to just ventral to the infraorbital foramen and from the caudal end of the longitudinal cut to just ventral to the medial angle of the eye. The dorsal ends of the transverse cuts should be ventral to the nasolacrimal duct. The cut edge of the maxilla is elevated at the facial crest. The oblique septum is cut. Elevation is continued until the maxilla breaks along a line connecting the dorsal ends of the transverse cuts. In

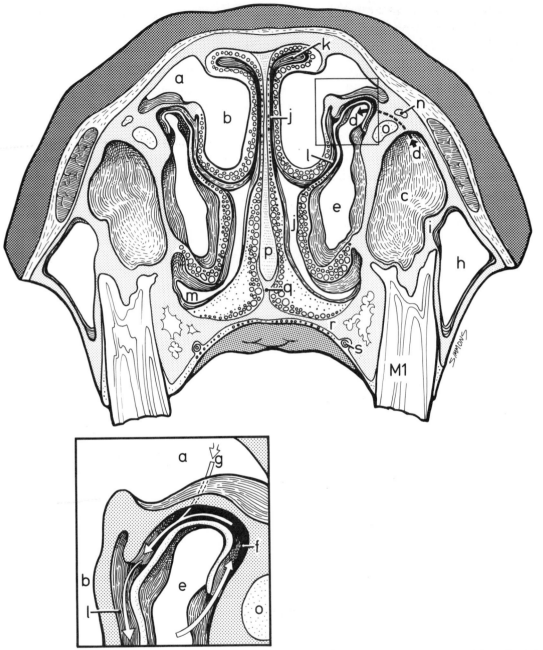

Figure 5–1. Paranasal sinuses, horse. Rostral surface of section through caudal part of the first molar. *a*, Frontal sinus; *b*, dorsal conchal sinus; *c*, rostral maxillary sinus; *d*, conchomaxillary opening; *e*, ventral conchal sinus; *f*, (inset) nasomaxillary opening of rostral maxillary sinus; *g*, (inset) nasomaxillary opening of caudal maxillary sinus; *h*, caudal maxillary sinus; *i*, oblique septum between rostral (*c*), and caudal (*h*) maxillary sinuses; *j*, common meatus; *k*, dorsal meatus; *l*, middle meatus; *m*, ventral meatus; *n*, lacrimal canal; *o*, infraorbital canal; *p*, nasal septum; *q*, vomer; *r*, hard palate; *s*, major palatine artery.

this procedure the levator labii superioris will be reflected dorsally, and the angularis oculi vein at the rostral end of the surgical site may need to be reflected or ligated.

In the horse over 5 years of age, the apices of the roots of lower P 2 to M 1 are just above the ventral border of the mandible. The trephination point for P 2 is in the transverse plane of the middle of the clinical crown; the points for P 3 and P 4 are in the plane of the caudal border of the crown of the same tooth. The point for M1 is 4 cm. rostral to the groove for the facial vessels, and the point for M 2 is 4 cm. above the ventral border of the mandible and 2 cm. caudal to the groove for the facial vessels. The point for M 3 is halfway from the rostral border of the crown to the middle of the angle of the mandible.

Medial View

The nasomaxillary openings in the middle meatus can only be demonstrated with wires or string.

Observe that the caudal part of the dorsal concha contains a sinus that is continuous with the frontal sinus. These sinuses can be drained by puncture of the dorsal concha (see Fig. 5–1:*a, b*).

The sinus in the ventral concha opens into the rostral maxillary sinus. Puncture of the ventral concha will provide drainage to the nasal cavity (see Fig. 5–1:*c, d, e*).

The sinuses in the dorsal and ventral conchae are separated rostrally from the bullae of these conchae by a bony septum. Bullae, like sinuses, are air-filled spaces that communicate with the nasal cavity. In the nasal conchae they are located rostral to the conchal sinuses and communicate by small openings with the nasal cavity.

5b. TRANSVERSE SECTIONS, HEAD, HORSE (Figs. 5–1 and 5–2)

On transverse sections of the head of a horse identify the following and understand their relationship to each other:

Frontal sinus. The rostral portion of the sinus in the horse is in the dorsal concha, but the whole cavity is known clinically as the frontal sinus.

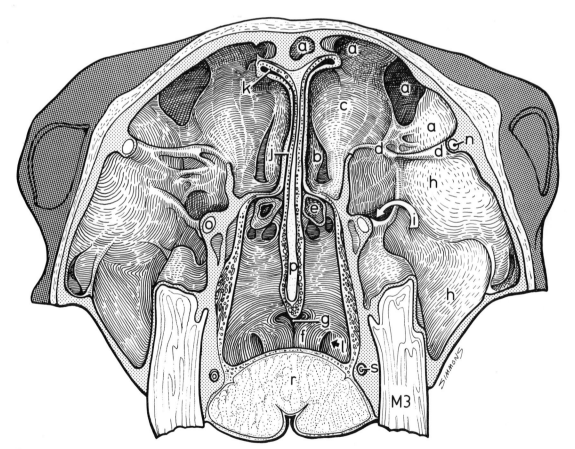

Figure 5–2. Paranasal sinuses, horse. Rostral surface of section through rostral part of third molar. *a*, Frontal sinus; *b*, dorsal conchal sinus; *c*, ethmoid labyrinth; *d*, caudal margin of frontomaxillary opening; *e*, middle nasal concha; *f*, nasopharynx; *g*, pharyngeal recess; *h*, caudal maxillary sinus; *i*, opening to sphenopalatine sinus; *j*, common meatus; *k*, dorsal meatus; *l*, orifice of auditory tube; *n*, lacrimal canal; *o*, infraorbital canal; *p*, nasal septum; *r*, soft palate; *s*, major palatine artery.

Frontomaxillary opening. This occurs only in the horse.

Maxillary sinuses. The rostral and caudal sinuses and the septum that divides them, the communication of the rostral sinus with the sinus in the ventral concha over the infraorbital canal, and the communication of the caudal sinus with the sphenopalatine sinus.

Infraorbital canal. Alveoli in septum ventrally.

Lacrimal canal. Bony canal containing the nasolacrimal duct.

Nasomaxillary openings to each maxillary sinus. These can be demonstrated with wire or string.

Ethmoid labyrinth.

Nasal septum. Caudal part between choanae, dorsal lateral cartilages arching laterally from its dorsal border.

Dorsal and ventral conchae and their sinuses.

5c. LATERAL DISSECTIONS, HEAD, HORSE

Identify the following:

The supraorbital nerve emerges from the supraorbital foramen to supply sensation to the forehead and upper eyelid (see Plate I).

The ramifications of the facial nerve.

Transverse facial vein and artery as they enter the origin of the masseter and the vein as it emerges at the end of the facial crest.

Arteries and veins on the levator labii superioris where it is reflected to expose the infraorbital foramen.

Check the external landmarks used to locate the following structures:

Limits of the rostral and caudal maxillary sinuses and the variable septum between them.

In the rostral sinus note the infraorbital canal and the septum that extends from the canal to the floor of the sinus. In young horses this septum contains the alveoli. Medial to the septum is the ventral conchal sinus, which may be drained through the ventral concha or, in old horses, it may be drained laterally through the septum into the trephined rostral maxillary sinus.

In the caudal sinus find the infraorbital canal and the medial part of the sinus, which opens freely into the sphenopalatine sinus.

The frontomaxillary opening, bounded laterally by the lacrimal canal.

The limits of the frontal sinus. The only outlet is the frontomaxillary opening. Rostral drainage is accomplished by puncture of the dorsal concha into the common nasal meatus.

Ethmoid labyrinth.

Invasion of the dorsal and common nasal meatuses. After removal of the plate of nasal bone, the dorsal lateral cartilage is encountered. Lining this is the thick mucosa and cavernous venous plexus. The dorsal concha occupies most of the field. The common meatus is the narrow slit next to the septum.

5d. LIVE HORSE

Maxillary Sinuses

Caudal limit. The rostral border of the orbit (for surgical purposes).

Rostral limit. A line from the rostral end of the facial crest to the infraorbital foramen. Palpate the infraorbital foramen under the levator labii superioris.

Dorsal boundary. A line from the infraorbital foramen parallel to the facial crest. The nasolacrimal duct runs dorsal to this line.

Ventral boundary (of the surgical field, but not of the sinuses): facial crest. The transverse facial vessels and branch of the auriculotemporal nerve run in the masseter just ventral to the crest, and the dorsal buccal branch of the facial nerve is subcutaneous there (see Plate I).

Estimate the positions of the roots of the upper teeth (see 5a). The rostral end of the facial crest reaches the caudal border of P 3 (second large cheek tooth) at 6 months, the caudal part of P 4 at 3 years, and the rostral part of M 1 after 5 years, i. e., the teeth move rostrally a little more than the width of P 4 relative to the end of the facial crest. The maxillary sinuses of most adult horses contain the roots of the last three cheek teeth.

Estimate the usual position of the ventral end of the oblique septum between the rostral and caudal maxillary sinuses, about 5 cm. from the end of the facial crest (see Plate I).

Frontomaxillary opening. In the dorsal plane of the lacrimal canal, midway between the medial angle of the eye and the median plane.

Frontal Sinus

Caudal limit. Surgically, the plane of the zygomatic processes of the frontal bones (see Plate I).

Rostral limit. Run the thumb and finger back along the horse's nose to the point where the nasal bones become abruptly wider. This point is midway between the orbit and the infraorbital foramen.

Supraorbital Foramen

The foramen is palpable in the base of the zygomatic process of the frontal bone. The supraorbital nerve may be blocked here to anesthetize the skin of a portion of the forehead and upper eyelid (see Plate I).

5e. DISSECTION, SINUSES, OX

Frontal sinuses (Fig. 5–3, see also Plate II):

Note the large frontal vein which ascends in a groove on the surface of the frontal bone from the angular vein of the eye to the supraorbital foramen, where it is continuous with the supraorbital vein. The foramen is 2 cm. caudal to the plane of the lateral angle of the eye.

The ox has one large caudal frontal sinus and two or three small rostral ones: the medial, the lateral, and the inconstant intermediate, rostral frontal sinuses. Right and left sinuses are separated by a median septum.

In the ox, the frontal bone comprises the entire dorsal portion of the calvaria. It meets the occipital bone caudally and the parietal bone lateroventrally in the temporal fossa.

The caudal limit of the caudal sinus is the occipital bone; the lateral limit of the caudal sinus is the temporal line; the rostral limit is an oblique septum that runs from the middle of the orbit caudomedially to join the median septum at the transverse plane of the caudal margin of the orbit. The oblique septum is variable in position, and in some specimens it is not completely osseous, leaving small areas where the rostral and caudal sinuses are separated only by mucous membrane. Nevertheless, the usual position of the septum must be taken into account in any operation for drainage of the caudal frontal sinus, which is the one that is invaded when its cornual diverticulum is opened in the dehorning of adult cattle.

The supraorbital canal conducts the supraorbital vein, which joins the ophthalmic venous plexus within the periorbita. The canal passes through the caudal sinus in an incomplete septum extending from the internal lamina of the frontal bone to the wall of the orbit. The postorbital diverticulum extends ventrally on both sides of the septum and is located between the cranial cavity, the orbit, and the temporal fossa. The nuchal diverticulum has numerous pockets, one of which extends into the paracondylar process in aged animals. The only opening to the caudal sinus is a small passage from the nasal cavity through an ethmoid meatus.

There is no frontomaxillary opening in any domestic animal except the Equidae. The rostral frontal sinuses lie between the rostral half of the orbit and the median septum. Each has an opening to an ethmoid meatus at its rostral extremity. A caudal diverticulum of the dorsal nasal concha projects backward between two of the rostral frontal sinuses.

Frontal sinusitis may be treated by lavage through trephine openings placed near the diverticula. The usual sites for trephining the caudal frontal sinus are: (1) laterally, 4 cm. caudal to the lateral angle of the eye, through the most lateral extent of the external lamina of the frontal bone, lateral to the supraorbital foramen; (2) caudally, over the nuchal diverticulum halfway from the midline to the base of the horn. If there is evidence of involvement of the rostral frontal sinuses (swel-

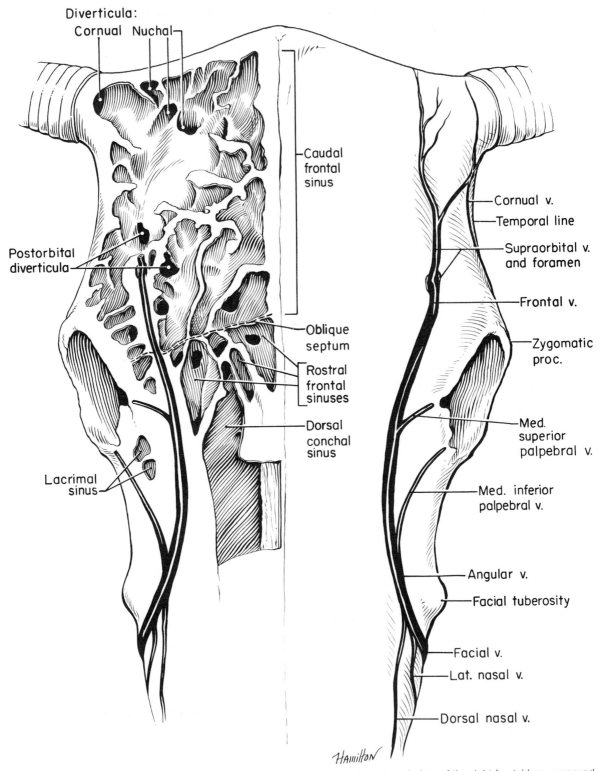

Diverticula:
Cornual   Nuchal

Caudal
frontal
sinus

Cornual v.

Temporal line

Supraorbital v.
and foramen

Frontal v.

Zygomatic
proc.

Postorbital
diverticula

Oblique
septum

Rostral
frontal
sinuses

Dorsal
conchal
sinus

Med.
superior
palpebral v.

Med. inferior
palpebral v.

Lacrimal
sinus

Angular v.

Facial tuberosity

Facial v.

Lat. nasal v.

Dorsal nasal v.

HAmilton

Figure 5–3. Dissection of the frontal sinus and frontal vein in the ox, with the external plate of the right frontal bone removed.

ling, pain, and dullness on percussion) they may be trephined medial to the orbit rostral to the oblique septum, avoiding the frontal vein.

Maxillary Sinus

The surgical field for the maxillary sinus extends from the orbit to a point slightly in front of the facial tuberosity. It is bounded ventrally by a line from the zygomatic arch to the facial tuberosity and dorsally by a line from the medial angle of the eye to the infraorbital foramen (see Plate II).

The maxillary sinus extends caudally into the lacrimal bulla. Look into the maxillary sinus and observe the large foramen over the infraorbital canal. It is the communication with the palatine sinus. Do not confuse the sinus with the nasal cavity. Farther back, between the planes of P 3 and M 3, there is a large defect in the bony wall between them. It is covered by mucous membrane. Note the caudodorsal diverticulum of the maxillary sinus, which extends into the medial wall of the orbit. It is called the lacrimal sinus. Note the nasolacrimal duct.

5f. LIVE COW

Outline the frontal sinuses on the surface of the head as described in 5e. Estimate the position of the septum between the rostral and caudal sinuses. Palpate the supraorbital groove containing the frontal vein; it runs rostrocaudally, about midway between the orbital margin and the median plane and ends at the palpable supraorbital foramen. The vein should be avoided in trephining the sinus.

Outline the surgical field for the maxillary sinus as described in 5e.

5g. DISSECTED HEAD, SHEEP

Note the large lateral and small medial frontal sinuses, the caudal diverticulum of the dorsal nasal concha, and the lacrimal sinus. Observe the openings from the nasal cavity through which *Oestrus ovis* larvae enter the sinuses. Treatment may be administered by puncturing the sinuses 5 mm. from the base of the horn, or, in polled sheep, near the median line in the transverse plane of the middle of the orbit. Avoid the frontal vein in the supraorbital groove. Note the maxillary and palatine sinuses. Note the position of the horn on the calvaria. In sheep and goats the parietal bone forms part of the dorsal surface of the calvaria between the frontal and occipital bones.

5h. SCULPTURED SKULL, PIG

The internal and external plates of the frontal bone are widely separated over the brain, rendering mechanical means of stunning for slaughter ineffective.

5i. SCULPTURED SKULL, DOG

On the medial surface of a sagittally sectioned specimen, identify the:

Large ventral concha, occupying most of the rostral half of the nasal cavity.

Narrow dorsal concha.

Middle concha between the dorsal concha and the caudal part of the ventral concha. The ethmoid labyrinth occupies the caudal part of the nasal cavity and forms a part of the floor of the frontal sinus.

Caudal to the ventral concha is the opening of the maxillary recess, which appears large in the skull, but is partially closed by the thickened mucosa containing the lateral nasal gland.[7] The duct from the gland opens on the lateral wall of the dorsal part of the vestibule. The recess is dorsal to the roots of the fourth premolar and caudal part of the third premolar. It is medial to the infraorbital canal and extends dorsally to the level of the medial angle of the eye. A swelling on the face in this region in the dog is usually caused by an apical abscess of the root of the fourth premolar.

On the dorsal surface of the sculptured specimen, identify the following:

The rostral, medial, and lateral frontal sinuses are seen, each with an opening from an ethmoid meatus. The lateral frontal sinus is much larger than the others. It occupies the zygomatic process of the frontal bone and extends caudally in a triangle bounded laterally by the temporal line and medially by the median septum. The caudal extent is greatest in dolichocephalic dogs, in which it reaches the transverse plane of the temporomandibular joints. The rostral frontal sinus lies between the median plane and the middle portion of the orbit. The ethmoid labyrinth forms a prominent dome-shaped elevation on the floor of the sinus. The medial frontal sinus is very small and may be absent. It lies in the triangle formed by the median septum and the walls of the other two frontal sinuses.

5j. RADIOGRAPHS, HEAD, DOG AND CAT

Locate the nasal cavities with their conchae, the sinuses, orbit, ethmoid bone (cribriform plate and labyrinth), maxillary recess (dog), and sphenoid sinus (cat).

5k. LIVE DOG

Outline the area occupied by the frontal sinuses. They form a rough triangle, with the longest side along the median plane and the opposite angle in the zygomatic process of the frontal bone. The rostral angle extends to the middle of the orbit. The caudal angle extends for a variable distance toward the plane of the temporomandibular joint. The lateral frontal sinus can be invaded surgically just caudal to the line connecting the zygomatic processes of the frontal bones (see Plate III).

5l. SKULL, CAT

Note the short nasal passages. The cat has frontal and sphenoid sinuses and a narrow maxillary recess. The frontal sinus of the cat can be opened between the median plane and the caudal half of the orbit. The objective is to visualize and irrigate the aperture, which is in the rostral wall of the sinus, about 4 mm. from the median plane. Note on the median section that a stiff cannula directed ventrally could enter the olfactory bulb or frontal lobe of the brain. The cannula should be directed rostrally.

The roots of upper premolars 3 and 4 are just ventral to the orbit and when abscessed may discharge pus into the conjunctival sac behind the lower lid (see Fig. 1–10).

References

1. Carpenter, J. L.: Diseases of the respiratory system. *In* Kirk, R. W. (ed.) Current Veterinary Therapy IV. Small animal practice. Philadephia: W. B. Saunders, 1971 pp. 121–123.
2. Cook, W. R.: Clinical observations on the anatomy and physiology of the equine upper respiratory tract. Vet. Rec. *79* (1966):440–446.
3. Günther, M., R. Krahmer and J. Schneider: Ein Beitrag zur Festlegung von Trepanationspunkten für die operative Entfernung der Backenzähne bei Pferden. Monatsh. Vet. Med. *22* (1967):891–895.
4. Hare, W. C. D.: Radiographic anatomy of the canine skull. JAVMA *133* (1958):149–157.
5. Hare, W. C. D.: Radiographic anatomy of the feline skull. JAVMA *134* (1959):349–356.
6. Murphey, H. S.: Some points on the surgical anatomy of the anterior part of the head, including a preliminary study of the teeth and sinuses of the horse. Iowa State Coll. Vet. Pract. Bull. *1* (1916):56–156.
7. Nickel, R., A. Schummer, E. Seiferle, and W. O. Sack: The Viscera of Domestic Mammals. New York: Springer, 1973.
8. Wheat, J. D.: Sinus drainage and tooth repulsion in the horse. Am. Assoc. Equine Pract. *19* (1973):171–176.

CHAPTER 6

EAR, HORN

OBJECTIVES

1. To be able to pass an endoscope through the pharyngeal orifice of the auditory tube and into the guttural pouch, utilizing the response of the orifice to respiration and swallowing.
2. To be able to diagnose a distention of the guttural pouch by palpation.
3. To be able to recognize the guttural pouches on radiographs.
4. To be able to open the guttural pouch surgically from the ventral or the caudal approach.
5. To understand the function of the auditory tube in any species and its relation to the guttural pouch in the horse.
6. To be able to open the guttural pouches at autopsy and know where to look for most mycotic infections.
7. To understand the relation of nerves and vessels to the guttural pouch and the signs produced when diseases of the pouch extend through the wall to affect the nerves and vessels.
8. To know the relationship of the external ear canal and tympanic bulla to the stylohyoid bone in the horse.
9. To understand the development and growth of the horn in order to prevent its development in the calf and to prevent regrowth after dehorning.
10. To be able to produce anesthesia and hemostasis for dehorning.
11. To appreciate the variations that can interfere with the cornual nerve block.
12. To be able to anesthetize the horn in the goat.
13. To be able to remove the horn glands from the goat.
14. To be able to do a venipuncture on the ear of the pig.
15. To be able to identify the surgical landmarks of the external ear of the dog.
16. To be able to trace the arteries and veins of the external ear of the dog. To know where a hematoma should be opened.
17. To be able to pass the otoscope tube through the external meatus and to recognize the eardrum when it is seen.
18. To be able to recognize all parts of the temporal bone on radiographs and to be able to position the animal in order to view the bullae separately.
19. To know the surgical anatomy for bulla osteotomy and to know the relationship of vessels and nerves to the bulla that must be avoided during surgery.
20. To be able to palpate the tympanic bulla externally in the cat and through the mouth of the dog and cat.

6a. DISSECTIONS AND CAST, GUTTURAL POUCH, HORSE

The auditory tube extends from the pharynx to the middle ear. The pharyngeal orifice is a slit about 3 cm. long on the lateral wall of the pharynx, directly caudal to the ventral nasal meatus and in the transverse plane of the lateral angle of the eye. The tube passes caudodorsally, becomes much smaller, enters the canal medial to the muscular process of the tympanic part of the temporal bone, and ends at the tympanic orifice in the rostral wall of the tympanic cavity. The lumen of the tube is a flat, sagittal slit, and the walls are stiffened by the cartilage of the tube, which consists of medial and lateral laminae joined dorsally. The medial lamina is much larger, so that the cartilage looks like an inverted J in cross section. The medial lamina extends into the medial flap that closes the pharyngeal orifice (Fig. 6–1, *13*). Normally the orifice opens during swallowing and is closed during inspiration.[3] Air enters and leaves during expiration and prior to inspiration.

In the horse, the auditory tube has a peculiar caudoventral diverticulum, the guttural pouch.[16] The opening between the tube and the pouch is a long slit in the caudoventral wall of the tube (Fig.

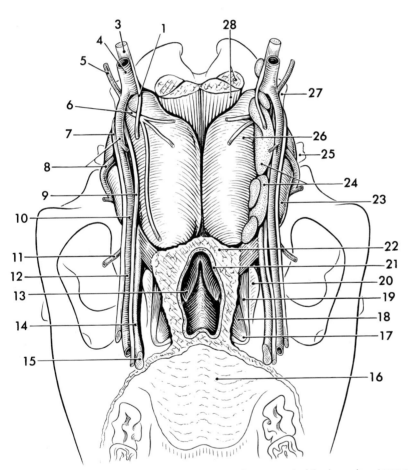

Figure 6–1. Ventral view of the guttural pouches after removal of the lower jaw, tongue, larynx, and oral and laryngeal parts of the pharynx. The upper border of the drawing is caudal. *1,* Cranial laryngeal n.; *3,* vagosympathetic trunk; *4,* common carotid a.; *5,* occipital a.; *6,* pharyngeal branch of vagus n.; *7,* hypoglossal n.; *8,* external carotid a.; *9,* glossopharyngeal n.; *10,* linguofacial a.; *11,* facial a.; *12,* lingual a.; *13,* ridge (torus tubarius) formed by the medial lamina of the cartilage of the auditory tube (the pharyngeal orifice of the tube is at the rostral end of the ridge, below the leader line in the drawing, and is foreshortened in this view); *14,* stylohyoid bone; *15,* cut surface where the keratohyoid was severed from the stylohyoid in removing the tongue (the epihyoid is rudimentary); *16,* soft palate; *17,* hamulus of pterygoid bone; *18,* m. pterygopharyngeus; *19,* m. tensor veli palatini; *20,* pyramidal (ptyerygoid) process of palatine bone; *21,* cut edge of pharyngeal mucosa; *22,* cut surface of pharyngeal muscles; *23,* right guttural pouch, lateral compartment; *24,* right medial retropharyngeal lymph nodes; *25,* external acoustic meatus; *26,* right guttural pouch, medial compartment; *27,* paracondylar process of occipital bone; *28,* m. rectus capitis ventralis (above) and m. longus capitis.

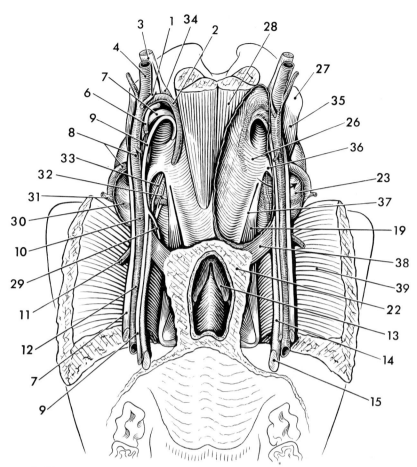

Figure 6–2. Same specimen as in Figure 6–1 after removal of the medial compartment of the left guttural pouch and the ventral wall of the right pouch. *1,* Cranial laryngeal n; *2,* internal carotid a.; *3,* vagosympathetic trunk; *4,* common carotid a.; *6,* pharyngeal branch of vagus n.; *7,* hypoglossal n.; *8,* external carotid a.; *9,* glossopharyngeal n., also shown on the right side enclosed with the hypoglossal n. in a fold of the pouch; *10,* linguofacial a.; *11,* facial a.; *12,* lingual a.; *13,* ridge (torus tubarius) formed by the medial lamina of the cartilage of the auditory tube (the pharyngeal orifice of the tube is at the rostral end of the ridge, below the leader line in the drawing, and is foreshortened in this view); *14,* stylohyoid bone; *15,* cut surface where the keratohyoid was severed from the stylohyoid in removing the tongue (the epihyoid is rudimentary); *19,* m. tensor veli palatini; *22,* cut surface of pharyngeal muscles; *23,* right guttural pouch, lateral compartment; *26,* medial compartment, (the pointer is on the bulla tympanica); *27,* paracondylar process of occipital bone; *28,* m. rectus capitis ventralis (above) and m. longus capitis (below); *29,* pharyngeal branch of glossopharyngeal n.; *30,* maxillary a.; *31,* masseteric a.; *32,* nerve of m. tensor tympani, a recurrent branch of the pterygoid n; the latter originates from the mandibular n. dorsal to the maxillary a.; *33,* chorda tympani; *34,* cranial cervical ganglion; *35,* m. occipitohyoideus; *36,* temporohyoid joint; *37,* slit in the ventral wall of the auditory tube through which it communicates with the guttural pouch; *38,* m. stylopharyngeus caudalis; *39,* m. pterygoideus medialis.

6–2, *37*). Lateral to this opening is the tensor veli palatini (Fig. 6–2, *19*), which in the horse originates mainly from the lateral lamina of the cartilage.[20] The condition of tympany of the guttural pouch in foals is considered to be caused by a functional disorder rather than by an organic defect.[7] It is corrected by various palliative operations, such as fenestration of the septum between the right and left pouches when the condition is unilateral or by removing the medial flap-like wall of the tube in the pouch.

An endoscope can be passed through the ventral nasal meatus, into the pharyngeal orifice of the tube, and into the guttural pouch. The pouch can be drained by passing a catheter in the same way. A urethral catheter for a mare has a curved tip that is helpful. The tip is pressed against the lateral wall of the pharynx as it is advanced and can be felt to slip across the caudal border of the pterygoid bone just before it enters the orifice.

Each pouch has a capacity of about 300 ml. and extends back to the atlas. It lies caudodorsal

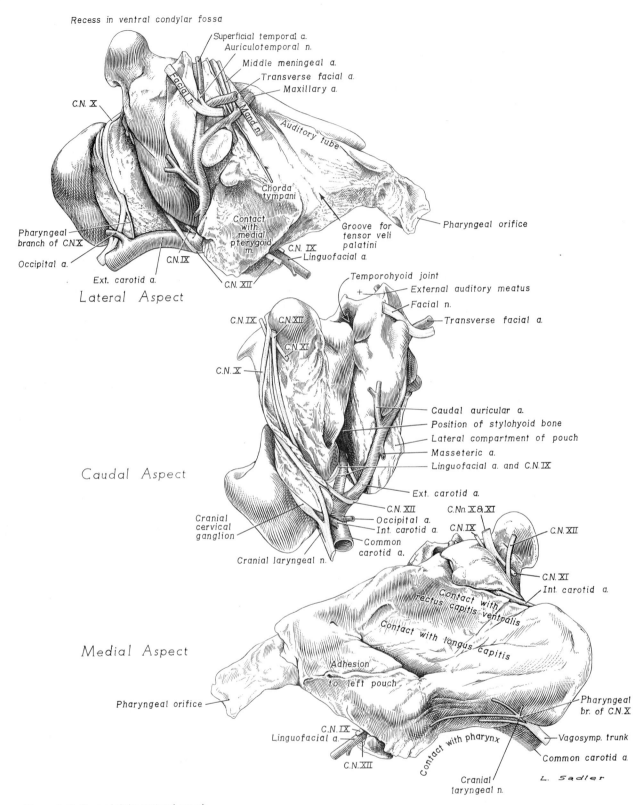

Figure 6–3. Cast of right guttural pouch.

to the pharynx and on the beginning of the esophagus. Its roof is in contact with the sphenoid bone, the tympanic bulla, the temporohyoid joint and the ventral condylar fossa.

The stylohyoid bone articulates by cartilage with the petrosal bone just lateral to the tympanic bulla. It invaginates the caudoventral surface of the pouch, dividing it into a large medial and a smaller lateral compartment (Fig. 6–3). The dorsal recess of the lateral compartment is attached to the styloid process of the auricular cartilage, which can be palpated in the live horse. It is also related to the external auditory meatus. The facial nerve passes around its lateral surface.

Laterally the pouch lies against the medial pterygoid muscle, the digastricus, and the parotid and mandibular salivary glands. Medially the two pouches are in contact rostrally, but caudally they lie on the longus capitis and rectus capitis ventralis muscles. The medial retropharyngeal lymph nodes are between the pharynx and ventral wall of the pouch. An abscess of these lymph nodes may invade the guttural pouch and cause empyema.

Because the guttural pouch and the auditory tube open into the nasopharynx, they are often involved in respiratory diseases. The mucosa of the pouch is secretory, covered by ciliated pseudo-stratified epithelium with goblet cells, and provided with glands. Therefore inflammations of the pouch are catarrhal. The copious exudate does not drain from the dorsally placed auditory tube when the head is held up. Feeding the patient off the floor may aid drainage. The enlarged pouch extends into the region of Viborg's triangle, formed by the mandible, the tendon of the sternocephalicus, and the linguofacial vein. A fluctuating swelling palpated here may be either a distended guttural pouch or an abscess of the retropharyngeal lymph nodes. Neither is palpable in the normal horse. Some surgeons prefer a more ventral approach than Viborg's. They make an incision between the linguofacial vein and the omohyoid and sternohyoid muscles.[10, 17]

Occasionally it is necessary to enter the caudal part of the pouch to remove solidified exudate. This is done through an incision at the ventrocranial margin of the wing of the atlas. The parotid gland is reflected forward, and the operator probes deep to the digastricus, sparing the occipital and internal carotid arteries and associated nerves. A fold of the pouch is grasped, drawn out, and opened.

A mycotic disease occurs in the guttural pouch in which a diphtheritic inflammation erodes the dorsal wall and produces a variety of signs by damage to the important vessels and nerves.[4, 5, 7] The most spectacular result is fatal epistaxis by rupture of the internal carotid artery (see Fig. 6–2). Dysphagia is the most common neurological sign. Paresis of the pharynx and soft palate is probably caused by lesions of the glossopharyngeal and vagus nerves, which lie in a caudodorsal fold of the pouch together with the hypoglossal nerve (see Fig. 6–3). Laryngeal hemiplegia has been associated with this condition. Signs of sympathetic nerve deficit—narrowed palpebral fissure, miosis, sweating, and hyperthermia on the same side of the face—have been attributed to damage to the cranial cervical ganglion or to the internal carotid nerve, which accompanies the artery. Facial paresis and extension of the lesion into the temporal bone to affect the inner ear and cause peripheral vestibular signs are rare. Figures 6–1 and 6–2 illustrate two stages in a method of postmortem examination for guttural pouch mycosis.[22] When the tongue, larynx, and esophagus are cut out of the head, the ventral walls of the pouches are usually incised, and the exposure will be similar to that shown in Figure 6–2.

Treatment of the epistaxis requires occlusion of the internal carotid artery on both sides of the site of bleeding into the dorsal aspect of the medial compartment.[14] If the artery is only ligated proximally along its course toward the pouch, bleeding can occur retrograde from the cerebral arterial circle through the distal end of the internal carotid artery. The latter can be occluded by passing a catheter with an inflatable balloon through the internal carotid artery, past the site of bleeding, and into the distal intracranial component of the artery. Inflation of the balloon will occlude this portion of the vessel.

6b. DISSECTION, CORNUAL NERVE AND ARTERY, OX

The best method of dehorning is to remove the horn bud from the calf or kid at 5 to 10 days of age. If this is properly done, no horn will regenerate. The reason is that the organizer for the development of all the tissues of the horn is the germinal epithelium of the horn bud, lying between the cornified layer and the dermis. If this entire area is removed, the defect will be filled by ingrowth of the surrounding haired skin, which is not capable of inducing development of horn dermis or a cornual process of the frontal bone.

At birth, the horn bud is covered by thickened stratum corneum in the shape of an inverted bowl. It has hair on it, but the follicles soon degenerate and the hair is rubbed off with the friable periderm. If allowed to develop, the papillae of the dermis elongate, so that the proliferating epidermal cells form horn tubules. The underlying bone proliferates and raises a cornual process, at first solid, but invaded by the frontal sinus at about 6 months. The horn grows from the whole surface of the cornual process in successive cones seen in the longitudinal section of a horn. The bases of these cones are marked by annular grooves caused by desquamation of soft horn produced during late pregnancy.

In the adult ox, the papillae on the sides of the cornual process are directed distally and are radially compressed so that they do not produce tubules, but layers of dense, solid horn. Tubules with medullae are formed only at the base and apex of the cornual process in the ox.

Since the cornual process is hollow and its bony wall is of equal thickness everywhere except at the tip, the easiest place to cut off the horn is through the skin at the base, proximal to the outer horn capsule.

Locate the cornual artery, a branch of the superficial temporal. It parallels the temporal line to the horn, where it divides into two branches. The smaller dorsal branch runs up over the base of the horn and supplies the dermis and bone. The ventral branch runs under the base, gives off branches to the dermis and the bony process, and upon reaching the caudal surface, runs medially to join the contralateral artery. It is important that the horn be amputated close enough to the head to cut the arteries before they enter the bone. Otherwise, the hemorrhage cannot be controlled with hemostatic forceps. In performing hemostasis, first pull the ventral branch directly caudal until it breaks. If the artery separates proximal to the dorsal branch, the latter will also stop bleeding.

Note the course of the cornual nerve, a branch of the zygomaticotemporal. It emerges from the orbit caudal to the zygomatic process of the frontal bone and runs just below the temporal line to the horn. Near the orbit it is deeply embedded in fat, but along the caudal half of the line the nerve is covered only by skin and the frontalis muscle (see Plate II). Injection of the cornual nerve in the usual site midway between the eye and the horn sometimes fails to anesthetize the horn. In one study it was concluded that of 62 halves of bovine heads dissected, the horns of 16 of them would not have been anesthetized by the standard block of the cornual nerve.[24] Failure can be caused by: (1) an abnormal course of the cornual nerve, under the periosteum or in the bone; (2) an abnormally long supraorbital or infratrochlear nerve, which can emerge from the dorsal margin of the orbit and run back over the frontal region; or (3) an abnormally long nerve of the frontal sinus. This small nerve normally arises in the orbit from the frontal or lacrimal nerve and passes through the orbital wall to the sinus. It may reach the cornual diverticulum, as in 3 of the 62 dissections. Superficial infiltration around the base of the horn will complete the anesthesia in the first two types of abnormal innervations but not in the third.

6c. LIVE COW

Palpate the temporal line. Determine the point of injection for cornual nerve anesthesia. It is midway between the eye and horn, just ventral to the line. The needle may be directed toward the horn for a fan-shaped subcutaneous injection or toward the orbit for a deeper injection in one spot. Palpate the dorsal margin of the bony orbit where the supraorbital and infratrochlear nerves emerge.

Palpation of the cornual artery is possible in a horned cow. Place the fingertips 1 cm. ventral to the caudal half of the temporal line. Try to take the pulse.

Examine the horn. Note the ring of soft horn (epikeras) that marks the transition between skin and horn. This corresponds to the periople on the hoof. The horn is amputated proximal to the epikeras for three reasons: (1) to make sure that no epidermis capable of producing horn is left; (2) to make hemostasis easier by exposing the arteries; and (3) to avoid cutting through the horny capsule.

6d. DISSECTION, INNERVATION OF HORN, GOAT

The cornual nerve is injected as close as possible to the caudal ridge of the root of the zygomatic process of the frontal bone to a depth of 1 to 1.5 cm. The infratrochlear nerve is injected at the dorsomedial margin of the bony orbit.[31]

The horn glands of male goats are patches of thick skin caudomedial to the base of the horn. The thickening is due to the presence of many large sebaceous and sudoriferous glands. They can be removed with the entire thickness of the skin by an elliptical incision, and this operation is said to eliminate the sexual odor.[9]

6e. EAR, CONVEX SURFACE, PIG

The lateral auricular vein near the lateral border is used for venipuncture.

6f. AURICULAR CARTILAGE, DOG

Examine a completely cleaned cartilage of the ear. Hold it with the concavity facing you. In the nomenclature, the convexity is regarded as the caudal surface. Note that the base of the cartilage is rolled to form a tube, which is curved strongly (110°). This makes examination of the dog's eardrum difficult without anesthesia.

Follow the margin (helix) of the cartilage from the apex toward the base on the medial side. About two-thirds of the way down is a triangular projection (spine of the helix) that rolls back on the convex surface. Proximal to this, the helix divides into two crura of which the medial is much larger. Now follow the helix proximally down the lateral border of the ear. It ends in the tail of the helix, which is separated by a notch from the sharp projection of the antitragus. The antitragus forms the lateral wall of the external end of the auditory meatus. It is separated by a small, rounded notch, the intertragic incisure, from the tragus. The tragus is a quadrilateral plate that completes the external end of the meatus in front and is overlapped by the larger crus helicis. The tragus is separated from the latter by the pretragic incisure.

In aural resection the rostral wall of the vertical portion of the external ear canal is removed. The dissection starts in the two incisures on either side of the tragus. The anthelix is a transverse ridge on the caudal wall of the auricular cartilage near the entrance to the external ear canal opposite to the tragus.

The annular cartilage is a quadrilateral plate rolled into a short tube. It connects the proximal end of the auricular cartilage to the bony meatus.

The scutiform cartilage is a flat L-shaped lever on the surface of the temporal muscle, rostromedial to the ear. It serves as attachment for several ear muscles (see Plate III).

6g. DISSECTION, ARTERIES, EAR, DOG

There are three arteries on the convex surface of the auricle: the medial, intermediate, and lateral auricular branches of the caudal auricular artery. The auricular cartilage has many foramina through which small branches of the arteries and veins perforate the cartilage to reach the concave surface. These are often ruptured by trauma, resulting in hematoma formation. In dogs the hematoma is usually on the concave surface. The blood is found in irregular cleavage spaces in the cartilage, between the cartilage and the perichondrium, or between the perichondrium and the skin.[23] The swelling appears on the concave side because the skin is thinner there. In cats, hematomata occur on either or both sides of the cartilage.[8]

6h. DISSECTION, VEINS, EAR, DOG

The caudal auricular vein comes from the maxillary and in the dog it gives off the lateral auricular vein and the small intermediate auricular vein. The superficial temporal gives off the rostral auricular, which supplies the medial auricular vein. The superficial temporal and rostral auricular veins curve around in front of the base of the ear and are endangered by the operation for drainage of the external meatus.

In the cat, the caudal auricular supplies the intermediate but not the lateral vein. The superficial temporal supplies the rostral auricular and the lateral auricular vein, which courses across the tragus and must be ligated in the operation to enlarge the external meatus.

6i. DISSECTION, BASE OF EAR, DOG

Identify the tragus and antitragus. Note the intertragic notch. Through an opening made in the bend in the external ear canal, pass a probe through the tympanum into the middle ear (tympanic cavity) medial to it. In the Zepp operation the horizontal portion of the external ear canal is opened directly onto the surface of the skin. Incisions are made on both sides of the tragus and continued down the vertical portion of the external ear canal. The flap so formed is turned down to expose the meatus below the bend. In aural resection for chronic proliferative otitis externa the cartilage and the lining of the external meatus are dissected out as far down as the bend and removed. The skin is closed over the wound except for a stoma formed by suturing the remaining horizontal meatus to the skin.[11, 30]

In aural resection or in other surgery involving the external ear canal, the major structures to be avoided are the parotid salivary gland, which covers the proximal one-third of the vertical portion of the canal; the facial nerve, which emerges from the stylomastoid foramen caudal to the external acoustic meatus and passes rostrally next to the bend in the external ear canal; the caudal auricular vessels caudal to the canal; and the superficial temporal vessels, the auriculopalpebral (motor) and the auriculotemporal (sensory) nerves rostral to the canal. The auricular muscles are innervated by the auricular branches of the facial nerve. Sensory innervation to the skin of the ear is complex and arises from the trigeminal, facial, vagus, and second cervical spinal nerves.[32] Stimulation of the ear to observe ear movement is a reliable test for the motor function of the facial nerve but not for fifth nerve anesthesia. The previously described areas of distribution of the trigeminal nerve sensory neurons should be used.

6j. SECTION THROUGH EAR, DOG

Observe the direction and length of the acoustic meatus from the cut edges where the tragus and antitragus were removed to the tympanic membrane. Visualize the proper angle for the otoscope if the depths of the canal are to be examined. Otoscope tubes of 5 to 7 cm. in length are required for various breeds of dogs. (Fig. 6–4).[30]

Examine the skull. The auditory tube is rostromedial to the tympanic bulla between the foramen lacerum and the oval foramen. Insert the otoscope into the external acoustic meatus and examine the middle ear. The ossicles have been removed. The tympanic orifice of the auditory tube can be seen in the rostral wall by inserting a wire from the rostral end. The orifice can be seen in the live dog when the eardrum is ruptured, as it usually is in otitis media. A catheter can be inserted through the otoscope into the orifice, and the auditory tube can be flushed into the pharynx. It is dangerous to apply pressure to the whole middle ear with a cannula that fits tightly in the external meatus, as this may rupture the secondary tympanic membrane in the cochlear window.[26] The cochlear window is seen at the caudal end of the promontory—a bulge of the dorsomedial wall of the middle ear formed by the cochlea. Dorsal to the promontory is the vestibular window, closed in life by the base of the stapes.

6k. DISSECTION, SURGICAL APPROACH TO THE TYMPANIC BULLA

The infected middle ear cavity can be drained laterally through the tympanum and external ear canal.[27] Drainage is facilitated by resection of the rostral wall of the vertical part of the canal. The

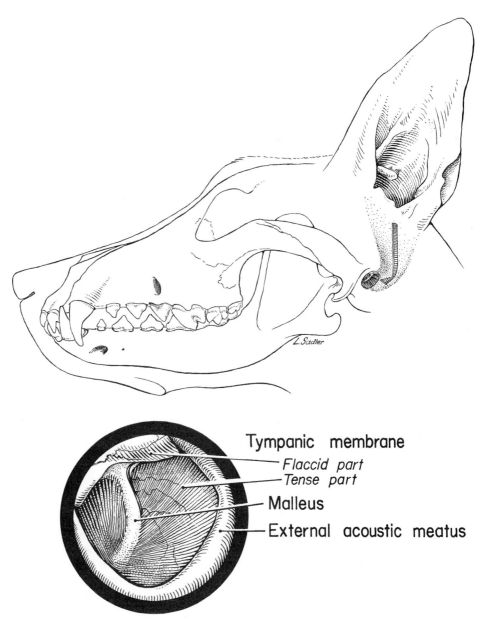

Figure 6–4. The canine tympanic membrane as seen with the otoscope.

middle ear cavity can be drained medially through a bulla osteotomy into the nasopharynx. An intramedullary bone pin is passed through the external ear canal and tympanum into the middle ear against the medial wall of the bulla. The pin should be directed rostrally, medially, and ventrally to avoid the vessels passing through the tympano-occipital fissure and carotid and petrobasilar canals.[26] For a ventral bulla osteotomy a longitudinal incision is made medial to the mandible, with the center of the incision at the angular process of the mandible.[1, 30] The cutaneous and mylohyoideus muscles are incised. An opening is made by blunt dissection dorsally between the digastricus and pterygoid muscles laterally and the hyoglossus and styloglossus medially. The hypoglossal nerve and lingual artery are displaced medially. The bulla can be palpated between the angular process of the mandible and the paracondylar process of the occipital bone. It is medial and just rostral to the articulation of the stylohyoid bone with the petrosal bone via the small tympanohyoid.

The stylohyoid can be followed dorsally as a guide to the bulla. The external carotid artery may overlie the bulla and need to be displaced.

6l. ANESTHETIZED DOG

Identify the parts of the auricular cartilage described in 6f. The lateral crus helicis is visible at the rostromedial margin of the concha, but the larger medial crus must be palpated under the skin. It forms the medial wall of the external part of the meatus and overlaps the tragus. Identify the intertragic notch, a surgical landmark. Find the helicine pouch in the skin on the lateral margin of the ear flap. Its only importance is that it is normal, and may be caught and torn. Palpate the scutiform cartilage (see 6f).

Palpate the cartilaginous meatus through the skin at the base of the ear. Note the sharp curve toward the skull. To use the otoscope, first draw the ear caudally. Insert the tube carefully in a rostroventral direction; always watch the progress of the tip by looking through the instrument. When the angle of the meatus is reached, draw the ear laterally and turn the tip of the instrument medially, thus straightening the meatus. The eardrum is a thin membrane with a white curved bone running from the dorsal margin rostroventrally (see Fig. 6–4). The bone is the handle of the malleus which is attached to the inner surface of the membrane. The eardrum is divided into a larger tense part and a smaller flaccid part in the dorsal quadrant. The tense part is dark because the dark cavity of the middle ear is seen through it. The flaccid part is opaque white with red blood vessels.

The appearance of the eardrum in normal dogs and in those with otitis externa has been described.[29] The eardrum could always be seen in normal dogs less than 1 year old. In one-third of normal adults it was difficult to see for a variety of reasons: it was too transparent, the tense part of the membrane was obscured by the flaccid part, it was concealed by projections of the lining of the meatus, the meatus was too narrow to reach the eardrum, or the eardrum was absent. In one-half the cases of chronic otitis externa the eardrum was ruptured.

Open the mouth and pass your hand caudally through the oropharynx, over the base of the tongue, and dorsolaterally caudal to the soft palate and palpate the tympanic bulla through the laryngopharynx. The bulla can be drained into the pharynx at this point.

6m. SKULL, CAT

The tympanic bulla is large in the cat and contains a nearly complete shelf of bone that divides the cavity into dorsal and ventral components. They communicate through a lateral opening. The ossicles, orifice of the auditory tube, and tympanum are in the dorsal compartment. The roof of the dorsal compartment is the petrosal bone, with its bony labyrinth and the cochlear window caudolaterally.

6n. LIVE CAT

Identify the cartilaginous components of the external ear. Palpate the external ear canal and the tympanic bulla medial to the mandible and digastricus muscle.

References

1. Ader, P. L. and H. W. Boothe: Ventral bulla osteotomy in the cat. J. Am. Anim. Hosp. Assoc. *15* (1979): 757–762.
2. Butler, W. F.: Innervation of the horn region in domestic ruminants. Vet. Rec. *80* (1967):490–492.
3. Cook, W. R.: Clinical observations on the anatomy and physiology of the equine upper respiratory tract. Vet. Rec. *79* (1966):440–446.
4. Cook, W. R.: Observations on the aetiology of epistaxis and cranial nerve paralysis in the horse. Vet. Rec. *78* (1966):396–406.
5. Cook, W. R., R. S. F. Campbell, and C. Dawson: The pathology and aetiology of guttural pouch mycosis in the horse. Vet. Rec. *83* (1968):422–428.
6. Cook, W. R.: Procedure and technique for endoscopy of the equine respiratory tract and Eustachian tube diverticulum. Eq. Vet. J. *2* (1970):137–152.
7. Cook, W. R.: Diseases of the ear, nose and throat of the horse. Part I: The ear. Vet. Annu.*12* (1971):12–43.
8. Ellet, E. W. and J. A. Bowen: Diseases of the ear. *In* Catcott, E. J. (ed.) Feline Medicine and Surgery. Wheaton, Ill.: Am. Vet. Public. 1964, pp. 378–383.

9. Ford, R. S.: Buck deodorizing. Dairy Goat J. *47/5* (1969):3–18.
10. Frank, E. R.: Veterinary Surgery, 7th ed. Minneapolis: Burgess, 1964.
11. Fraser, G., W. W. Gregar, C. D. Mackenzie, et al.: Canine ear disease. J. Small Anim. Pract. *10* (1970):725–754.
12. Freeman, D. E.: Diagnosis and treatment of diseases of the guttural pouch. Part I. Comp. Cont. Ed. *2* (1980):S3–S11.
13. Freeman, D. E.: Diagnosis and treatment of diseases of the guttural pouch. Part II. Comp. Cont. Ed. *2* (1980):S25–S30.
14. Freeman, D. E. and W. J. Donawick: Occlusion of internal carotid artery in the horse by means of a balloon-tipped catheter: clinical use of a method to prevent epistaxis caused by guttural pouch mycosis. JAVMA *176* (1980):236–240.
15. Getty, R., H. L. Foust, E. T. Presley, et al.: Macroscopic anatomy of the ear of the dog. Am. J. Vet. Res. *17* (1956):364–375.
16. Getty, R.: Sisson and Grossman's The Anatomy of the Domestic Animals, 5th ed. Philadelphia: W. B. Saunders, 1975.
17. Guard, W. F.: Surgical Principles and Technics. Columbus, Ohio: Guard, 1953.
18. Heffron, C. J. and G. J. Baker: Endoscopic observations on the deglutition reflex in the horse. Eq. Vet. J. *11* (1979):137–141.
19. Heffron, C. J., G. J. Baker, and R. Lee: Fluoroscopic investigations of pharyngeal function in the horse. Eq. Vet. J. *11* (1979):148–152.
20. Himmelreich, H. A.: Der M. tensor veli palatini der Säugetiere unter Berücksichtigung seines Aufbaus, seiner Funktion und seiner Entstehungsgeschichte. Anat. Anz. *115* (1964):1–26.
21. Howard, P. E., T. M. Neer, and J. S. Miller: Otitis media. Part II. Surgical considerations. Comp. Cont. Ed. *5* (1983):18–21.
22. King, J. M., D. C. Dodd, and M. E. Newson: Gross Necropsy Technique for Animals. Ithaca, New York: Dept. of Pathology, N.Y.S. College of Vet. Med., 1982.
23. Larsen, S.: Intrachondral rupture and hematoma formation in the external ears of dogs. Path. Vet. *5* (1968):442–450.
24. Lauwers, H. and N. R. De Vos: Innervatie van de hoorn bij het rund in verband met het verloop van de N. ophthalmicus. Vlaams Dierg. Tijd. *35* (1966):451–464.
25. Neer, T. M., and P. E. Howard: Otitis media. Comp. Cont. Ed. *4* (1982):410–418.
26. Ott, R. L.: Diagnosis and correction of chronic otitis media. Mod. Vet. Pract. *45/6* (1964):39–42.
27. Parker, A. J., A. G. Schiller, and P. K. Cusick: Bulla curettage for chronic otitis media and interna in dogs. JAVMA *168* (1976):931–933.
28. Siemering, G. H.: Resection of the vertical ear canal for treatment of chronic otitis externa. J. Am. Anim. Hosp. Assoc. *16* (1980):753–758.
29. Spreull, J. S. A.: Treatment of otitis media in the dog. J. Small Anim. Pract. *5* (1964):107–122.
30. Spreull, J. S. A.: Otitis media of the dog. *In* Kirk, R. W. (ed.) Current Veterinary Therapy IV. Small Animal Practice. Philadelphia: W. B. Saunders, 1971 pp. 486–493.
31. Vitums, A.: Nerve and arterial blood supply to the horns of the goat with reference to the sites of anesthesia for dehorning. JAVMA *125* (1954):284–286.
32. Whalen, L. R. and R. L. Kitchell: Electrophysiologic and behavioral studies of the cutaneous nerves of the concave surface of the pinna and external ear canal of the dog. Am. J. Vet. Res. *44* (1983):628–634.
33. Whalen, L. R. and R. L. Kitchell: Electrophysiologic studies of the cutaneous nerves of the head of the dog. Am. J. Vet. Res. *44* (1983):615–627.

CHAPTER 7

POLL, NECK

OBJECTIVES

1. To be able to locate the cranial nuchal (atlantal) bursa in the horse and to understand why it develops there. It prevents friction between which two structures? To appreciate the consequences of injuring the structures ventral to the bursa during surgery for poll evil.
2. To know which of the ventral structures of the neck are covered by deep fascia and which are covered only by superficial fascia. To know the significance of these fascial sheaths for the drainage of pus from wounds in the various organs of the ventral part of the neck.
3. To be able to find the fused right and left sternohyoideus muscles and to separate them on the midline for tracheotomy.
4. To be able to identify the normal thyroid gland by palpation in the horse and to know its location in other species.
5. To be able to palpate the muscles bordering the jugular groove in any species, to raise the external jugular vein, and to know the relationship of the carotid artery to the external jugular in order to avoid the artery during venipuncture and drug injection.
6. To be able to differentiate between a normal jugular pulse and an abnormal one and to be able to evaluate them clinically.
7. To be able to identify the common carotid and axillary arteries by palpation. The object of this exercise is not to count the pulse rate but to appreciate the vulnerability of these arteries to trauma and to avoid them in surgery.
8. To be able to avoid the recurrent laryngeal nerves and the vagosympathetic trunks in operations on the neck.
9. To be able to follow the course of a stomach tube in the cervical esophagus.
10. To be able to take a blood sample from the cranial vena cava in the pig.
11. To understand the surgical and radiological anatomy of the cervical vertebrae, their ossification centers, and their intervertebral discs.
12. To be able to identify the cervical vertebrae, larynx, and trachea in radiographs and by palpation.
13. To be able to identify the landmarks for obtaining CSF from the cerebellomedullary cistern.
14. To be able to palpate the transverse processes of the cervical vertebrae in all species.

7a. DISSECTION, POLL, HORSE

Note the thick, fatty crest on the dorsal surface of the neck. The funiculus nuchae and the splenius, semispinalis capitis, and rectus capitis dorsalis muscles attach to the occipital bone. In the connective tissue between the arch of the atlas and the funiculus nuchae is the cranial nuchal (atlantal) bursa, which may be very small in the normal state. In poll evil the bursa is greatly distended by pus, and the funiculus nuchae is necrotic. The incision required for débridement and drainage extends to the nuchal crest. Note the structures deep to the operative field. The rectus capitis dorsalis muscles cover the dorsal atlanto-occipital membrane and the atlanto-occipital joint capsules. The membrane covers the vertebral canal and blends laterally with the joint capsules. Branches of the occipital and vertebral arteries supply the area. Farther caudally, over the spine of the axis, is the caudal nuchal bursa, which is also difficult to find in the normal horse. It lies between the funiculus nuchae and the large digitation of the lamina nuchae that is attached to the spine of the axis. The laminar attachments of the ligamentum nuchae provide support for the neck, and indirectly for the head after the funiculus has been severed.

7b. DISSECTION, CERVICAL FASCIA, HORSE

Note on the nomenclature: species differences in the muscles of the neck of domestic quadrupeds are given below.

Brachiocephalicus, all species
    Cleidobrachialis, all species
    Clavicular intersection, all species
    Cleidocephalicus, all species
        Cleidomastoideus, all species
        Cleido-occipitalis, swine, ruminants
        Cleidocervicalis, cat, dog
Sternocephalicus, all species
    Sternomastoideus, cat, dog, swine, ruminants
    Sterno-occipitalis, cat, dog
    Sternomandibularis, ox, goat,
Omotransversarius, all species

Identify the structures that are encountered in passing from superficial to deep layers (Fig. 7–1 see also Plate I). Those covered only by superficial fascia and skin are:
    Cervical part of trapezius.
    Rhomboideus cervicis.
    Omotransversarius (formerly cleidotransversarius in the horse).
    Cleidomastoideus.
    The ventral branches of cervical nerves 2 to 6 emerge between the omotransversarius and the cleidomastoideus.
    Sternocephalicus.
    External jugular vein. Enclosed in the superficial fascia between the cleidomastoideus and sternocephalicus.
    Omohyoideus. Deep to the external jugular vein and superficial to the deep fascia that forms the carotid sheath. It passes under the external jugular vein and the sternocephalicus to its termination. This muscle and the sternocephalicus, sternohyoideus, and sternothyroideus are resected in Forssell's operation to prevent cribbing. Bilateral neurectomy of the ventral branch of the accessory nerve to the sternocephalicus muscle where it enters at the musculotendinous junction has given variable results in the treatment of cribbing.[4, 7] This is approximately 5 cm. caudal to the bifurcation of the external jugular into the linguofacial and maxillary veins. A combination of bilateral neurectomy with excision of portions of the omohyoideus, sternohyoideus, and sternothyroideus improved the results with minimal cosmetic defect.[17]
    The following structures ventral to the vertebrae are covered by deep fascia. The clinical importance of the fascial layers of the neck lies in the fact that the deep fascia is attached caudally at the

first rib, sternum, and endothoracic fascia. A septic process in one of the structures that are deep to the deep fascia may gravitate to the thoracic cavity (see Fig. 7–1).

Common carotid artery.

Vagosympathetic trunk.

Recurrent laryngeal nerve. These three structures are enclosed in the carotid sheath formed by

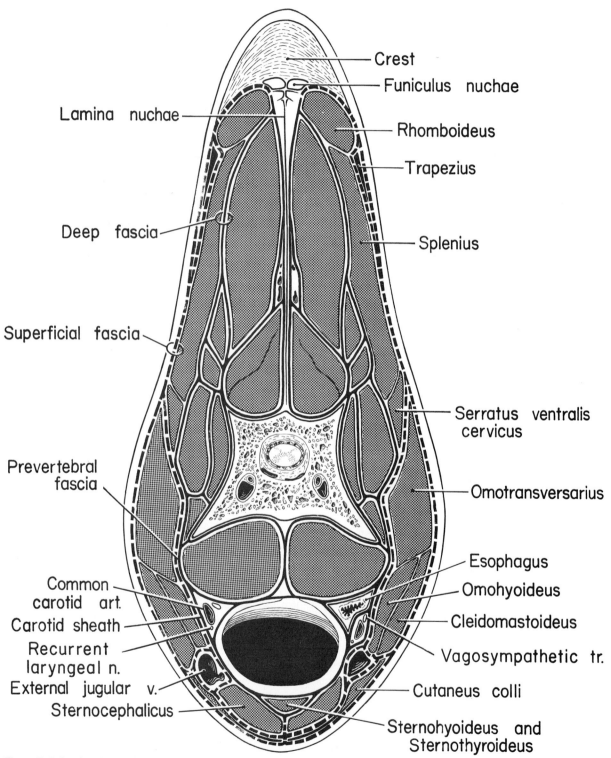

Figure 7–1. Section through the fifth cervical vertebra of a horse.

the deep fascia. The sheath has been opened at the caudal end. The deep surface of the carotid sheath blends with the fascia of the trachea and esophagus, so that the recurrent laryngeal nerve is sometimes described as a companion structure of the carotid, sometimes of the trachea or esophagus.

Trachea, with the lobe of the thyroid gland near the larynx. The isthmus is very narrow.

Esophagus. On the left side.

Sternothyroideus and sternohyoideus. Trace these to their terminations. The right and left sternohyoidei are fused on the midline, and the sternothyroidei are fused to them up to the middle of the neck. Resection of 4 to 6 cm. of the bilaterally fused sternothyroideus and sternohyoideus muscles in the midcervical region has been recommended for treatment of dorsal displacement of the soft palate.[9]

Deep muscles of the neck which lie upon the vertebrae. The layer of deep fascia that covers the longus colli ventral to the vertebrae is the prevertebral fascia.

7c. RADIOGRAPHS, CERVICAL VERTEBRAE, HORSE

Identify the cervical vertebrae on lateral view. The lateral vertebral foramen of the axis is not closed until 2 years. The cranial growth plates usually close by 2 years. Caudal growth plates close later, and the ventral part may persist for 5 to 6 years. In young animals an extra ossification center may be present at the end of the cranial portion of the transverse processes and ventral to the caudal epiphysis of the axis.[15]

Identify the borders of each vertebral foramen. In lateral view estimate the smallest distance between the dorsal and ventral wall in each vertebral foramen. This is the minimum sagittal diameter of that foramen. In a lateral view of a flexed neck estimate the change in position of the adjacent vertebrae at each joint by measuring the distance from the most craniodorsal portion of the vertebral body of the caudal vertebra to the caudal end of the dorsal wall of the vertebral foramen of the cranial vertebra. This is the minimum flexion diameter. Note the range of normal movement between these vertebrae on flexion of the neck. In a normal myelogram the ventral dye line normally is thin over the intervertebral disc between flexed vertebrae, but the dorsal dye line does not attenuate.

7d. LIVE HORSE

Palpate the wing of the atlas and note on the skeleton that the cranial angle is in the transverse plane of the atlanto-occipital space where CSF can be obtained on the midline. The caudal angle is in the transverse plane of the atlantoaxial joint. Palpate the transverse processes of the remaining cervical vertebrae as far caudally as possible, which is usually C 5.

Extend the head and palpate the entire length of the sternocephalicus. Find the point of divergence of the right and left muscles.

On the ventral surface of the trachea find the thin muscular sheet formed by the right and left sternohyoideus and sternothyroideus muscles and trace them to their hyoid and laryngeal terminations. Count the tracheal rings caudally from the larynx to rings 4 to 6, the area for tracheotomy.

Palpate the lobe of the thyroid gland on the lateral surface of the trachea, just caudal to the larynx. It is covered by the sternocephalicus. Push your fingers dorsally between the trachea and the sternocephalicus. At the same time push the sternocephalicus laterally with the back of your fingers and grasp the thyroid lobe on the side of the trachea. It feels like half of a plum, is freely movable, and slips easily out from under your fingers.

Find the ventral border of the brachiocephalicus at the shoulder and follow it to the head. Distend the entire external jugular vein to see its course between the brachiocephalicus and sternocephalicus. Venipuncture is usually performed above the middle of the neck, where the external jugular vein is separated from the carotid artery by the omohyoideus, although this thin muscle offers little protection. Always examine the color of the blood and the force of the flow from the needle before injecting intravenous drugs. Many drugs will cause seizures and death if they are inadvertently injected into the carotid artery.[5] Inadvertent injection into the carotid sheath can cause a sympathetic paralysis of the head (Horner's syndrome) and laryngeal hemiplegia.

In the caudal 10 to 13 cm. of the jugular groove, palpate the common carotid artery dorsolateral to the trachea on the ventral surface of the longus colli. It will be felt as a surprisingly large soft tube. In fat or very muscular horses it cannot be palpated. On the left side, the esophagus can also be palpated in the jugular groove. Farther cranially these structures are deep to the omohyoideus.

7e. DISSECTION AND CROSS SECTION, NECK, CALF

The external jugular vein courses in the jugular groove formed by the sternomandibularis ventromedially and cleidocephalicus dorsolaterally throughout most of the neck. The sternomastoideus forms the deep or medial wall of the groove and separates the external jugular vein from the carotid artery except for a small area near the first rib, where there is no muscle between the two vessels. These muscles are covered by superficial fascia of the neck.

The thymus is large in calves and lies in the deep fascia deep to the sternomastoideus along the trachea. Lateral reflection of the thymus exposes the carotid sheath on the dorsolateral aspect of the trachea. In addition to the carotid artery, the sheath contains the large vagosympathetic trunk and the internal jugular vein, which joins the external jugular vein close to the thorax. The esophagus lies on the left side beween the carotid artery and the trachea. The thyroid lobe is flat and triangular and lies on the trachea caudal to the larynx. The isthmus is wide and glandular.

7f. LIVE COW

Palpate the sternomandibularis from the sternum. Find the mandibular termination.

Locate the ventral border of the cleidomastoideus. The jugular groove between the cleidomastoideus and sternomandibularis is rather wide in the ox (see Plate II).

Observe the degree of fullness of the external jugular vein and apply the venous stasis test by compressing the cranial end of the vein.[16] If the blood drains out of the vein toward the heart, the result is normal, or negative, for venous stasis. If the vein does not drain immediately but is continuously distended, the result is positive for venous stasis, which is caused by obstruction of venous return to the thorax or heart and is associated with congestion and edema. Pericarditis is the most common cause.

In normal cattle a slight undulation may be seen near the thorax. It is synchronous with respiration, the vein distending during expiration. This is more pronounced when animals are dyspneic from respiratory disease.

In some cattle a normal (negative, false) jugular pulse can be observed. This is a brief interruption in the flow of blood to the heart that is synchronous with atrial systole. It appears as a dilation of the vein near the thoracic inlet. Both the respiratory undulation and the normal jugular pulse are obliterated by compressing the cranial end of the vein and abolishing the column of blood from that point to the thoracic inlet, as in a negative venous stasis test.

In some normal cattle the carotid pulse can be seen in the jugular groove. This can be identified by palpation, timing, and its persistence when the column of blood in the external jugular vein disappears after compression.

When the right atrioventricular valve is incompetent owing to heart disease, blood will be ejected back into the atrium and major veins during ventricular systole. This causes an abnormal (positive, true) jugular pulse, which cannot be obliterated by compressing the cranial end of the vein; that is, the venous stasis test is positive. It can be obliterated by compressing the vein at the thoracic inlet. If the jugular pulse is observed at a 30° angle from the thoracic inlet, a normal pulse is undulating and an abnormal pulse is bounding.

Finding:	Synchronous with:	Venous stasis test:
Undulation	Respiration	Negative
Venous pulse (normal)	Atrial systole	Negative
Venous pulse (abnormal)	Ventricular systole	Positive
Venous distention	Continuous	Positive

Palpate the common carotid artery in the thoracic inlet.

Palpate the first rib at the thoracic inlet and the axillary artery as it rounds the first rib.

Palpate the esophagus and wait for a swallow or an eructation.

Palpate the caudal cervical lymph nodes on the first rib. This may be difficult. The normal bovine thyroid gland is too soft and flat to palpate.

Palpate the transverse processes of the cervical vertebrae and the landmarks for obtaining CSF from the cerebellomedullary cistern (see 7d). Make the same palpations in a small ruminant. Appreciate the more caudal position of the wings of the atlas and the site of the cerebellomedullary cistern relative to the position of the horns.

7g. DISSECTION, NECK, PIG

The following cervical muscles originate on the manubrium sterni:

Cutaneus colli.

Sternomastoideus. The pig has only the sternomastoid part of the sternocephalicus.

Sternohyoideus. This muscle is large and, unlike the condition in other species, its origin is separate from that of the sternothyroideus. It arises from the tip of the manubrium.

Sternothyroideus. The point of origin is the angle between the manubrium and the first rib. Another peculiarity of the pig is that the sternothyroideus divides into two branches; one terminates rostroventrally on the thyroid cartilage, and the other terminates caudolaterally.

The jugular groove is short and lies between the brachiocephalicus dorsally and sternomastoideus ventrally. The sternomastoideus passes medial to the external jugular vein, where the

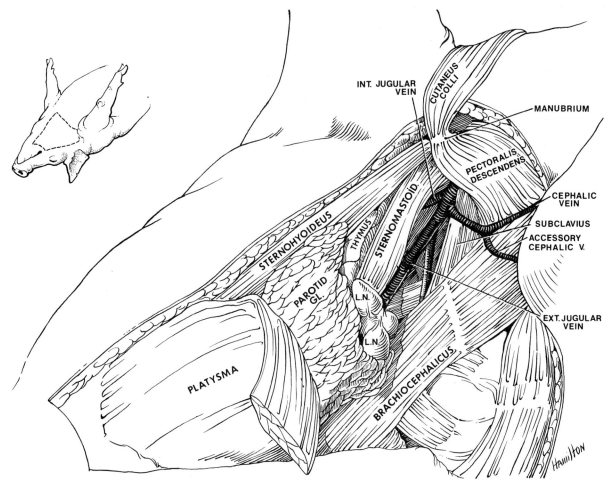

Figure 7–2. Veins and muscles of the neck in the pig. L.N., ventral superficial cervical lymph nodes.

latter divides into maxillary and linguofacial veins. Throughout the neck the external jugular vein is covered by the thick cutaneus colli muscle. There is a depression on the surface of the caudal cervical region that is bounded caudolaterally by the descending pectoral and subclavius and medially by the sternomastoideus. In this hollow the external and internal jugular veins originate from the brachiocephalic vein. This depression can be palpated in the live pig a short distance craniolateral to the manubrium (Fig. 7–2). For venipuncture, the needle is inserted here and directed toward the dorsal border of the opposite scapula. The operation should be performed on the right side, where the phrenic nerve is less vulnerable and there is no thoracic duct.[10]

The thyroid gland is farther caudal to the larynx than in other domestic animals and is found near the thoracic inlet. Its right and left lobes are fused to the massive isthmus and pyramidal lobe ventral to the trachea. The thymus gland is large and extends throughout the neck of the young pig lateral to the larynx and trachea.

7h. DISSECTION, NECK, DOG

The jugular groove clearly lies between the cleidocephalicus and sternocephalicus at the caudal end. Cranially it is less distinct, as the sternocephalicus crosses deep to the vein. There is no sternomandibularis to continue the ventral border of the groove (see Plate III). The common carotid artery, vagosympathetic trunk, and internal jugular vein can be identified in the carotid sheath deep to the sternocephalicus muscle. The subclavian artery is continued by the axillary artery, which crosses the cranial surface of the first rib in its course to the thoracic limb.

The lobe of the thyroid gland is dark, elongated, and flattened on the trachea caudal to the larynx. It is covered by the sternocephalicus, sternothyroideus, and the carotid sheath.

7i. BONES AND RADIOGRAPHS, NECK, CAT AND DOG

Examine a typical cervical vertebra, for example, the fourth. The cranial end of the body is convex and the caudal end is concave, and this conformation should be kept in mind during curettage of the disc. Notice the prominent tubercle at the caudal end of the crest on the ventral surface of the body. This is a reference point for the ventral approach to disc fenestration. The diseased disc is identified by number in a lateral radiograph. One approach is to make a ventral midline incision between the right and left sternomastoideus and sternohyoideus muscles to expose the trachea. The trachea and esophagus are retracted to the left, with careful attention to the protection of the right recurrent laryngeal nerve on the trachea and the contents of the right carotid sheath, which is retracted to the right. The longus colli muscles are now exposed. Their cervical muscle bundles originate from the transverse processes and converge from right and left to terminate on the ventral crest of the preceding vertebra in a V shape pointing cranially.

The ventral tubercles of the vertebrae can be palpated and counted caudally from the atlantoaxial joint. This is in the transverse plane of the caudal angle of the wing of the atlas. The disc is caudal to the tubercle.[14]

The arch is composed of two pedicles that arise from the body and two laminae that extend from the pedicles to the median plane, where they fuse. The laminae are removed in laminectomy, the dorsal approach to the vertebral canal. The important processes are the transverse, spinous, and articular. The foramina are: the vertebral foramen, which is formed by the body and arch and contains the spinal cord; the intervertebral foramen, which is formed by the cranial and caudal vertebral notches in the arches of adjacent vertebrae and transmits the spinal nerve and vessels; the lateral vertebral foramen, which is formed in some vertebrae by enclosure of a vertebral notch, as in the atlas; the transverse foramen, which runs longitudinally through the root of the transverse process (except C 7) and transmits the vertebral artery, vein, and nerve; and in the atlas the alar foramen, or notch in the cat and dog, which transmits the ventral branch of the first cervical nerve ventrally and the vertebral artery dorsally.

A typical cervical vertebra has three ossification centers at birth: one in the centrum of the body and one in each half of the arch.[8] Centers for epiphyses on the ends of the body appear in the third week, and all five are fused by 7 to 14 months.[8]

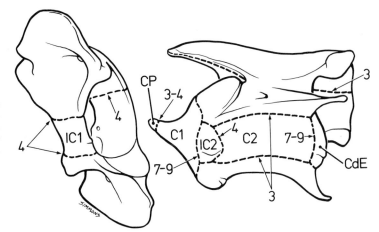

Figure 7–3. Diagram of canine atlas and axis showing ossification centers and approximate time in months of closure of growth plates observed radiographically, ventrolateral aspect. *C1,* Centrum one; *C2,* centrum two; *CP,* centrum of proatlas; *CdE,* caudal epiphysis; *IC7,* intercentrum one; *IC2,* intercentrum two.

The atlas is composed of two lateral masses bearing the transverse processes (wings) and articular fossae, a dorsal arch, and a ventral arch. It has three ossification centers at birth, one for each lateral mass and half of the dorsal arch and one for the ventral arch (intercentrum 1). These are fused at 4 months (Fig. 7–3).[8]

The axis is unusual in having four ossification centers at birth. The extra one (centrum 1) includes most of the dens and part of the cranial articular surfaces.[12] Note that centrum 1 is incorporated in the axis rather than in the atlas. In the third week the caudal epiphysis and intercentrum 2 (cranial part of the body) appear. The latter forms between centrum 1 and centrum 2 and is comparable to the cranial epiphysis of other vertebrae. The arch and centrum 2 unite at 3 months. Intercentrum 2 fuses with centrum 2 at 4 months, and the center for the dens and the cranial articular surfaces fuses with the intercentrum at 7 to 9 months, at the same time the fusion of the caudal epiphysis occurs. There is an additional center for the apex of the dens. It appears and fuses at 3 to 4 months and may or may not be separated in atlantoaxial subluxation. Thus the axis has seven ossification centers.[8, 18, 19]

Atlantoaxial stability is maintained in carnivores by the transverse ligament of the atlas, which is dorsal to the dens, the apical and alar ligaments passing from the dens to the occipital bone, and the dorsal atlantoaxial ligament between the spine of the axis and the arch of the atlas.

In the radiographs identify the following structures:

Larynx and trachea.

Clavicle in the cat. It is also evident on dorsoventral views of many dogs.

Occipital condyles.

Wing of the atlas.

Transverse foramen of the atlas.

Lateral vertebral foramen of the atlas.

Dens of the axis. On lateral view the transverse processes of the atlas are superimposed on the dens. Slight lateral rotation of the head will displace these processes and allow visualization of the dens.

Spinous process of the axis. Note relationship to the arch of the atlas on lateral view. The space between these enlarges in subluxations. It overlaps part of the dens in dorsoventral view.

Processes of other cervical vertebrae:

    Transverse.

    Cranial and caudal articular.

    Spinous.

    Intervertebral discs.

Identify the ossification centers of the vertebral body in young dogs and differentiate growth plates from intervertebral discs. On dorsoventral view of some dogs younger than 4 months, the median growth plate between the halves of the dorsal arch of the atlas may be confused with a fracture.

Observe the relationship between cervical vertebrae on lateral views of the neck in full flexion and full extension. Consider the effect of these positions on lesions that compress the spinal cord. Flexion will exacerbate the spinal cord compression if there is intervertebral laxity and subluxation and if there is a firm non-movable mass ventrally, such as a mineralized intervertebral disc. A soft movable mass such as proliferation of the dorsal longitudinal ligament will be stretched out and narrowed by neck flexion, decreasing the compression. A similar effect will occur with a proliferation of the ligamentum flavum dorsally. Extension of the neck will exacerbate the compression caused by ventral or dorsal soft tissue proliferations and excessive cranial growth of the vertebral arch or craniomedial growth of the cranial articular processes. Normally, there is often less movement between the sixth and seventh cervical vertebrae on neck flexion or extension.[2]

7j. LIVE DOG

Palpate the brachiocephalicus. It stands out clearly if the paw is raised and released. The dog lets the paw down slowly, tensing the muscle. The sternomastoideus may be traced to the mastoid insertion, but the sterno-occipitalis is too thin to palpate.

Distend the external jugular vein by pressure at the caudal end of the jugular groove. This is the best place to obtain large blood samples in the cat[11] and often in the dog also.

Palpate the sternohyoideus and sternothyroideus and try to palpate the thyroid gland (see 7h). Lightly stroke the dorsolateral aspect of the trachea just caudal to the larynx. The normal gland cannot be felt.

Palpate the landmarks for cerebellomedullary cistern puncture. Under general anesthesia the head is flexed to open the atlanto-occipital aperture but not enough to kink an endotracheal tube. The needle is inserted in the median plane (palpate the external occipital protuberance) at the intersection of a line drawn across the cranial extremities of the wings of the atlas. A styleted needle is inserted perpendicular to the skin, directed toward a line connecting the angular processes of the mandibles, and advanced cautiously until cerebrospinal fluid is obtained. Find these features in lateral and dorsoventral radiographs and on the skeleton.

Palpate the transverse processes of the cervical vertebrae.

References

1. Cechner, P. E.: Ventral cervical disc fenestration in the dog: a modified technique. J. Am. Anim. Hosp. Assoc. 16 (1980):647–650.
2. Conrad, C. R.: Motion of the canine cervical vertebral column in the median plane—a radiographic method of analysis. Master's Thesis, Cornell University, 1972.
3. Cook, J. R. and J. E. Oliver, Jr.: Atlantoaxial luxation in the dog. Comp. Cont. Ed. 3 (1981):242–250.
4. Firth, E. C.: Bilateral ventral accessory neurectomy in windsucking horses. Vet. Rec. 106 (1980):30–32.
5. Gabel, A. A. and A. Koestner: The effects of intracarotid artery injection of drugs in domestic animals. JAVMA 142 (1963):1397–1403.
6. Geary, J. C., J. E. Oliver, and B. F. Hoerlein: Atlantoaxial subluxation in the canine. J. Small Anim. Pract. 8 (1967):577–582.
7. Greet, T. R. C.: Windsucking treated by myectomy and neurectomy. Equine Vet. J. 14 (1982):299–301.
8. Hare, W. C. D.: Radiographic anatomy of the cervical region of the canine vertebral column. JAVMA 139 (1961):209–220.
9. Haynes, P. F.: Dorsal displacement of the soft palate and epiglottic entrapment: Diagnosis, management, and interrelationship. Comp. Cont. Ed. 5 (1983): S379–S389.
10. Hoerlein, A. B., E. P. Hubbard, and R. Getty: The procurement and handling of swine blood samples on the farm. JAVMA 119 (1951):357–362.

11. Hovell, G. J. R., K. J. O'Reilly, and R. C. Povey: A method of venipuncture in the cat. Vet. Rec. 87 (1970):184–185.
12. Jenkins, F. A.: The evolution and development of the dens of the mammalian axis. Anat. Rec. 164 (1969):173–184.
13. Monen, T.: Surgical management of crib biting in the horse. Comp. Cont. Ed. 4 (1982):S69–S74.
14. Piermattei, D. L. and R. G. Greeley: Approach to the cervical vertebrae and intervertebral disks through a ventral incision. In: An Atlas of Surgical Approaches to the Bones of the Dog and Cat, 2nd ed. Philadelphia: W. B. Saunders, 1979, pp. 38–41.
15. Rendano, V. T. and C. B. Quick: Equine radiology—the cervical spine. Mod. Vet. Pract. 59 (1978): 921–927.
16. Rosenberger, G. (ed): Circulation. In: Clinical Examination of Cattle. Berlin: Verlag Paul Parey, 1979, pp. 116–118.
17. Turner, A. S., N. White, and J. Ismay: Modified Forssell's operation for crib biting in the horse. JAVMA 184 (1984):309–312.
18. Watson, A. G. and H. E. Evans: The development of the atlas-axis complex in the dog. Abstract. Anat. Rec. 184 (1976):558.
19. Watson, A. G.: The phylogeny and development of the occipito-atlas-axis complex in the dog. PhD Thesis, Cornell University, 1981.

CHAPTER 8

WITHERS, SHOULDER, AND ARM

OBJECTIVES

1. To be able to diagnose paralyses and sensory deficits caused by injury to the six main nerves of the thoracic limb or the segments of the spinal cord from which they originate.
2. To be able to palpate the superficial cervical lymph node in all species and to be able to treat abscesses of the node (especially in the horse) without cutting the underlying artery.
3. To gain access to a supraspinous bursitis, remove necrotic tissue, and provide bottom drainage without making a hole in the dorsoscapular ligament that would admit pus to the deeper tissues.
4. To be able to diagnose lameness caused by inflammation of the shoulder joint, intertubercular bursa, or infraspinatus bursa and to be able to insert a needle into these structures, using palpable landmarks.
5. To be able to diagnose shoulder lameness in the dog due to abnormal laxity or contracture of supporting structures.
6. To be able to palpate and identify the skeletal prominences of the region as an aid to diagnosis of fractures and dislocations and to the interpretation of radiographs.
7. To be able to distinguish between a fracture, a normal epiphyseal cartilage, and a separated epiphysis.
8. To be able to anesthetize the paw in the dog by blocking the nerves in the brachium. To be able to locate the brachial artery for the injection of antivenin.
9. To be able to avoid surgical complications caused by the suprahamate process and the supracondylar foramen in the cat.
10. To be able to make the best surgical approach to the shoulder joint, the distal part of the shaft of the humerus, and the medial side of the condyle in the dog.

Note on the Nomenclature. Rotation of a limb or a segment of a limb on its long axis is designated by the direction of movement of its cranial or dorsal surface. For example, in medial rotation of the thigh, the femoral trochlea is turned medially. Rotation of the forearm and manus and of the pes, movements that do not occur normally in ungulates, are designated by the special terms, pronation (medial rotation) and supination (lateral rotation).

Nerves Of the Thoracic Limb

Knowledge of the origin and distribution of the six clinically important nerves is necessary for the diagnosis of injuries to the spinal cord and nerves. The following table shows the major contributions of the spinal nerves to the nerves of the limb. In a few dogs the brachial plexus has neurons from C 5, and in most dogs from T 2, but the number from these two nerves is insignificant.[3] In the horse the origins are slightly more caudal and the contribution of T 2 is larger.

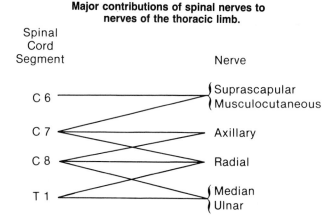

Major contributions of spinal nerves to nerves of the thoracic limb.

The clinical signs of section of these nerves have been described.[37, 40] The loss of motor neurons can be determined by observation of the gait and depression of tone and reflexes, and palpation of muscle atrophy from denervation. The loss of sensory neurons is best determined by the loss of painful response to noxious stimuli—analgesia. The cutaneous area is the total area of skin supplied by a specific peripheral nerve. The autonomous zone is the area of skin supplied by *only* that specific peripheral nerve (Figs. 8–1 and 8–2).[13] Overlap of sensory innervation by adjacent peripheral nerves is extensive. Knowledge of the autonomous zones of peripheral nerves is critical in the assessment of neurologic deficits. Both motor and sensory neurons contribute to spinal reflexes. Loss of either will result in a decrease in or a loss of spinal reflexes.

Suprascapular Nerve. Section causes no change in the gait in the dog. Lateral buckling of the shoulder joint sometimes occurs in the acute stage in the horse. It is best seen from the front. There is a marked and rapid atrophy of the supraspinatus and infraspinatus muscles, with resultant prominence of the spine of the scapula (sweeny).

Musculocutaneous Nerve. Section causes little change in gait despite paralysis of the biceps brachii and brachialis. Difficulty in flexing the elbow is seen when the dog tries to raise the paw to place it on a table. Anesthesia of the medial side of the forearm in the autonomous zone of the medial cutaneous antebrachial nerve is seen (see Fig. 8–1).

Axillary Nerve. Although this nerve supplies a group of flexors of the shoulder—teres major, teres minor, and deltoideus—paralysis does not cause much loss of flexion. The long head of the triceps and the latissimus dorsi also have this action. There is a small area of anesthesia caudal to the scapula and shoulder and on the lateral side of the arm. This is the autonomous zone of the cranial lateral cutaneous brachial nerve.

Radial Nerve. Radial paralysis is the most characteristic paralysis in the forelimb. If the nerve is severed above the branches to the triceps, the limb will support no weight (not even in the horse; the vaunted stay apparatus will not replace the triceps). The extensors of all the joints except the shoulder are paralyzed, and the limb is carried in a flexed position. If the toes touch the ground, they flex and rest on the dorsal surface (knuckling).

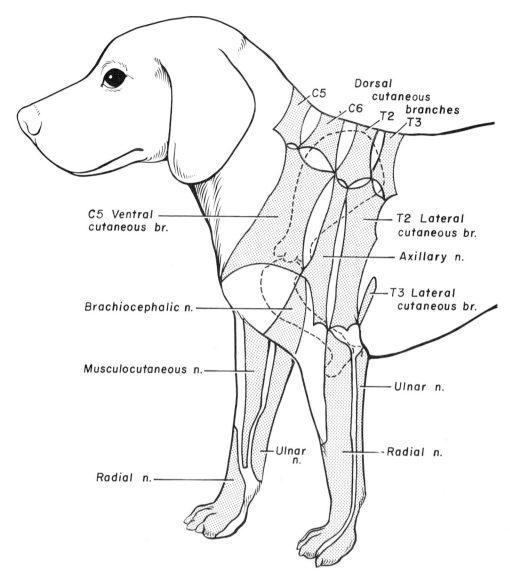

Figure 8–1. Autonomous zones of the cutaneous innervation of the canine thoracic limb. (Reprinted by permission from de Lahunta, A.: *Veterinary Neuroanatomy and Clinical Neurology,* 2nd. Ed., Philadelphia, W. B. Saunders Co., 1983, p. 171.)

The most common serious injury of the nerves of the forelimb is avulsion of the roots of the spinal nerves whose ventral branches form the brachial plexus. This results from severe abduction or retraction of the forelimb caudally along the trunk and is usually associated with automobile trauma. Avulsion of all the roots from C 6 through T 1 or T 2 causes complete paralysis with a fully extended flaccid limb that is unable to support weight and is dragged on the dorsal surface of the paw. There is usually analgesia distal to the elbow. If only the caudal roots that contribute to the brachial plexus (C 8, T 1, T 2) are avulsed, the limb will be carried with the elbow and shoulder flexed owing to the function of neurons in the suprascapular, musculocutaneous, and axillary nerves. By 10 to 14 days after the injury the distribution of denervation atrophy will help in determining which spinal nerves have been injured.

If the radial nerve is damaged distal to the branches to the triceps, all species soon compensate for the loss of extensor function in the carpus and digits by flipping the foot forward, so that it lands on the pads or sole surface, and the gait is restored to its normal appearance. In the dog, the loss of sensation in the field of the superficial branch on the distal cranial and the lateral surfaces of the forearm and the dorsal surface of the manus is diagnostic.

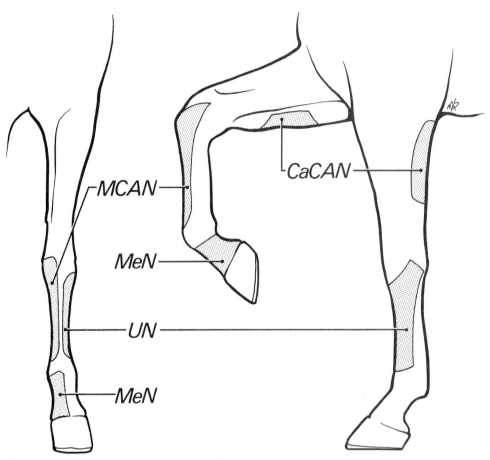

Figure 8–2. Autonomous zones of cutaneous innervation of the equine thoracic limb distal to the elbow. Medial cutaneous antebrachial nerve (*MCAN*), caudal cutaneous antebrachial nerve (*CaCAN*), median nerve (*MeN*), ulnar nerve (*UN*). (Reprinted by permission from Blyth, L. L., and R. L. Kitchell: Electrophysiologic studies of the thoracic limb of the horse. Am. J. Vet. Res. *43*(1982):1511–1524.)

The axillary nerve overlaps with the radial nerve in the cutaneous innervation of the skin of the proximal one-half to two-thirds of the cranial surface of the forearm and rarely the entire cranial surface; therefore, the most reliable skin area to test for radial nerve function is the mid-dorsal surface of the paw.[13] A common cause of injury distally in the radial nerve is a fracture of the distal shaft of the humerus. Because of the skeletal injury and associated swelling and pain, the motor function of the radial nerve cannot usually be tested; therefore, only the function of the nociceptive neurons to the autonomous zone can be relied on to determine if any function persists in the radial nerve.

The horse is unusual among domestic animals in having a short superficial branch of the radial nerve that supplies only the craniolateral surface of the arm and forearm. No area of anesthesia occurs if this nerve is injured because of the overlap of cutaneous innervation from adjacent nerves (see Fig. 8–2). A common cause of forelimb paralysis in horses is related to prolonged anesthesia. This is thought to be due to a myopathy from pressure-induced ischemic hypoxia to portions of muscle in the downside limb that are restricted from swelling because of their fascial sheaths.[16, 39] Muscles most commonly affected are the triceps brachii, quadriceps femoris, middle gluteal, and masseter. As a rule this does not involve sensory components of nerves. Atrophy of the extensor muscles in the forearm 1 month after injury differentiates radial nerve damage from transient ischemic paralysis caused by surgical restraint in the horse.[17]

Median Nerve. There is little change in gait when this nerve is cut in the dog. When the animal is standing on the limb, the carpus and metacarpophalangeal joints sink into overextension. The claws are raised off the ground, and the foot spreads so that the track is larger. If a dog in sternal recumbency is dragged backward, the claws of the normal paw dig in, but the claws of the paralyzed paw do not. If the dog is required to dig for food, the flexor paralysis of the affected paw will be evident.[4] The median and ulnar nerves are sensory to the palmar surface of the paw, but no deficit is seen unless both are severed together with the communicating branch from the musculocutaneous to the median proximal to the elbow.

Ulnar Nerve. Section causes no change in gait or digging function. There is a slight spreading of the digits. There is anesthesia in the caudal antebrachial region and in the lateral surface of the fifth digit.

8a. DISSECTION, WITHERS, HORSE

At the base of the neck, the sternocephalicus and external jugular vein are concealed by the cutaneus colli and brachiocephalicus. The omohyoideus is dorsal to the jugular here but passes medial to the vein farther cranially.

The superficial cervical (prescapular) lymph nodes lie along the cranial border of the subclavius muscle. The chain of small lymph nodes extends across the omohyoideus, lying between that muscle and the deep surfaces of the brachiocephalicus and omotransversarius. The prescapular branch of the superficial cervical artery runs between the lymph nodes and the subclavius and is endangered by surgical treatment of abscesses of the lymph nodes.

Fistulous withers is a suppurative infection of the supraspinous bursa, which is located between the funiculus nuchae and the second to fourth thoracic spinous processes. Knowledge of its anatomical boundaries is important in the treatment. The trapezius muscle is the most superficial, arising from the funiculus nuchae and the adjacent supraspinous ligament. The rhomboideus cervicis is deep to the trapezius and also arises from the funiculus nuchae. It attaches laterally to the medial surface of the scapular cartilage. The dorsoscapular ligament is deep to the rhomboideus and extends ventrolaterally from the summits of the cranial thoracic vertebral spines to the scapula and first few ribs. The rhomboideus thoracis originates from the lateral surface of the thick dorsal part of the ligament. The splenius arises from its cranial border. Two thin longitudinal lamellae originate from the deep surface and pass beween epaxial muscles to the vertebrae and ribs. A third gives origin to the serratus dorsalis cranialis muscle. The ventral part is thin and elastic and gives rise to transverse elastic lamellae that extend laterally between bundles of the serratus ventralis to the scapula. The floor of the supraspinous bursa can be reached for drainage by blunt dissection between the rhomboideus cervicis and the superficial surface of the dorsoscapular ligament.[9] It is important that the bursa is normally superficial to the dorsoscapular ligament. Large branches of the costocervical trunk supply this area.

8b. DISSECTION, DETACHED SHOULDER AND ARM, HORSE

Deep to the supraspinatus, the suprascapular nerve crosses the cranial border of the scapula with the artery of the same name (see Plate I).

The brachiocephalicus covers the lateral side of the biceps brachii. The intertubercular bursa is between the tendon of origin of the biceps and the humerus.

Reflection of the lateral head of the triceps will uncover the radial nerve in its course around the caudolateral surface of the humerus with the brachialis and the collateral radial vessels. The latter are branches of the deep brachial artery and vein. The radial nerve also passes under the origin of the extensor carpi radialis (see Plate I).

The bursa under the tendon of the long head of the triceps can be exposed by reflecting the distal stump of the lateral head. The subcutaneous bursa may not be present, but it is the one affected in capped elbow.

The infraspinatus bursa is between the long tendon of termination of the muscle and the major tubercle. The short termination is on the caudal part of the major tubercle. The tendon is a landmark for injection of the shoulder joint (see Plate I).

8c. SECTION, WITHERS, HORSE

The following should be observed on a cross section through the region of the supraspinous bursa in the horse:

Funiculus nuchae. Two flattened halves dorsal to the muscles.

Summit of second thoracic spinous process.

Origin of laminae nuchae, yellow elastic tissue on both sides of the summit of the second and third thoracic spinous processes.

Supraspinous bursa. Between the funiculus above, and the dorsoscapular ligament, second spinous process, and laminae nuchae below. Rarely, a bursa may occur between the spine of the second thoracic vertebra and the laminae nuchae deep to the dorsoscapular ligament.

Trapezius. Thin, lateral to scapula. Originates from funiculus nuchae.

Rhomboideus. Between the scapular cartilage and the dorsoscapular ligament.

Supraspinatus and infraspinatus.

Serratus ventralis. Thick at this level.

Subscapularis. Thin, ventral to the serratus.

Dorsoscapular ligament.

Epaxial muscles between the dorsoscapular ligament and the ribs and vertebrae.

The cartilage of the scapula and the dorsal end of the spine of the scapula. Correlate this with the relations of the scapula and thoracic spinous processes on a skeleton.

8d. RADIOGRAPHS, HORSE

Identify the skeletal features associated with the adult shoulder and the ossification centers in the young animal.[19, 20] The scapula has four ossification centers: scapular cartilage, body of scapula, supraglenoid tubercle and coracoid process, and the cranial part of the ventral angle. The body of the scapula unites with the distal ossification centers by 10 to 12 months. The ossified scapular cartilage joins the scapula sometime after 3 years. The proximal humerus develops from two ossification centers, which unite with the shaft (diaphysis) from 18 to 30 months. These two centers are the major tubercle and the proximal epiphysis. The latter forms the head and the minor tubercle. (See table 1 of Appendix.)

8e. LIVE HORSE

The first anatomical problem in diagnosing lameness is to decide which of the four limbs is sore. Limping is basically a means of shifting the center of gravity to ease the load on the sore limb when it is bearing weight and to shorten the period of weight-bearing. The center of gravity in the standing horse is about 43 percent of the distance from the shoulder joint to the tuber ischiadicum. In a horse with a trunk length of 160 cm. the center of gravity lies in a transverse plane 38 cm. caudal to the olecranon.[21] Raising the head shifts the center of gravity caudally and eases the weight on the forelimbs. This is the reason for the old rule that in forelimb lameness the horse "nods on the sound foot." The nod is the necessary reciprocating action that allows him to raise his head at the next step when the sore foot is on the ground. Lowering the head shifts the center of gravity forward and takes some of the weight off a sore hind limb when it is on the ground. With hind limb lameness, a trotter nods on the forelimb opposite to the lame hind limb and a pacer nods on the forelimb on the same side as the lame hind limb. Lameness in a hind limb is best recognized by the characteristic "hitch," "hip hike," or elevation of the hindquarters when the sound limb pushes off the ground. Other abnormalities of the gait and stance must also be considered. On the track a horse tends to move away from the unsound limb. With a left forelimb lameness, the horse will "bear out" or tend to move away from the rail. With a left hind limb lameness, the hindquarters may be to the right of the forequarters, and the left hind limb will land closer to the midline. For trotters and pacers the hindquarters will be carried next to the shaft on the side of the sound hind limb.

When observations from a distance have been made, the detailed examination begins with the hoof. This procedure saves time in general practice because the incidence of lameness is greater in the parts of the limb that are closest to the ground. The anatomical study of the limbs, however, must follow the proximodistal sequence because of the branching of the vessels and nerves.

One cause of lameness is inflammation of a subtendinous synovial bursa. Such a bursa will cause pain when the tendon that crosses it exerts pressure or friction on the bursa. Diagnosis of a bursitis requires anatomical knowledge of the location and action of the tendon involved so that three kinds of signs can be utilized.

1. How the animal avoids pain in the gait. The animal refuses to perform the action of the muscle. For example, if the intertubercular bursa is painful, the animal takes a short stride, because it is reluctant to use the biceps brachii to extend the shoulder.

2. How the animal avoids pain in standing. The animal uses other muscles to adopt a posture that eases tension on the tendon by placing the termination closer to the origin of the muscle. For example, if the infraspinatus bursa is painful, the body is eased away from the affected limb, leaving it in abduction at the shoulder joint.

3. How the clinician manipulates the joint to elicit pain. He moves the joint in the direction opposite to the action of the muscle. For example, in intertubercular bursitis, the foot is picked up and the carpus is drawn caudally. This flexes the shoulder and extends the elbow, both actions opposing the biceps brachii. The clinician also employs his knowledge of the location of the bursa to apply direct pressure to the tendon over it.

Not all synovial bursae are of constant occurrence. The subcutaneous ones develop with age and trauma over skeletal prominences such as the tuber olecrani and the tuber calcanei. They are subject to inflammation, but usually do not involve underlying tendons. The synovial bursae of the horse have been described.[22]

Locate the following structures:

Rhomboideus cervicis. Turn the head to the other side to make the muscle stand out. Do not confuse it with the crest.

Second thoracic spinous process. The first is not palpable; see the skeleton. The normal location of the supraspinous bursa is in the space between the funiculus and the lamina nuchae over the second to fourth spinous processes. It is greatly enlarged in disease (see Plate I).

Highest spinous process. This is the fourth or fifth.

Bilateral expansions of the funiculus at the high point of the withers.

Scapula. Spine, caudal angle, cranial angle. The ventral angle is at the shoulder.

Supraspinatus muscle.

Subclavius muscle. It lies along the cranial border of the supraspinatus.

Superficial cervical lymph nodes. A long chain of small nodes.

Infraspinatus muscle and its broad long tendon of termination on the major tubercle of the humerus. This is partly cartilaginous and can be grasped and moved over the infraspinatus bursa. This will elicit a painful response if the bursa is inflamed. The shoulder joint capsule can be exposed surgically by retracting the deltoideus caudally, incising the infraspinatus tendon longitudinally, and retracting the halves.[8]

Major tubercle of the humerus. Palpate the notch between the cranial and caudal parts of the major tubercle. Anesthetic injection into the shoulder joint can be made by inserting a needle cranioproximal to the caudal part of the major tubercle and cranial to the edge of the infraspinatus tendon. It is directed medioventrally to a depth of 5 cm. If the needle is directed too far forward, it will enter the intertubercular bursa. The joint capsule and the bursa are separate in the horse, cow, and goat.

The origin of the biceps and the intertubercular bursa are deep to the subclavius and brachiocephalicus. Find the terminations of the biceps on the radial tuberosity and on the tendon of the extensor carpi radialis (lacertus fibrosus).

Deltoid tuberosity. To inject the intertubercular bursa, insert the needle in front of the proximal end of the deltoid tuberosity and direct it proximally between the biceps and the bone.[38]

Brachialis muscle. Palpable on the humerus below the deltoid tuberosity.

Triceps muscle. Outline the long and lateral heads. Palpate the termination.

8f. LIVE COW, SHEEP, GOAT

Locate the following structures:

Rhomboideus cervicis.

Scapula. Spine, caudal angle, cranial angle, acromion.

Supraspinatus muscle.

Superficial cervical lymph node. In the cow, the node is very large, about 3×10 cm., and lies in the groove on the cranial border of the supraspinatus, covered by the brachiocephalicus and the omotransversarius. The best technique of palpation is to place the palm of the hand on the cow's neck with the finger tips against the supraspinatus and to draw the tissues in the groove cranially. The node will pop out from under the fingers toward the groove. Other approaches usually push the node farther under the supraspinatus, where it cannot be palpated (see Plate II).

Termination of the infraspinatus muscle. There is a large bursa under the long tendon of termination.

Note the great extent of the major tubercle of the humerus (see the skeleton).

Palpate the notch in the proximal border of the major tubercle. The shoulder joint of small ruminants can be injected distal to the midpoint of a line between this notch and the acromion.[27] The needle is directed mediodistally and slightly cranial. The shoulder joint capsule and intertubercular bursa communicate in sheep but not in cattle and goats. The greater tubercle projects dorsal to the level of the head; therefore, the needle must be placed medial to the tubercle.

Tendon of origin of biceps. Easier to find than in the horse because the subclavius is rudimentary.

Deltoid tuberosity.

Brachialis muscle. Important as an indication of the course of the radial nerve in the arm.

Triceps.

8g. SCAPULA AND HUMERUS, CAT AND DOG

Observe the following features of the scapula:

Spine.

Acromion. In the cat this has two parts—the distal, hooked, or hamate process and the suprahamate process that curves back over the infraspinous fossa. The suprahamate process could cause trouble in freeing the infraspinatus muscle for retraction.

Scapular notch.

Caudal angle.

Neck.

Glenoid cavity.

Supraglenoid tubercle. This is the point of origin of the biceps.

Humerus:

Head.

Neck.

Major tubercle.

Termination of supraspinatus.

Termination of infraspinatus.

Minor tubercle.

Intertubercular groove for the biceps tendon.

Shaft with spiral groove for the brachialis. Most fractures of the humerus are in the shaft. See the supracondylar foramen in the cat. This contains the median nerve and brachial artery (see Fig. 8–4).

Condyle. The humerus has but one condyle, comprising the whole distal end except the epicondyles. In man and cat, the distal articular surface is divided into a medial trochlea for the ulna and a lateral capitulum for the radius. In the dog, the capitulum is smaller, and the radius also articulates with the trochlea. In the ungulates, the radius articulates with the capitulum and the whole width of the trochlea, which is the wide grooved portion, separated by a ridge from the capitulum on the lateral side.

Radial and olecranon fossae meet in the dog to form a supratrochlear foramen, which is not present in any other domestic mammal, except occasionally in the pig.

Coronoid fossa. This term has been used erroneously in veterinary anatomy to refer to the radial fossa. A true coronoid fossa occurs in the cat and accommodates the medial coronoid process of the ulna when the elbow is flexed.

Lateral (extensor) epicondyle.

Medial (flexor) epicondyle.

8h. RADIOGRAPHS, HUMERUS AND SCAPULA, DOG AND CAT

In connection with the radiology and surgery of the limbs it is essential to have an understanding of the anatomy of a long bone as an organ. The diaphysis is the shaft. An epiphysis is a part of a bone formed from a secondary center of ossification, as at the ends of long bones and at some tubercles and processes. It is separated from the rest of the bone during growth by the epiphyseal cartilage or growth plate. The metaphysis is a zone of transformation of calcified cartilage to spongy bone at the end of the diaphysis. The epiphyseal cartilage is radiolucent. When growth ceases and the epiphysis unites with the shaft, the radiolucent zone disappears, and the blood vessels inside the diaphysis anastomose with those of the epiphysis. This is referred to as closure of the growth plate.

Identify the structures listed:

Spine of the scapula.

Acromion.

Supraglenoid tubercle.

Humeral head.

Major and minor tubercles.

Deltoid tuberosity.

Groove for the brachialis.

Crest of the major tubercle.

Condyle.

Medial and lateral epicondyles.

Supratrochlear foramen.

Supracondylar foramen (cat).

Identify the ossification centers where they are still present. The time of fusion of ossification centers with the rest of the bone is as determined by radiographs. (See Table 2 in Appendix.)

The scapula has two ossification centers—the body and the supraglenoid tubercle. These unite at 3 to 7 months in dogs and 3 ½ to 4 months in cats. The head and tubercles of the proximal humerus develop from a single ossification center, the proximal epiphysis, which unites with the shaft or diaphysis at 10 to 15 months in dogs and at 18 to 24 months in cats. The distal humerus arises from four ossification centers—the medial and lateral parts of the condyle and the medial and lateral epicondyles. In the cat, all four are present after birth. In the dog, the lateral epicondyle is usually fused before birth. The three ossification centers observed are the prominent medial epicondyle and the medial and lateral parts of the condyle. In the cat, these ossification centers usually fuse with each other and the diaphysis by 3½ to 4 months. In the dog, the medial and lateral parts of the condyle unite at 5 months and the medial epicondyle fuses with the condyle by 5 to 6 months. This distal epiphysis fuses with the diaphysis at 5 to 8 months. It is necessary to examine both lateral to medial and cranial to caudal views to study these centers.

On an arthrogram of the shoulder note the extent of the joint and its communication with the intertubercular bursa around the tendon of the biceps brachii.[32]

8i. DISSECTION, SHOULDER AND ARM, DOG

Four surgical approaches are described for the shoulder joint: lateral, caudolateral, craniomedial, and craniolateral. The superficial veins of the region require some explanation because they must be retracted or ligated (see Fig. 8–3). The cephalic vein is a branch of the external jugular. It runs laterodistally across the terminations of the superficial pectoral muscles and deep to the brachiocephalicus to the groove between the brachiocephalicus and brachialis. Here it is connected by a large anastomosis, the axillobrachial vein, with the axillary vein behind the shoulder joint. The axillobrachial was formerly considered part of the cephalic, but this was not consistent with the course of the cephalic vein in other species. The axillobrachial vein is connected to the external jugular by the omobrachial, which runs obliquely across the superficial surface of the brachiocephalicus.

In the lateral approach[26] the spine of the scapula is exposed by severing the attachments of the trapezius, omotransversarius, and the scapular part of the deltoid. The acromial part of the deltoid is isolated, sparing the deltoid branch of the axillary nerve in the space between the two parts of the muscle and the axillobrachial vein at the distal end of the incision. The origin of the acromial part of the deltoid is transected or the acromion is cut off to reflect the muscle. The supraspinatus and infraspinatus are freed and retracted from the spine of the scapula, sparing their branches of the suprascapular nerve, which passes across the neck of the scapula under the acromion. The tendon of termination of the infraspinatus is transected, and sometimes also that of the teres minor, to expose the joint.

The caudolateral approach is preferred for treatment of osteochondrosis, as it exposes the caudal portion of the humeral head.[25] There are many variations of this procedure.[5] It is not necessary to transect the acromial deltoid. In some dogs, adequate exposure can be obtained without any tenotomy. The joint can be exposed between the infraspinatus and teres minor by cranial retraction of the acromial deltoid, craniodorsal retraction of the infraspinatus, and cranial or caudal retraction of the teres minor.

If tenotomy of the infraspinatus or teres minor is necessary, caudal retraction of the acromial deltoid will permit these tenotomies. In all approaches, medial rotation of the limb will help expose the humeral head.

The cranial exposures are used to treat luxations. Luxations of the shoulder are not common. The medial and lateral glenohumeral ligaments in the wall of the joint capsule prevent this.[35] Adjacent supporting muscles also contribute to its stability. The tendon of origin of the biceps may be diverted to form a medial collateral ligament, or less often a lateral collateral ligament, to prevent recurrent luxation of the shoulder. In medial luxation of the humerus, the medial border of the brachiocephalicus is separated from the superficial pectoral muscles and retracted laterally (see Fig. 8–3). It may be necessary to ligate the omobrachial vein. The terminations of the superficial pectoral muscles are partially transected by an incision that extends from the cranial border to the cephalic vein. The vein is accompanied by an artery, the deltoid branch of the superficial cervical. The termination of the deep pectoral muscle is transected and reflected to expose the shoulder joint and the coracobrachialis muscle. The termination of the subscapularis, deep to the tendon of the coracobrachialis, is detached from the minor tubercle if not already ruptured. The biceps tendon is freed from the intertubercular groove by opening the diverticulum of the joint capsule that ensheaths it and cutting the transverse humeral retinaculum. The tendon is placed in a groove, curetted under a bone flap of the minor tubercle. The bone flap is pinned down. The capsule is repaired and the joint is covered and reinforced by drawing the muscle stumps somewhat beyond their terminations and suturing them to the fascia on the humerus. The subscapularis then passes over the transplanted biceps tendon.

Another procedure for treating medial luxation diverts the medial half of the supraspinatus tendon, along with the portion of greater tubercle where it terminates, to an area on the lesser tubercle from which the cortex has been removed.[7] The surgical approach is the same. It's important to reef the medial joint capsule along with the medial glenohumeral ligament.

In lateral luxation of the humerus the brachiocephalicus is retracted medially, exposing the minations of the supraspinatus, deltoideus, and pectoral muscles. The terminations of the superficial and deep pectoral muscles are incised as for the craniomedial approach and the termination of the deltoid is transected similarly. In order to transplant the tendon of origin of the biceps brachii laterally the part of the major tubercle with the supraspinatus attached is cut off and pinned back in place after moving the biceps tendon to the lateral side of the major tubercle. The biceps tendon then passes deep to the supraspinatus and lateral to the major tubercle. It is sutured in position, the capsule is repaired, and the muscles are reattached.

In exposing the distal shaft of the humerus from the lateral side, the axillobrachial vein must be avoided at the proximal end of the incision and the radial nerve at the distal end. The brachiocephalicus and distal termination of the superficial pectoral are detached from the bone and

Figure 8–3. Craniomedial approach to the canine shoulder. The stump of the deep pectoral is retracted by forceps and the subscapularis is transected at its termination.

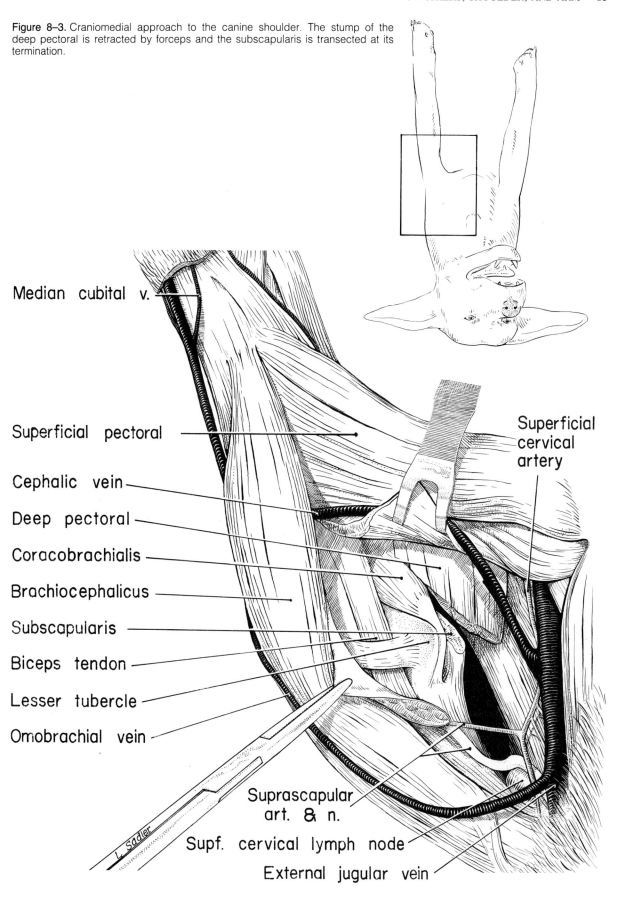

Median cubital v.

Superficial pectoral

Cephalic vein

Deep pectoral

Coracobrachialis

Brachiocephalicus

Subscapularis

Biceps tendon

Lesser tubercle

Omobrachial vein

Superficial cervical artery

Suprascapular art. & n.

Supf. cervical lymph node

External jugular vein

L. Sadler

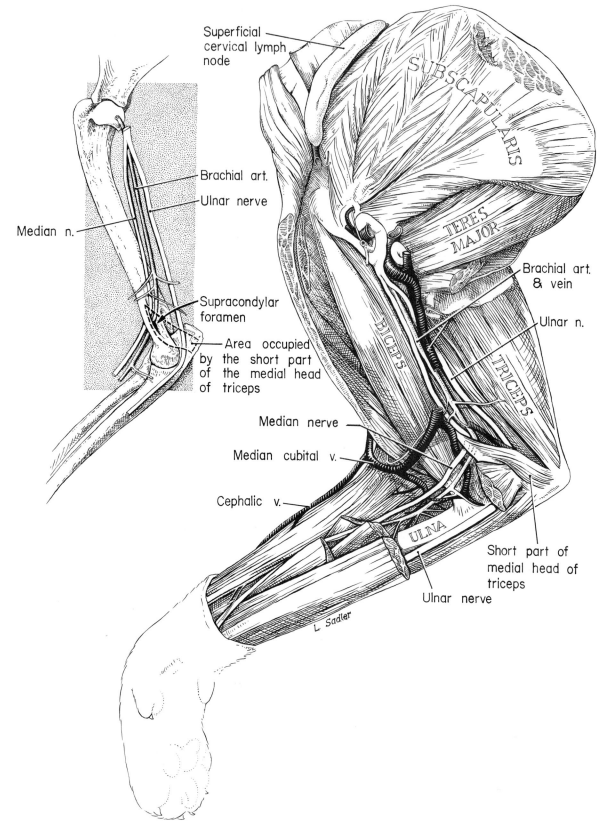

Superficial
cervical lymph
node

Brachial art.

Ulnar nerve

Median n.

Supracondylar
foramen

Area occupied
by the short part
of the medial head
of triceps

SUBSCAPULARIS

TERES
MAJOR

Brachial art.
& vein

Ulnar n.

BICEPS

TRICEPS

Median nerve

Median cubital v.

Cephalic v.

ULNA

Short part of
medial head of
triceps

Ulnar nerve

L. Sadler

Figure 8–4. Medial aspect of thoracic limb of cat. The musculocutaneous nerve is concealed by the biceps.

retracted cranially. The lateral head of the triceps is retracted caudally, and the brachialis and radial nerve are retracted either cranially or caudally, depending on the location of the fracture. The brachialis protects the radial nerve from injury by fracture of the shaft.

In the approach to the distal shaft of the humerus from the medial side,[26] the biceps and triceps are retracted cranially and caudally along with the vessels and nerves.

In the cat, the supracondylar foramen hinders retraction of the median nerve and brachial artery (Fig. 8–4). In approaching the medial side of the condyle, the short part of the medial head of the triceps must be carefully separated from the bone to avoid damage to the underlying ulnar nerve, lying caudal to the epicondyle. There is no omobrachial vein in the cat.

Nerve Blocks. Infiltration of four nerves in the brachium will anesthetize the paw.

Radial Nerve. It curves around the shaft of the humerus on the caudal surface of the brachialis. It can be palpated and stimulated on the lateral side of the humerus between the middle and distal thirds of the bone, deep to the lateral head of the triceps.[33] The superficial branch emerges at the distal border of the lateral head of the triceps and gives off the lateral cutaneous antebrachial nerve and the lateral and medial branches, which go to their respective sides of the cephalic vein and supply the cranial surface of the forearm and the dorsum of the paw. They are best blocked by a single injection of the superficial branch, which is palpable as it emerges at the border of the triceps (see Plate III).

Musculocutaneous, Median, and Ulnar Nerves. These may be blocked by one injection. They lie in craniocaudal order in the groove between the biceps and triceps on the medial surface of the middle of the humerus. The brachial artery is deep to the musculocutaneous and median nerves, and the pulse can be palpated at the point of injection. The needle must penetrate the deep fascia.[38] The brachial artery is the site for intra-arterial injection of antivenin for snake bites in the forelimb. Other sites are the femoral and common carotid arteries.[14]

8j. LIVE DOG

The principles of diagnosing lameness are the same for all species. In the dog, the tail may elevate when the lame hind limb is placed on the ground. This is similar to a "hip hike."[15]

Careful palpation is important in the differential diagnosis of three bone diseases that are common in young rapidly growing dogs of the large breeds. Osteochondrosis is a disturbance of endochondral ossification that affects articular cartilage.[18] The caudal part of the head of the humerus is a common site, and pain can be elicited from a dog when the diseased joint is manipulated. Other sites of predilection for this disease are the medial side of the trochlea of the humerus and the medial coronoid process of the ulna at the elbow, the medial side of the trochlea of the talus in the tarsus, and the lateral condyle of the femur at the stifle.

Hypertrophic osteodystrophy primarily affects the metaphyseal region of long bones. The distal metaphyses of the radius, ulna, and tibia are most commonly affected. The enlarged metaphysis may be visible, and the dog with this disease may show pain when the swollen metaphysis is palpated.

Panosteitis affects the endosteum and the marrow cavities of long bones along with the foramen for the nutrient artery.[34] The initial lesion begins in the medulla near the nutrient foramen. Pain may be elicited when the region of the nutrient foramen in the diaphysis is palpated. There is at least one major nutrient foramen in the diaphysis of each long bone. The following is a list of bones and the approximate position of the nutrient foramen in decreasing order of involvement with this disease.

Ulna. Proximal third, cranial (interosseous) surface.

Radius. Middle, caudal (interosseous) surface.

Humerus. Middle, caudal surface.

Femur. Proximal third, caudal surface.

Tibia. Proximal third, caudal surface.

Loss of stability of the shoulder from injury or abnormal forces from muscle contracture will be evident in the gait by the abnormal position of the elbow and may be confirmed by the abnormal response to medial or lateral rotation of the humerus. Normally the humerus is prevented from rotation around its longitudinal axis by the terminations of the infraspinatus and teres minor laterally and the subscapularis and teres major medially. The lateral supporting muscles prevent excessive medial rotation of the humerus and the medial supporting muscles prevent excessive lateral rotation. When a dog begins to walk following an injury that tears the termination of the infraspinatus or teres minor or both, the elbow will abduct as weight is placed on that limb. This is a reflection of the excessive medial rotation of the humerus that results from the loss of these lateral supporting muscles. If the arm of each forelimb is grasped and rotated medially, there will be excessive movement on the affected side.

Hunting dogs occasionally suffer acute trauma to the infraspinatus, causing incomplete rupture with hemorrhage.[12, 24] This is followed by fibrosis and contracture, which cause persistent lateral rotation of the humerus and some shoulder extension. After 7 to 10 days these dogs begin to bear weight on the limb and as they do the elbow adducts. During the full support phase of the gait the elbow adducts and during protraction (the swing phase) the paw abducts in compensation. There is moderate atrophy of the infraspinatus muscle and there is decreased ability to rotate the humerus medially. The humerus is kept in a position of partial lateral rotation. This can be corrected by cutting the tendon of the infraspinatus.

The denervation atrophy of the supraspinatus and infraspinatus muscles (sweeny) associated with suprascapular nerve injury does not affect the rotatory stability of the shoulder.

In palpating muscles to determine atrophy it is important to have the animal support its weight equally on both forelimbs and hind limbs. If the animal shifts its weight away from one limb, those muscles will decrease in tone and may feel smaller than normal. For the forelimbs it helps to stand over the dog, facing in the same direction, and palpate the muscles of both limbs simultaneously from proximal to distal. As the following muscles are palpated, their innervation should be kept in mind.

Muscle(s)	Nerve
Supraspinatus, infraspinatus	Suprascapular
Deltoideus, acromial part	Axillary
Superficial pectoral	Cranial pectoral
Deep pectoral	Caudal pectoral
Triceps brachii	Radial
Biceps brachii, brachialis	Musculocutaneous
Cranial forearm	Radial
Caudal forearm	Median, ulnar
Latissimus dorsi	Thoracodorsal

Palpate the following structures: On the scapula: spine, acromion, caudal angle, cranial border, supraglenoid tubercle.

Tendon of origin of the biceps brachii.

On the humerus: Crest of the major tubercle, which is the most cranial aspect of the proximal third of the humerus, major and minor tubercles, intertubercular groove, deltoid tuberosity, brachialis muscle, brachial artery.

Radial, musculocutaneous, median, and ulnar nerves. Palpate the sites of injection as described in section 8i.

Retract the arm and palpate the superficial cervical (prescapular) lymph node deep to the brachiocephalicus and cranial to the supraspinatus. It is slightly dorsal to the level of the acromion. (see Plate III, 98).

To puncture the shoulder joint, flex it to 110° and rotate the humerus slightly medially to open the gap between the acromion and the caudal part of the greater tubercle (see Plate III, 25 and 26). Insert the needle midway between them.

Palpate the long head of the triceps to its termination. The bursa is not palpable unless affected.

References

1. Adams, O. R.: Lameness in Horses, 3rd ed. Lea & Febiger. Philadelphia, 1974.
2. Blythe, L. L. and R. L. Kitchell: Electrophysiologic studies of the thoracic limb of the horse. Am. J .Vet. Res. *43* (1982):1511–1524.
3. Bowne, J. G.: Neuroanatomy of the Brachial Plexus of the Dog. PhD Thesis, Iowa State University, 1959.
4. Cermak, K.: Untersuchungen einiger Nervenlähmungen am Vorderbein, mit besonderer Berücksichtigung der Pfotenfunktion beim Hund. Tierärztl. Umschau. *26* (1970):378–384.
5. Chaffee, V. W. and C. D. Knecht: A modified posterior approach to the canine scapulohumeral joint. J. Am. Anim. Hosp. Assoc. *12* (1976):782–783.

6. Chapman, W. L.: Appearance of ossification centers and epiphyseal closures as determined by radiographic techniques. JAVMA *147* (1965):138–141.

7. Craig, E., R. B., Hohn and W. D. Anderson: Surgical stabilization of traumatic medial shoulder dislocation. J. Am. Anim. Hosp. Assoc. *16* (1980):93–102.

8. DeBowes, R. M., P. C.; Wagner and B. D. Grant: Surgical approach to the equine scapulohumeral joint through a longitudinal infraspinatus tenotomy. Vet. Surg. *11* (1982):125–129.

9. Guard, W. F.: Surgical Principles and Technics. Columbus, Ohio: Guard, 1953.

10. Hare, W. C. D.: Radiographic anatomy of the canine pectoral limb. JAVMA *135* (1959):264–271, 305–310.

11. Hohn, R. B. et al.: Surgical stabilization of recurrent shoulder luxation. Orthopedic surgery in small animals. Vet. Clin. North Am. *1* (1971):537–548.

12. Hufford, T. J., M. L. Olmstead, and L. C. Butler: Contracture of the infraspinatus muscle and surgical correction in two dogs. J. Am. Anim. Hosp. Assoc. *11* (1975):613–618.

13. Kitchell, R. L., L. R. Whalen, C. S. Bailey, et al.: Electrophysiologic studies of the cutaneous nerves of the thoracic limb of the dog. Am. J. Vet. Res. *41* (1980):61–76.

14. Knowles, R. P. et al.: Bites of venomous snakes. *In* Kirk, R. W. (ed.) Current Veterinary Therapy IV. 1971.

15. Leach, D., G. Sumner-Smith, and A. I. Dagg: Diagnosis of lameness in dogs: a preliminary study. Can. Vet. J. *18* (1977):58–63.

16. Lindsay, W. A., W. McDonell, and W. Bignell: Equine postanesthetic forelimb lameness: intracompartmental muscle pressure changes and biochemical patterns. Am. J. Vet. Res. *41* (1980):1919–1924.

17. Marolt, J. et al.: Untersuchungen über Funktionsstörungen des Nervus radialis und des Kreislaufes in der Arteria axillaris beim Pferd. Deutsche tierärztl. Wschr. *69* (1962):181–189.

18. Milton, J. L.: Osteochondritis dissecans in the dog. Vet. Clin. North Am. Small Anim. Pract. *13* (1983):117–134.

19. Myers, V. S. and J. K. Burt: The radiographic location of epiphyseal lines in equine limbs. Proc. Am. Assoc. Equine Pract. *12* (1966):21–39.

20. Myers, V. S. and M. A. Emmerson: The age and manner of epiphyseal closure in the forelegs of two Arabian foals. J. Am. Vet. Rad. Soc. *7* (1966):39–47.

21. Nickel, R., A. Schummer, and E. Seiferle: Lehrbuch der Anatomie der Haustiere. Vol. I, Bewegungsapparat, 4th ed. Berlin: Parey, 1977.

22. Ottaway, C. W. and A. N. Worden: Bursae and tendon sheaths of the horse. Vet. Rec. *52* (1940):477–483.

23. Paul, H. A.: Lameness in young large breed dogs. Proc. Am. Anim. Hosp. Assoc. *49* (1982):325–327.

24. Pettit, G. D., C. C. Chatburn, G. A. Hegreberg, et al.: Studies of the pathophysiology of infraspinatus muscle contracture in the dog. Vet. Surg. *7* (1978):8–12.

25. Piermattei, D. L.: Surgical approaches to the joints. Am. Anim. Hosp. Assoc. Proc. 38th mtg. (1971):368–378.

26. Piermattei, D. L. and R. G. Greeley: An Atlas of Surgical Approaches to the Bones of the Dog and Cat, 2nd ed. Philadelphia: W. B. Saunders, 1979.

27. Sack, W. O. and W. Cottrell: Puncture of shoulder, elbow and carpal joints in goats and sheep. JAVMA *185* (1984):63–65.

28. Smith, R. N. and J. Allcock: Epiphyseal fusion in the Greyhound. Vet. Rec. *72* (1960):75–79.

29. Smith, R. N.: Fusion of ossification centers in the cat. J. Small Anim. Pract. *10* (1969):523–530.

30. Stromberg, B.: A review of the salient features of osteochondrosis in the horse. Equine Vet. J. *11* (1979):211–214.

31. Sumner-Smith, G.: Observations on epiphyseal fusion of the canine appendicular skeleton. J. Small Anim. Pract. *7* (1966):303–311.

32. Suter, R. F. and A. V. Carb: Shoulder arthrography in dogs—radiographic anatomy and clinical application. J. Small Anim. Pract. *10* (1969):407–413.

33. Thomson, F. K. and J. M. Bowen: Electrodiagnostic testing: mapping and clinical use of motor points in the dog. JAVMA *159* (1971):1763–1770.

34. Van Sickle, D. C.: Canine panosteitis: a skeletal disease of unknown etiology. Proc. Kal Kan Symp. *4* (1980):67–71.

35. Vasseur, P. B., D. Moore, and S. A. Brown: Stability of the canine shoulder joint: an in vitro analysis. Am. J. Vet. Res. *43* (1982):352–355.

36. Vasseur, P. B.: Clinical results of surgical correction of shoulder luxation in dogs. JAVMA *182* (1983):503–505.

37. Vaughan, L. C.: Peripheral nerve injuries: an experimental study in cattle. Vet. Rec. *76* (1964):1293–1300.

38. Westhues, M. and R. Fritsch: Animal Anesthesia Vol. I. Local anesthesia. A. D. Weaver, Trans., Edinburgh: Oliver and Boyd, 1964.

39. White, N. A.: Postanesthetic recumbency myopathy in horses. Comp. Cont. Ed. *4* (1982):S44–S50.

40. Worthman, R. P.: Demonstration of specific nerve paralyses in the dog. JAVMA *131* (1957):174–178.

CHAPTER 9

ELBOW, FOREARM, AND CARPUS

OBJECTIVES

1. To be able to recognize ossification centers and their respective growth plates in the dog and horse.
2. To know the contribution of the epiphyses to growth in length of the radius and ulna in the dog and understand radius curvus.
3. To be able to palpate the extremities of the radius and ulna in the dog and cat for the diagnosis of fractures.
4. To be able to overcome the blocking effect of the anconeal process in the reduction of luxations of the elbow. To understand the problem of non-union of the anconeal process in some breeds of large dogs.
5. To be able to make the recommended surgical approaches to the bones of the elbow joint.
6. To be able to identify the bones of the carpus in radiographs, especially in the dog and horse, and to recognize the various radiographic views.
7. To be able to diagnose ruptured collateral ligaments of the elbow in the dog.
8. To be able to diagnose a hyperextension injury of the carpus and to palpate the collateral ligaments of the carpus to find injuries and inflammations.
9. To understand the causes of angular deformities of the forelimb of foals.
10. To be able to find the joint cavities of the carpus and to know which ones communicate and which are separate.
11. To be able to make a surgical approach to the radiocarpal joint without injury to the tendon sheaths.
12. To be able to palpate the pulse in the brachial artery at the elbow in all species, as a landmark and as a convenient means of correlating the heart sounds with the pulse in large animals.
13. To be able to trace the cephalic vein in all species and to distinguish it from the accessory cephalic vein. It is a landmark for nerves, a surgical hazard, and must be raised for venipuncture in small animals.
14. To be able to identify the muscles of the forearm by palpation, as landmarks, and to diagnose diseases of their tendons and tendon sheaths and paralysis caused by nerve damage.
15. To be able to examine the axillary lymph node in meat inspection.
16. To be able to block the median, ulnar, and medial cutaneous antebrachial nerves in the horse and the median, ulnar, and superficial branches of the radial nerve in the dog.
17. To understand the two different purposes of nerve blocks and the contraindications.
18. To be able to recognize the clinical signs of a fracture of the olecranon.
19. To be able to place a needle in the elbow joint of a horse.
20. To be able to predict the skeletal injuries that often occur with falls from "high rise" buildings.

9a. BONES AND RADIOGRAPHS, HORSE

The distal end of the humerus develops from two ossification centers, one for the entire condyle and lateral epicondyle and a separate one for the medial epicondyle. These unite with each other and with the diaphysis between 10 and 18 months. The proximal epiphysis of the radius unites with the diaphysis around 14 months. The diaphysis of the ulna includes the shaft, trochlear notch, and anconeal process. The ossification center of the olecranon tuber joins the diaphysis around 27 to 30 months.

Fractures of the olecranon result in a dropped position of the elbow. The triceps attachment to the olecranon displaces it proximally. This is most evident in the standing large animal. It cannot support weight on the limb but can extend the carpus and digit.

Note the rough depressions on the proximal articular surface of the radius and the trochlear notch of the ulna. These are normal synovial fossae, which are not covered by cartilage, occur in many joints, and should not be mistaken for lesions.

Examine the grooves on the cranial surface of the distal end of the radius. From medial to lateral they lodge the tendons of the extensor carpi obliquus, extensor carpi radialis, and common digital extensor. Far around on the lateral surface is the groove for the lateral extensor (see Plate I).

On the distal articular surface of the radius, the lateral styloid process is marked off from the rest by a groove. It is the distal epiphysis of the ulna. Radiographs of most horses under 2 years of age show incomplete fusion of this epiphysis. About 40 percent of horses 2 to 4 years old still show incomplete fusion, as do 30 percent of horses over 4 years old.[19]

Radiological union of the distal epiphysis of the radius is usually complete at 22 to 32 months but may be delayed until almost 3 years.[1]

Examine the eight carpal bones in an articulated skeleton. The first carpal is inconstant and must be recognized as a normal bone rather than a fragment. Chip fractures of the bones of the carpal joint occur on the dorsal surface and in the following order of frequency: distal border of the radial carpal, third carpal, radius, proximal border of the radial carpal, intermediate carpal.[30] Many different views are usually required for diagnosis.[21] Try the dorsolateral-palmaromedial oblique view on the skeleton to see how the dorsal surface of the radial carpal bone can be exposed with little interference from the others.

The standardized nomenclature for radiographic views is discussed in the Introduction to this book. The four routine views of the equine carpus are: dorsopalmar (DP), lateromedial (LM), dorsolateral-palmaromedial oblique (DLPMO), and dorsomedial-palmarolateral oblique (DMPLO).

All the carpal bones should be identified on the various views of the equine carpus, and the following features should be noted.[29] Direct comparison with the articulated carpal bones will help you appreciate the radiographic anatomy.

Dorsopalmar View
> Distal radius.
>> Medial styloid process with a prominent medial projection for attachment of the medial collateral ligament.
>> Lateral styloid process, which is the distal epiphysis of the ulna fused to the radius.
>> Note the line of junction of the articular surface with the cranial surface.
> Accessory carpal.
>> Superimposed over most of intermediate carpal, part of ulnar carpal, and part of radius.
>> Articulates with radius and ulnar carpal.
> Second carpal.
>> Mostly palmar to the wide third carpal except for its medial surface.
> Third Carpal.
>> Note distinct palmar process.
> First carpal.
>> Inconstant.
> Fifth carpal.
>> Rare.

Lateromedial View

Distal radius.

> The transverse crest on the caudal surface is on the epiphyseal line. The trochlea is concave cranially and convex caudally; the medial part projects more distally.

Radial carpal.

> Dorsal surface superimposed on intermediate carpal and extends slightly distal to intermediate carpal.

Third carpal.

> Projects most dorsally in distal row.

Fourth metacarpal.

> Palmar to third and second metacarpals.

Flexed Lateromedial View

> Radiocarpal joint has the largest opening, and the midcarpal joint shows a smaller gap. If the horse falls on the flexed carpus, these joints may be punctured by sharp objects.

Carpometacarpal joint.

> No visible flexion.

Distal radius.

> Distal projection of medial part of trochlea.

Radial carpal is distal to intermediate and ulnar carpals. Flexion of the carpus increases the distance between the radial and intermediate carpals and is helpful in locating chip fractures on the distal edge of their dorsal surface.

Dorsolateral-Palmaromedial Oblique View

Accessory carpal.

> Least superimposed in this oblique view. Articulates with radius and ulnar carpal.

Radial carpal and third carpal.

> Dorsomedial surfaces not superimposed on adjacent bones.
>
> Preferred view for fractures of distal border of the dorsomedial surface of radial carpal.

Distal Radius.

> May show incomplete fusion of lateral styloid process. Large medial portion of trochlea on dorsal surface.

Fourth Metacarpal.

> Not superimposed.

Second Metacarpal.

> Articulation with second carpal superimposed over third metacarpal and third carpal articulation.

Dorsomedial-Palmarolateral Oblique View

Distal radius.

> Prominent projection of medial styloid process.

Accessory carpal.

> Dorsal portion superimposed on radius and radial carpal.

Intermediate carpal or ulnar carpal.

> Dorsal surfaces are usually superimposed—depends on angle of obliquity.

Third carpal or fourth carpal.

> Dorsal surfaces are usually superimposed—depends on angle of obliquity.

Second carpal.

> Not superimposed, articulation with second metacarpal.

Fourth metacarpal.

> Superimposed on third metacarpal.

Angular deformities often occur at the carpus of foals due to a developmental abnormality of carpal bones, abnormal growth, and injuries.[3, 4, 18, 22] The terms valgus and varus are often used for these deformities as well as for other joints in the body. In present usage a valgus deformity refers to a lateral deviation of a bone distal to a joint. Varus refers to a medial deviation of a bone distal to a joint. Most angular deformities at the carpus in the foal are valgus deformities. The various causes include laxity of the medial collateral ligament, slower growth in the lateral side of the epiphyseal cartilage at the distal radial epiphysis, hypoplasia of the ulnar and intermediate carpal bones, delayed ossification of the ulnar and fourth carpal bones, and osteochondrosis of the ulnar carpal or third and fourth carpal bones with compression of these bones. Based on the theory that the periosteum resembles a fibroelastic tube uniting the proximal and distal epiphyses and is under tension as growth occurs in opposite directions at these epiphyses, hemicircumferential transection of the periosteum proximal to the growth plate releases this tension and results in increased growth.[2, 5] This procedure has been used to treat valgus deformities of the carpus in foals.

9b. DISSECTION, FOREARM AND CARPUS, HORSE

The large radiocarpal and midcarpal joints are readily aspirated or injected medial to the tendon of the extensor carpi radialis when the joint is flexed.[33] The radiocarpal joint capsule also bulges proximal to the accessory carpal bone between the tendons of the lateral digital extensor and the ulnaris lateralis. It can be punctured here as well, but the carpal tendon sheath of the flexor tendon must be avoided. It is separate from the other carpal joints. The carpometacarpal joint capsule is tight, but it may be injected via the midcarpal joint, with which it communicates. The midcarpal joint can also be injected on either side of the common digital extensor tendon.

Identify the medial and lateral collateral carpal ligaments as well as the distal ligament of the accessory carpal bone.

Identify the nine muscles of the forearm, their tendons, and the seven carpal synovial sheaths. The extent of the sheaths may be approximated as follows. They begin about 7 cm. above the carpus. The distal extent of the sheath of the extensor carpi radialis is the middle of the carpus, but there is also a bursa under the tendon at the level of the third carpal bone. The distal extent of the sheath of the digital flexors is the middle of the metacarpus. The other five sheaths extend to the proximal end of the metacarpus.

Extensor Carpi Radialis. This is the most cranial muscle on the lateral surface. The tendon is in the middle groove of the distal end of the radius and terminates on the tuberosity of the third metacarpal.

Extensor Carpi Obliquus (abductor pollicis longus). The tendon passes over that of the extensor carpi radialis to the groove on the medial side of the cranial surface of the distal end of the radius. It terminates on the second metacarpal.

Flexor Carpi Radialis. On the medial surface, behind the subcutaneous border of the radius, terminating on the second metacarpal.

Flexor Carpi Ulnaris. The most caudal muscle of the medial surface. It has no tendon sheath (see Plate I), and it terminates on the accessory carpal.

Digital Flexors. They are palpable medially between the tendons of the flexor carpi radialis and flexor carpi ulnaris; laterally, between lateral digital extensor and ulnaris lateralis.

Ulnaris Lateralis. The sheath is on the long termination, which runs in the groove on the lateral surface of the accessory carpal to the fourth metacarpal. The short termination is on the accessory carpal.

Lateral Digital Extensor. The tendon is in the groove on the lateral styloid process of the radius.

Common Digital Extensor. The tendon is in the lateral groove on the cranial surface of the radius (see Plate I).

Before the nerve blocks of the forearm are described, the following general principles of the use of nerve blocks should be considered. There is a fundamental difference between the block used to anesthetize a field for surgery and the diagnostic block. To obtain surgical anesthesia, one tries to block all the nerves in the limb below a certain point. Collateral branches given off the nerve above the block may by-pass it and make the anesthesia ineffective. Therefore it is necessary to block the nerves far above the surgical field. For example, to operate in the metacarpus the nerves are blocked in the forearm.

Diagnostic blocks, on the other hand, begin with the anesthesia of the smallest possible distal field; for example, that of the palmar digital nerve. If the horse is sound after this, the lesion has been located in a small area. If the horse is still lame, it is necessary to make successively more proximal blocks affecting larger areas until the horse goes sound. The nerves should never be blocked above their muscular branches for diagnostic purposes. The resulting disturbance of muscular function would distort the gait so much that the analgesic effect on the lameness could not be evaluated. Diagnostic blocks should be used with caution and only in chronic, obscure lamenesses that cannot be diagnosed by other methods. The danger is that the block, by abolishing the protective pain, will allow the animal to put full weight on the limb and pound a slight lesion until it becomes a major one. For example, a hairline fracture of a phalanx, diagnosed by sudden onset, acute pain, and a radiograph, should not be confirmed by a diagnostic block.

Locate the median, medial cutaneous antebrachial, and ulnar nerves, all of which must be blocked to anesthetize the metacarpus and fetlock. The median and ulnar nerves supply the digit.

Find the median nerve and brachial artery, on the medial surface of the elbow, cranial to the origin of the flexor carpi radialis. The muscular branches to the flexor carpi radialis and the deep digital flexor should be identified.

A short distance below the elbow joint the nerve and artery pass between the radius and the flexor carpi radialis and run distally on the deep surface of the muscle. In the distal half of the forearm, the nerve is accessible from the groove between the radial and ulnar flexors of the carpus (see Plate I).

The medial cutaneous antebrachial nerve (termination of the musculocutaneous) is cranial to the junction of the cephalic and median cubital veins. It emerges between the distal ends of the biceps and brachialis and crosses the lacertus fibrosus of the biceps from lateral to medial where it can be palpated. The branches of the nerve accompany the cephalic and accessory cephalic veins.

The ulnar nerve is between the flexor carpi ulnaris and ulnaris lateralis. Do not confuse the nerve with the tendon of the ulnar head of the deep flexor. Note the dorsal branch as it emerges from the groove between the muscles and turns forward around the lateral surface of the tendon of the ulnaris lateralis; it can be palpated here. It supplies the dorsolateral surface from the carpus to the region of the fetlock joint (see Fig. 10–1).[26]

Anesthesia of the carpus can be obtained by blocking the three nerves above plus the continuation of the deep branch of the radial on the deep surface of the tendon of the common digital extensor just above the carpus.[14] A simpler method for the interior of the joint is to inject the joint capsules.

Find the axillary and cubital lymph nodes.

9c. LIVE HORSE

Locate the elbow joint by palpating the lateral epicondyle of the humerus and the lateral collateral ligament that attaches to it. Injections are made into the joint just cranial to the ligament and caudal to the common digital extensor at the palpable articular surface of the condyle.

Take the pulse from the brachial artery where it passes over the medial surface of the elbow joint and enters the groove between the radius and the flexor carpi radialis. Palpate this groove and follow it proximally until the pulse is felt through the transverse pectoral muscle. The median nerve is superficial and caudal to the artery. The nerve may also be blocked in the middle of the forearm, well below the muscular branches. The needle is inserted 10 cm. above the chestnut on the caudal border of the flexor carpi radialis and directed toward the back of the radius across the deep surface of the muscle.[35]

Find the site of the ulnar nerve block in the groove between the flexor carpi ulnaris and ulnaris lateralis 10 cm. proximal to the accessory carpal bone. The dorsal branch can be palpated as it runs obliquely across the lateral surface of the tendon of the ulnaris lateralis. Blocking the median and ulnar nerves will anesthetize the digit. If it is desired to anesthetize the fetlock and metacarpus also, the medial cutaneous antebrachial nerve must be blocked. This is palpable on the proximal part of the lacertus fibrosus of the biceps, cranial to the accessory cephalic and cephalic veins.

Note on the Nomenclature. The carpus is not the knee; it is the wrist.

Palpate the medial and lateral collateral carpal ligaments and the distal ligament of the accessory carpal bone.

Flex and extend the carpus to find the level of the radiocarpal joint capsule, which is the largest one in the carpus. This capsule, when distended, puffs out between the tendons on the dorsal surface, and laterally, proximal to the accessory carpal bone, between the tendons of the lateral digital extensor and the ulnaris lateralis. Palpate also the midcarpal joint.

Palpate the nine muscles of the forearm and their tendons as described in section 9b.

9d. RADIOGRAPHS, OX

In each view of the carpus identify the carpal bones and the following features.[28] The second and third carpal bones are normally fused in the ox and the first carpal is usually absent.

Dorsopalmar View
    Accessory Carpal.
        Small and superimposed on ulnar carpal.
    Ulnar Carpal.
        Large with palmar process superimposed on fourth carpal.
    Intermediate Carpal.
        Medial extension palmar to radial carpal.
        Styloid processes of radius and ulna superimposed on radial and ulnar carpal, respectively.
Lateromedial View
    Accessory Carpal.
        Articulates only with ulnar carpal.
    Ulnar Carpal.
        Palmar process extends distally.
    Second and Third Carpals.
        Clear view of dorsal surface in distal row.
    Fourth Carpal.
        Clear view of palmar surface in distal row.
Flexed Lateromedial View
    Antebrachiocarpal and midcarpal joints open.
    Radial Carpal.
        Projects distally in proximal row.
    Fourth Carpal.
        Projects proximally in distal row.
Dorsolateral-Palmaromedial Oblique View
    Ulna.
        Styloid process projects on lateral surface.
    Accessory Carpal.
        Exposed.
    Ulnar Carpal.
        Palmar process prominent.
    Radial and Second and Third Carpals.
        Dorsomedial surface exposed.
    Fifth Metacarpal.
        Articulates with fourth metacarpal.
Dorsomedial-Palmarolateral Oblique View
    Accessory Carpal
        Superimposed on radial carpal.
    Ulnar Carpal
    Dorsal surface usually exposed.
    Distal Row.
        Fourth carpal exposed on dorsal side. Second and third carpals exposed on palmar side.

9e. DISSECTION, FOREARM AND CARPUS, OX

The axillary lymph node is in the angle between the subscapular and thoracodorsal veins, at the end of the axillary vein. The node is on the medial surface of the distal end of the teres major. In the hanging split carcass, the node is drawn cranially by the weight of the forelimb and may be conveniently found by an incision from the inside of the thoracic wall in the middle of the first intercostal space. There is no cubital node.

The termination of the transverse pectoral muscle must be reflected to see the median nerve between the biceps in front and the origin of the flexor carpi radialis behind. The skeletal prominence caudal to the nerve is the medial epicondyle of the humerus. The brachial artery is cranial and deep to the nerve.

The medial cutaneous antebrachial nerve emerges on the flexion surface of the elbow, crosses deep or superficial to the median cubital vein, and runs distally on the craniomedial surface of the limb to the fetlock.

The superficial branch of the radial nerve emerges at the distal border of the lateral head of the triceps. It runs down the craniolateral surface of the forearm. In the distal third of the forearm, there is a complex communication with the medial cutaneous antebrachial nerve. The radial nerve supplies the axial dorsal nerves to both digits and the abaxial dorsal nerve to the third digit.

In the incision between the flexor carpi ulnaris and ulnaris lateralis, the ulnar nerve is seen to divide. The dorsal branch emerges near the carpus and supplies the abaxial dorsal nerve to the fourth digit. The median nerve and the palmar branch of the ulnar supply the palmar digital nerves.

9f. LIVE COW

Palpate the median nerve as it crosses the medial surface of the elbow joint cranial to the medial epicondyle of the humerus and the origin of the flexor carpi radialis. Push the nerve forward or backward and take the pulse from the brachial artery, which lies deep and a little cranial to the nerve.

Palpate the muscles of the forearm and trace their tendons across the carpus. There are two differences from the horse: (1) The common digital extensor has two palpable tendons in a common sheath; one bifurcates just above the fetlock and terminates on both main digits; the other terminates entirely on the third digit and has been called the medial digital extensor. (2) The superficial flexor has two tendons; one descends through the carpal canal and the other passes between two layers of the flexor retinaculum. They join in the metacarpus.

Hygroma of the carpus is a large sac that develops from an inconstant subcutaneous bursa on the dorsal surface. It should be dissected off the underlying synovial structures with care, but it usually does not communicate with the tendon sheaths, subtendinous bursae, or joint capsules.

9g. LIVE SHEEP AND GOAT

Palpate the condyle of the humerus and the olecranon at the elbow joint. The elbow joint of sheep and goats can be injected in the angle between the caudal surface of the humerus and the cranial border of the olecranon.[27] The needle is directed mediodistally and slightly cranial.

Flex the carpus and palpate the radiocarpal and midcarpal joint spaces and the extensor carpi radialis tendon where it crosses these joints. The radiocarpal joint is best injected lateral to the extensor carpi radialis tendon and the midcarpal joint medial to this tendon.[27] The latter injection also serves the carpometacarpal joint because of their communication.

9h. BONES AND RADIOGRAPHS, DOG AND CAT

Articulate the radius and ulna and rotate the radius. Articulate the humerus with the radius and ulna. The anconeal process of the ulna lies in the olecranon fossa of the humerus in such a way that medial or lateral luxation of the elbow is prevented unless the elbow is flexed to 45°. Lateral luxation of the radius and ulna is more common because the lateral epicondyle is smaller. Reduction should not be attempted without flexing the joint to 45°.

Fractures of the condyle are most common laterally.[11] The radius bears most of the weight of the body between the elbow and carpus. At the elbow it articulates with the capitulum and the lateral part of the trochlea in the dog. The lateral part of the condyle projects laterally from the shaft of the humerus and is partly separated from it by the supratrochlear foramen. Therefore, the lateral portion of the condyle is commonly fractured when upward stress occurs; this type of injury is associated with animals falling long distances and attempting to land on extended forelimbs. The weight-bearing part of the ulna is the medial coronoid process, which also may fracture in these "high rise" falls. With fractures of the distal shaft of the humerus, the condyle is often displaced cranially and distally by the extensor muscles of the forearm and digit.

"High rise" falls also account for hyperextension injuries of the carpus, which result from tearing of the palmar carpal ligaments, especially those that support the carpometacarpal and midcarpal joints.[12] There are numerous ligaments on the palmar aspect of the carpus that contribute to the support of this joint and are involved in these injuries. The palmar carpal fibrocartilage attaches to most of the carpal bones but is especially thick distally, where it attaches the distal row of carpal bones to metacarpals three through five. The accessory carpal and radial carpal bones have long palmar ligaments that attach to the fourth and fifth metacarpals and second and third metacarpals, respectively.

In the radiographs, identify the anconeal process and the medial and lateral coronoid processes of the ulna and note that the medial coronoid process is longer than the lateral. Osteochondrosis occurs in the medial coronoid process and in the medial side of the trochlea of the humerus.[6] In lateral view note the difference in the caudal projection of the medial and lateral epicondyles. Distinguish the medial epicondyle from the anconeal process in radiographs of young and adult dogs. Table 9–1 and Table 2 of the appendix show to the nearest month the ages when the epiphyses unite with the diaphyses.

The radius forms from three ossification centers—a diaphysis, a proximal epiphysis, and a distal epiphysis. The proximal epiphyseal cartilage accounts for about 30 to 40 percent of the growth in length of the radius and the distal epiphyseal cartilage for 60 to 70 percent. The ulna forms from a diaphysis, a proximal epiphysis for the olecranon tuber, and a distal epiphysis. The proximal epiphysis contributes less than 15 percent to the length of the bone. The distal epiphyseal cartilage provides about 85 percent of the growth in length of the bone and all the growth in length distal to the elbow. Because of the close relationship of these two bones, their shape is dependent on their synchronous growth.[20]

Injury to the distal epiphyseal cartilage of the ulna causes premature closure between the diaphysis and distal epiphysis.[8–10] This stops the growth in length of the ulna. The radius continues to grow in length but the asynchronous growth causes the bones to curve, with their convexity cranial. This is most evident in the radius and is called radius curvus. Proximally the growing radius causes a subluxation at the elbow by separating the trochlea from the trochlear notch of the ulna. Distally the paw will deviate laterally (valgus deformity) and be partially supinated. Inherited premature closure of the distal ulnar epiphyseal growth plate is reported.[16] Injuries to the distal epiphyseal cartilage of the radius can also cause premature closure and inhibit growth in length of the radius.[32] If the ulna continues to grow in length, the radius will be separated from the humeral condyle at the elbow, the

Table 9–1. EPIPHYSEAL FUSION IN THE FOREARM AND CARPUS (AGE IN MONTHS)

Location	Dogs	Cats
Proximal radius	5–11	5–7
Tuber olecrani	5–10	9–13
Anconeal process	3–5	—
Distal radius and ulna	6–12	14–25
Radial carpal bone	3–4	—
Accessory carpal bone	3–6	4

ulna will curve with its convexity lateral, and the paw may deviate medially (varus deformity) if the premature closure is asymmetrical.

In the puppy, the shape of the distal ulna is much different than in the adult. At 4 to 5 months the distal ulna is wide and cone-shaped. It is twice as wide as the distal radius. The epiphyseal cartilage is also conical, which may make it more susceptible to compression injuries. By 7 to 9 months the distal radius and ulna are the same width.

A center of ossification for the anconeal process is present in only a few breeds of dogs. It appears in the Greyhound and German Shepherd at 12 weeks.[34] It unites with the ulna at 14 to 15 weeks in the Greyhound and causes no trouble in that breed. It normally fuses at 16 to 20 weeks in the German Shepherd, but may become separated and cause serious lameness. This may be a result of osteochondrosis in some dogs.

Occasionally a sesamoid bone is found on the lateral side of the elbow articulating with the head of the radius. This is in the tendon of origin of the supinator muscle from the lateral collateral ligament.

In young animals the distal epiphysis of the radius is sometimes mistaken for a carpal bone by the unwary. There are only two rows of carpal bones. In the dorsopalmar view, the radial and ulnar carpal bones are easily identified in the proximal row, but the accessory carpal is superimposed on the ulnar carpal. The ulnar carpal extends distally on the palmar surface of the fourth carpal bone.

The carpus is entirely cartilaginous at birth. The radial (intermedioradial) carpal bone is formed by the fusion of three ossification centers:[24] the radial and the intermediate in the proximal row and the central carpal distal to the junction of the radial and intermediate centers. The intermediate is the largest and is first to appear. All these are apparent by 4 weeks of age and are fused by 3 to 4 months. The two centers of the accessory carpal bone fuse by 3 to 6 months. In the distal row, the second, third, and fourth carpal bones are seen in the dorsopalmar view, but the first carpal is often obscured by the second metacarpal. The fourth carpal bone articulates distally with the fourth and fifth metacarpals.

The small round bone medial to the radial carpal in some of the radiographs is of clinical interest only because it is normal—a sesamoid bone at one insertion of the abductor pollicis longus.

9i. DISSECTION, FOREARM AND CARPUS, DOG AND CAT

Blood from the cephalic vein flows to both medial and lateral sides of the arm. At the elbow the median cubital vein connects the cephalic and brachial veins. Just distal to the deltoid tuberosity is the V-shaped junction of the cephalic and axillobrachial veins. From here the cephalic vein conducts blood medially, deep to the brachiocephalicus, to the external jugular vein, and the axillobrachial passes laterally around the arm to the axillary vein.

In the dog, the axillobrachial vein at the level of the deltoid tuberosity gives off the omobrachial vein, which courses craniomedially superficial to the brachiocephalicus to enter the external jugular vein. Therefore, to raise the cephalic vein for venipuncture in the forearm it must either be compressed below the elbow or the lateral, cranial, and medial surfaces of the arm must be compressed. Above the carpus the cephalic vein gives off the accessory cephalic to the dorsum of the paw and passes obliquely over the medial surface to the palmar side of the paw (Fig. 9–1).

Although nerve-block anesthesia of the paw is seldom used, general anesthesia being preferred, it becomes necessary if general anesthesia is contraindicated, or if the patient persists in tearing off a bandage and chewing a lesion of the paw. A long-lasting local anesthetic will prevent the irritation and permit healing.

The paw can be anesthetized by blocking the following nerves (Fig. 9–1):

Superficial branch of the radial nerve. It emerges at the distal border of the lateral head of the triceps, giving off the lateral cutaneous antebrachial nerve, and dividing into medial and lateral branches, which accompany the cephalic and accessory cephalic veins to the dorsal surface of the paw. It is blocked as described in section 8i by palpating and injecting it subcutaneously, where it

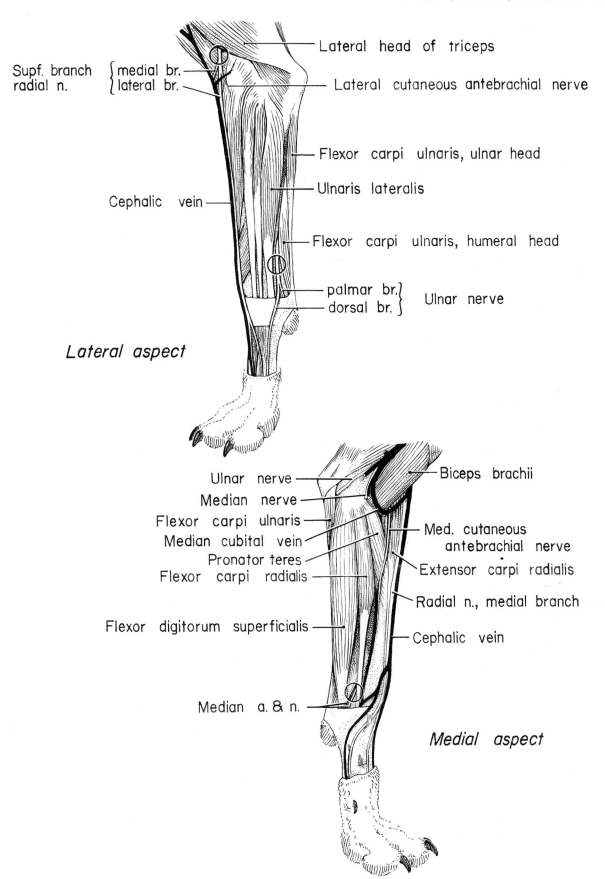

Lateral head of triceps

Supf. branch radial n. { medial br. { lateral br.

Lateral cutaneous antebrachial nerve

Flexor carpi ulnaris, ulnar head

Ulnaris lateralis

Cephalic vein

Flexor carpi ulnaris, humeral head

palmar br. } dorsal br. } Ulnar nerve

Lateral aspect

Ulnar nerve
Median nerve
Flexor carpi ulnaris
Median cubital vein
Pronator teres
Flexor carpi radialis

Biceps brachii

Med. cutaneous antebrachial nerve
Extensor carpi radialis
Radial n., medial branch
Cephalic vein

Flexor digitorum superficialis

Median a. & n.

Medial aspect

Figure 9–1. Nerve blocks (circled) to anesthetize the forepaw of the dog.

emerges. It can also be blocked by injections on both sides of the cephalic vein in the middle of the forearm.

Dorsal and palmar branches of the ulnar nerve. Palpate the styloid process of the ulna and the accessory carpal bone. With the carpus extended, palpate the tendon of the flexor carpi ulnaris, at its termination on the accessory carpal bone, and the tendon of the ulnaris lateralis, passing distally over the styloid process. Insert the needle distally under the skin in the deep groove between these tendons, about one-fifth of the length of the forearm proximal to the accessory carpal bone. Block the dorsal branch of the ulnar nerve subcutaneously at this point. To block the palmar branch, advance the needle to the carpal canal on the medial surface of the accessory carpal bone and inject. The ulnar nerve can also be blocked on the medial side of the elbow just caudal to the epicondyle. It is palpable there.

Median nerve. Extend the carpus and palpate the taut tendon of the flexor carpi radialis behind the distal third of the radius and proximal to the cephalic vein. Insert the needle along the caudal border of the tendon to its deep surface and block the nerve, which lies in front of the large median artery.

There are many surgical approaches to the elbow and bones of the forearm.[23] The elbow joint can be approached from the lateral side for removal of a separated anconeal process by undermining and retracting the lateral head of the triceps and transecting the anconeus.

A more radical exposure of the elbow and humeral condyle can be made by retracting the triceps proximally off the caudal surface of the joint. To do this, the cranial borders of the medial and lateral heads of the triceps are undermined. The ulnar nerve and collateral ulnar vessels must be spared and retracted distally as the border of the medial head is freed. In the cat, the ulnar and median nerves and the brachial artery are covered by the short part of the medial head of the triceps, which does not exist in the dog (see Fig. 8–4). This part originates from the flat bar of bone enclosing the supracondylar foramen and from a line continuing to the medial epicondyle. It should be cut carefully near the olecranon—not elevated from the humerus. The triceps can be detached from the olecranon by cutting the tendon in the young dog, or, if the epiphysis is fused, by cutting off the tuber olecrani and reattaching it. The joint is opened by cutting the anconeus and the capsule off the medial epicondylar ridge of the humerus.

The head of the radius is approached from the lateral side between the common and lateral digital extensors. When they are separated and retracted, the supinator muscle will be seen. In the cat, the radial nerve crosses the superficial surface of the supinator; in the dog, the nerve crosses deep to the aponeurosis of origin of the muscle and emerges at the caudal border. Its branches to the digital extensors can be seen. The nerve must be protected while the supinator is being transected near its origin. The proximal stump is reflected to expose the joint cavity. The head of the radius is covered laterally by the collateral ligament. Incision of the lateral collateral ligament and tendon of the lateral digital extensor provides more exposure laterally. Incision and reflection of the common digital extensor and part of the extensor carpi radialis will provide access to the cranial part of the joint.

A medial approach to the elbow is used for access to the medial coronoid process and medial side of the condyle.[15, 17] The ulnar nerve courses caudal to the palpable medial epicondyle, and the median nerve, brachial artery, and brachial vein are just cranial to it. These should be identified and retracted. From cranial to caudal the muscles that arise from the medial epicondyle are the pronator teres, flexor carpi radialis, humeral head of the deep digital flexor, superficial digital flexor, and the humeral head of the flexor carpi ulnaris. Identify the pronator teres and flexor carpi radialis. Transect their origin from the epicondyle and reflect them distally to expose the medial collateral ligament. Spare the brachial vessels and median nerve that are beneath their proximal ends. The medial collateral ligament is transected and reflected to expose the medial coronoid process and the medial part of the trochlea of the elbow joint. The distal attachment of the ligament is primarily to the radius.

An alternative method is to identify the pronator teres, flexor carpi radialis, and humeral head of the deep digital flexor, which all arise from the most medial prominence of the medial epicondyle. This portion of the medial epicondyle is cut off the condyle with an osteotome and reflected distally with its attached medial collateral ligament.[15] Abduction of the forearm will help expose the joint.

The radiocarpal joint can be entered on the dorsal surface between the tendon sheaths. The incision is lateral and parallel to the accessory cephalic vein and midway between the tendons of the extensor carpi radialis and the common digital extensor. It extends from the abductor pollicis longus to the distal border of the radial carpal bone. It is deepened down to the bone, and the periosteum is elevated and retracted laterally and medially with the joint capsule and tendon sheaths.

Palpate the prominent medial epicondyle of the humerus. The ulnar nerve can be palpated as it courses caudal to the epicondyle. The median nerve and brachial artery are just cranial to the epicondyle.

Palpate the radius and ulna from one end to the other. With the carpus flexed to 90°, pronate and supinate the forearm while palpating the radius and ulna. The bones are crossed, so that the rotation of the head of the radius is palpated on the lateral surface of the elbow, and the styloid process of the ulna is palpated on the lateral side at the carpus.

Rupture of the collateral ligaments of the elbow can be diagnosed by the degree of pronation and supination permitted (Fig. 9–2). To estimate this, the elbow and carpus are flexed to 90°, and the paw is used as the indicator of the degree of rotation. The normal limit of supination is 60 to 70°; with the lateral ligament cut, it is 120 to 140°. The normal limit of pronation is 40 to 50°; with the medial ligament cut, it is 90 to 100°.[7]

For injection of the elbow joint, locate the lateral collateral ligament by palpating the area distal to the lateral epicondyle while flexing and extending the joint. Insert the needle cranial to the ligament at the level of the joint (see Plate III).

Locate the radiocarpal articulation. Palpate the accessory carpal bone, which is lateropalmar. The prominent tendon of the flexor carpi ulnaris is inserted on it. The structures palpable medial to the accessory carpal are the tendons of the flexor carpi radialis and superficial digital flexor.

Trace the cephalic vein from the carpus to the flexion surface of the elbow. In raising the vein, one should be aware of the fact that the blood is drained medially and laterally at the flexion surface of the elbow.

Palpate the points of injection of the ulnar and median nerves and the superficial branch of the radial given in section 9i.

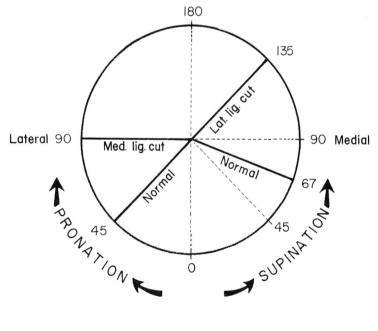

Figure 9–2. Degrees of rotation of the right forearm viewed from the distal end, with the elbow and carpus flexed 90°.

References

1. Adams, O. R.: Lameness in Horses, 3rd ed. Philadelphia: Lea & Febiger, 1974.
2. Auer, J. A. and R. J. Martens: Periosteal transection and periosteal stripping for correction of angular limb deformities in foals. Am. J. Vet. Res. *43* (1982):1530–1534.
3. Auer, J. A., R. J. Martens, and E. L. Morris: Angular limb deformities in foals. Part I. Congenital factors. Comp. Cont. Ed. *4* (1982):S330–S340.
4. Auer, J. A., J. Martens, and E. H. Williams: Periosteal transection for correction of angular limb deformities in foals. JAVMA *181* (1982):459–467.
5. Auer, J. A., J. R. Martens, and E. L. Morris: Angular limb deformities in foals. Part II. Developmental factors. Comp. Cont. Ed. *5* (1983):S27–S35.
6. Berzon, J. L. and C. B. Quick: Fragmented coronoid process: anatomical, clinical, and radiographic consideration with case analyses. J. Am. Anim. Hosp. Assoc. *16* (1980):241–252.
7. Campbell, J. R.: Nonfracture injuries to the canine elbow. JAVMA *155* (1969):735–744.
8. Carrig, C. B., D. F. Merkley, and U. V. Mostosky: Asynchronous growth of the canine radius and ulna: effects of different amounts of ulnar growth retardation: J. Am. Vet. Radiol. Soc. *19* (1978):16–23.
9. Carrig, C. B. and J. A. Wortman: Acquired dysplasias of the canine radius and ulna. Comp. Cont. Ed. *3* (1981):557–565.
10. Carrig, C. B.: Growth abnormalities of the canine radius and ulna. Vet. Clin. North Am.—Small Anim. Pract. *13* (1983):91–115.
11. Denny, H. R.: Condylar fractures of the humerus in the dog: a review of 133 cases. J. Small Anim Pract. *24* (1983):185–197.
12. Gambardella, P. C. and R. C. Griffiths: Treatment of hyperextension injuries of the canine carpus. Comp. Cont. Ed. *4* (1982):127–131.
13. Garner, H. E., L. E. St. Clair, and H. J. Hardenbrook: Clinical and radiographic studies of the distal portion of the radius in race horses. JAVMA *149* (1966): 1536–1540.
14. Getty, R., J. A. Sowa, and R. L. Lundvall: Local anesthesia and applied anatomy as related to nerve blocks in horses. JAVMA *128* (1956):583–587.
15. Henry, W. B., P. L. Wadsworth, and C. J. Mehlhaff: Medial approach to elbow joint with osteotomy of medial epicondyle. Vet. Surg. *8* (1979):46–50.
16. Lau, R. E.: Inherited premature closure of the distal ulnar physis. J. Am. Anim. Hosp. Assoc. *13* (1977):609–613.
17. McCurnin, D. M., R. Slusher, and R. L. Grier: A medial approach to the canine elbow joint. J. Am. Anim. Hosp. Assoc. *12* (1976):475–481.
18. McLaughlin, B. G., C. E. Doige, P. B. Fretz, et al.: Carpal bone lesions associated with angular limb deformities in foals. JAVMA *178* (1981):224–230.
19. Myers, V. S.: Confusing radiologic variations at the distal end of the radius of the horse. JAVMA *147* (1965):1310–1312.
20. Noser, G. A., C. B. Carrig, D. F. Merkley, et al.: Asynchronous growth of the canine radius and ulna: effects of cross pinning the radius to the ulna. Am. J. Vet. Res. *38* (1977):601–611.
21. Park, R. D., J. P. Morgan, and T. O'Brien: Chip fractures in the carpus of the horse: a radiographic study of their incidence and location. JAVMA *157* (1970): 1305–1312.
22. Pharr, J. W. and P. B. Fretz: Radiographic findings in foals with angular limb deformities. JAVMA *179* (1981): 812–817.
23. Piermattei, D. L. and R. G. Greeley: An Atlas of Surgical Approaches to the Bones of the Dog and Cat, 2nd ed. Philadelphia. W. B. Saunders, 1979.
24. Pomriaskinsky-Kobozieff, N. and Kobozieff, N.: Etude radiologique de l'aspect du squelette normal de la main du chien aux divers stades de son évolution de la naissance à l'âge adulte. Rec. Méd. Vét. *130* (1954):617–646.
25. Riser, W. H. and J. F. Shirer: Normal and abnormal growth of the distal foreleg in large and giant dogs. J. Am. Vet. Radiol. Soc. *6* (1965):50–64.
26. Sack, W. O.: Die Endausbreitung der Nerven in Metacarpus und Zehe des Pferdes gewonnen an Serienschnitten foetaler Gliedmassen. Berl. Münch. Tierärztl. Wschr. *87* (1974):136–143.
27. Sack, W. O. and W. Cottrell: Puncture of shoulder, elbow, and carpal joints in goats and sheep. JAVMA *185* (1984):63–65.
28. Shively, M. J. and J. E. Smallwood: Normal radiographic and xeroradiographic anatomy of the bovine manus. Bovine Pract. *14* (1979):74–83.
29. Smallwood, J. E. and M. J. Shively: Radiographic and xeroradiographic anatomy of the equine carpus. Equine Pract. *1* (1979):22–38.
30. Thrall, D. E., J. L. Lebel, and T. R. O'Brien: A five-year survey of the incidence and location of equine carpal chip fractures. JAVMA *158* (1971):1366–1368.
31. Turner, T. M. and R. B. Hohn: Craniolateral approach to the canine elbow for repair of condylar fractures on joint exploration. JAVMA *176* (1980):1264–1266.
32. Vandewater, A. and M. L. Olmstead: Premature closure of the distal radial physis in the dog. A review of eleven cases. Vet. Surg. *12* (1983):7–12.
33. Van Pelt, R. W.: Intra-articular injection of the equine carpus and fetlock. JAVMA *140* (1962):1181–1190.
34. Van Sickle, D.: The relationship of ossification to elbow dysplasia. Animal Hosp. *2* (1966):24–31.
35. Westhues, M. and R. Fritsch: Animal Anesthesia. Vol. I. Local Anesthesia. A. D. Weaver, (trans.) Edinburgh: Oliver and Boyd, 1964.

CHAPTER 10

METACARPUS AND FETLOCK JOINT

OBJECTIVES

1. To be able to identify by palpation, in the horse, the small metacarpal (splint) bones as landmarks and as the site of fractures.
2. To be able to palpate and gain surgical access to the proximal sesamoid bones, which are sometimes fractured in the horse and dog. To understand the tension applied to these bones by the tendons and ligaments attached to them.
3. To understand the difference in ossification centers between metacarpal bones and phalanges.
4. To be able to insert a needle into the equine fetlock joint from the proximal and distal approaches.
5. To be able to relate the metacarpophalangeal joints to the exterior of the canine paw.
6. To understand the anatomy involved in inflammation of the ligaments between the metacarpal bones in the horse.
7. To be able to diagnose inflammation of the accessory (check) ligament of the deep digital flexor tendon.
8. To be able to examine the collateral ligaments of the fetlock joint.
9. To be able to identify the tendons of the metacarpus in the horse and ox by palpation. The grooves between them are landmarks, and they are themselves affected by injury and inflammation. To recognize distention of the tendon sheaths.
10. To understand the terminations of the tendons and their action on the digits for diagnostic and surgical purposes.
11. To know the course of the main artery of the metacarpus and how it supplies the digital arteries in all species, including the remarkable peculiarity in the cat.
12. To be able to avoid the large veins of the metacarpus in surgery of the region and to be able to use these veins in the ox for intravenous local anesthesia or antibiotic therapy.
13. To know how to produce anesthesia of the digit or digits by nerve blocks in the metacarpus of the horse and ox.
14. To be able to make diagnostic nerve blocks to diagnose lameness in the horse.
15. To understand the anatomy of the various fetlock deformities that occur in young horses and their surgical correction.

10a. BONES AND LIGAMENTOUS PREPARATIONS, HORSE

METACARPAL LIGAMENTS

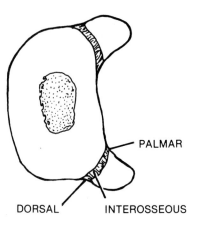

Examine the following structures:

Metacarpal bones. The large (third) metacarpal bone bears most of the weight, but the small second and fourth bones (splint bones) also bear weight from the carpus even though they have no distal means of support. They are attached to the large metacarpal bone by short metacarpal ligaments that allow little movement. At 3 to 5 years of age many horses undergo an acute inflammation, also called a "splint," of the dorsal metacarpal ligament and adjacent periosteum. It is usually on the medial side in the upper third of the metacarpus, and the swelling is easily seen from the front. After the inflammation subsides, the small bone is attached to the large bone by synostosis and a bony swelling often remains. This may be seen on skeletal specimens.

The third metacarpal bone is formed from three ossification centers. The proximal epiphysis unites with the diaphysis before birth. The distal epiphysis unites at 6 to 12 months. A nutrient foramen is on the palmar surface at the junction of the proximal and middle thirds. The second and fourth metacarpals vary in length and shape. Usually the second is longer. Fractures of the small metacarpals occur most commonly in the 5- to 7-year-old Standardbred, and they usually occur in the distal third of the bone.[3]

Identify a small transverse ridge on the head of the third metacarpal bone. This blends in the middle with the prominent sagittal ridge. In the normal standing position, the surface of the head dorsal to the transverse ridge articulates with P I, and the palmar surface articulates with the proximal sesamoid bones. A shallow synovial fossa is often found on the palmar side of this transverse ridge adjacent to the sagittal ridge. These are often the sites of ulcerative or subchondral bone lesions in racing Thoroughbreds.[15, 22]

Note on the Nomenclature: "Fetlock joint" is a perfectly good English term for the metacarpophalangeal joint. There is no reason for anyone, layman or veterinarian, to call it the ankle. The human ankle is homologous to the hock. The term sesamoid bone in this discussion means the proximal sesamoid bone. The distal sesamoid bone is commonly called the navicular bone in the horse.

Interosseus. This tendinous muscle originates from the palmar surface of the proximal end of the large metacarpal bone and divides into two branches, which are attached to the concave abaxial surfaces of the sesamoid bones. The tension of the interosseus on the sesamoid bones is transmitted to the palmar surface of the proximal and middle phalanges (P I and P II) by the sesamoid ligaments (to be discussed in Chapter 11). Thin, narrow extensor branches of the interosseus pass around the sides of the proximal phalanx to the common digital extensor tendon. They have two actions when the weight is on the limb and the fetlock joint is overextended: they stiffen the digit, resisting the tendency of the deep digital flexor tendon to flex the coffin joint when it is stressed by the descending fetlock joint, and they form part of the interosseus-sesamoid suspensory apparatus that supports the fetlock joint.

Deep digital flexor tendon. The second structure supporting the fetlock is the deep flexor tendon. Its accessory (check) ligament is a continuation of the deep palmar carpal ligament, and it lies between the interosseus and the deep flexor tendon. The latter terminates on the distal phalanx.

Superficial digital flexor tendon. The third tendinous structure supporting the fetlock is the superficial flexor tendon. It has an accessory (check) ligament attached to the medial caudal border of the radius. In most species, each digital branch of the tendon forms a sleeve (manica) around the corresponding branch of the deep flexor tendon and terminates entirely on the middle phalanx. It acts as a flexor of the proximal interphalangeal joint. In the horse, it divides distal to the sleeve into medial and lateral branches, each of which divides and terminates on the distal end of P I, as well as the proximal end of P II. Therefore, the superficial flexor in the horse has a secondary, paradoxical action when stressed by the weight of the fetlock joint—it resists flexion or buckling forward of the pastern joint because the hoof is planted on the ground.

The tendinous structure of the interosseus and the attachment of the accessory ligaments of the superficial and deep digital flexors to their respective tendons provide the thoracic limb with a series of ligaments that act as a passive spring system between bones.[16] They are a major component of the stay apparatus that provides primary resistance to overextension of joints during the support phase of the gait. Transection of the deep digital flexor tendon proximal to its accessory ligament has no effect on the fetlock angulation at the walk or trot. Cutting the accessory ligament of this tendon does not affect the fetlock joint angulation.[19] If the three tendinous structures supporting the fetlock joint—interosseus, deep flexor, and superficial flexor—are cut one at a time proximal to the fetlock in the standing horse under local anesthesia, the amount of overextension increases as each is severed until, when the last one is cut, the fetlock joint is resting on the ground.

Similar studies have concluded that the interosseus-sesamoidean suspensory apparatus absorbs the initial concussion when the hoof strikes the ground. As the fetlock joint starts to hyperextend, the digital flexor tendons act to prevent excessive hyperextension and to maintain normal fetlock joint angulation.

In the young horse, the metacarpophalangeal joint may be nearly straight rather than in the normal position of overextension. This is part of a syndrome referred to as flexor deformity; it is also called by the misnomer contracted tendons.[9, 29] It may be congenital or acquired. Shortening of the superficial digital flexor relative to the bone length causes the fetlock joint to flex while the hoof is in its normal position flat on the ground. This may be the result of a discrepancy between rapid bone growth at the distal radius and the capacity for similar lengthening of the accessory ligament of the superficial digital flexor. This is difficult to treat successfully. Surgery to transect the accessory ligament of the superficial digital flexor may be effective in mild cases. This is done on the medial side of the distal forearm, where the ligament is found at its radial attachment deep to the flexor carpi radialis tendon. In severe cases, transection of the accessory ligament of the deep digital flexor and of the interosseus may be necessary. Shortening of the deep digital flexor alone causes excessive flexion of the distal interphalangeal joint. This produces a boxy or club-like hoof, elevates the bulbs of the hoof off the ground, and causes a concavity on the dorsal surface of the wall. This may be treated surgically by transection of the accessory ligament of the deep digital flexor in the proximal metacarpus, where it is found between the interosseus and the deep digital flexor tendon. These muscle-joint abnormalities often occur together. If only the superficial digital flexor is involved, flexion of the carpus will permit more extension of the fetlock joint. If only the deep digital flexor is involved, carpal flexion will not affect the range of motion in the distal interphalangeal joint because of the location of its accessory ligament distal to the carpus. As a rule, acquired fetlock flexion is more common in horses 6 weeks to 6 months old and acquired distal interphalangeal joint flexion occurs at 10 to 14 months.

Varus or valgus angular deformity of the fetlock joint is less common than at the carpus. Growth at the epiphyseal plate at the distal end of the metacarpal bone slows by 90 days and virtually ceases by 120 days.[12] It only contributes about 4 percent to the total growth in length.[5] Therefore, treatment that depends on differential growth of the distal end of the metacarpal bone is often unsuccessful.

The flexor tendons are subject to various diseases and injuries and also serve as landmarks for the nerves, vessels, and synovial structures. Refer to section 10b and Figures 10–1 and 10–2 for the importance of the grooves between the large metacarpal bone and the interosseus and between the interosseus and the deep flexor tendon.

The collateral ligaments of the fetlock joint run straight from the large metacarpal bone to the proximal collateral tubercles of P I. The collateral sesamoid ligaments are triangular, attaching the sesamoid bones to the metacarpal bone and to P. I. The intersesamoid ligament connects the sesamoid bones and extends proximal to them, augmenting the flexor surface. The palmar annular ligament passes from one sesamoid bone to the other around the palmar surface of the flexor tendons.

The ligamentous attachments of a sesamoid bone are important when it is fractured and a fragment must be removed. The fractures in the Thoroughbred are usually in the base of the sesamoid bone of a forelimb and are thought to be caused by external force. Those in the Standardbred are usually apical, in the lateral sesamoid bone of the hind limb and are thought to be caused by stress when the fetlock goes into extreme overextension resulting from fatigue. These are more common in 2- to 3-year-old Standardbreds when first training at race speeds.[28]

If the fracture is apical and the fragment is not more than one third of the bone, it can be removed by an approach through the joint capsule pouch in the groove between the large metatarsal bone and the interosseus. The fragment is dissected free from the intersesamoid ligament and the interosseus, sparing as much of the latter as possible. Small basal fragments can also be removed. If the fracture is transverse, leaving fragments too large to remove, a compression lag screw can be inserted from base to apex.[8]

10b. DISSECTION OR MODEL, METACARPUS AND FETLOCK JOINT, HORSE

Note on the Nomenclature. The present system of naming the vessels and nerves on the metacarpus and metatarsus is based on the human nomenclature. The superficial metapodial vessels and nerves are called common digital, whereas the deep vessels and nerves are called metacarpal or metatarsal. There are four sets of blood vessels in the metacarpus: dorsal common digital, dorsal metacarpal, palmar common digital, and palmar metacarpal. The blood vessels of the metatarsus are: dorsal common digital, dorsal metatarsal, plantar common digital, and plantar metatarsal. The nerves have the same names, but one set of nerves is missing—there are no dorsal metacarpal nerves; only the dorsal common digital nerves are present in the metacarpus. In the horse, because the superficial branch of the radial nerve does not extend distal to the forearm, only the dorsal branch of the ulnar nerve and the medial cutaneous antebrachial nerve from the musculocutaneous are present. Also in the horse, because there is only one digit, the terms palmar and plantar common digital are simplified to palmar and plantar, e.g., the term medial palmar nerve is adequate to designate palmar common digital nerve II. Another principle is that only vessels have anastomotic branches; nerves have communicating branches.

Identify the following on the dissections or models provided.

Interosseus. Trace it from the carpus to the attachment on the sesamoid bones and extensor tendon.

Flexor tendons.

Extensor tendons.

Palmar annular ligament of the fetlock joint, which covers the flexor tendons and sesamoids.

Distal ends of small metacarpal bones.

Proximal pouch of the fetlock joint capsule. It extends proximally between the interosseus and the large metacarpal bone for about one fourth of the length of the metacarpus. For another means of access to the fetlock joint, see section 11b.

Proximal extent of the digital sheath of the flexor tendons.

Distal extent of the carpal sheath of the flexor tendons. Note the level of the area that is free of tendon sheaths. It is the fourth of the metacarpus distal to the middle. This is important for tenotomy for if a tendon is divided in a sheathed segment, the ends will not reunite spontaneously but will become rounded.

Medial palmar artery. This is on the medial side in the groove between the interosseus and the deep flexor tendon (see Fig. 10–2). The medial palmar artery is the largest and most important artery supplying blood to the foot. It is a continuation of the median artery in the antebrachium. In the distal fourth of the metacarpus, between the interosseus and deep flexor tendon, it divides into medial and lateral digital arteries that cross the sesamoid bones. The lateral palmar artery is insignificant.

Metacarpal arteries. Dorsal metacarpal arteries from the dorsal rete are small and located in the grooves between the large and small metacarpal bones. The small palmar metacarpal arteries, branches of the deep palmar arch, course distally on the palmar surface of the third metacarpal bone covered by the interosseus.

Veins. Medial and lateral palmar veins and digital veins accompany the arteries. The medial and lateral palmar veins anastomose proximal to the sesamoid bones between the interosseus and the deep flexor tendon. The medial palmar vein is the continuation of the radial vein, which is joined by the cephalic vein in the antebrachium. The lateral palmar vein is a continuation of the median vein in the antebrachium.

Medial and lateral palmar nerves. These arise by the bifurcation of the median nerve above the carpus and course in the groove between the interosseus and deep flexor tendon. The lateral palmar nerve is fused for a short distance with the palmar branch of the ulnar nerve at the carpus and exchanges fibers with it. Distal to this communication the deep palmar branch of the ulnar is given off and passes to the palmar surface of the interosseus, while the lateral palmar nerve, composed of fibers from the median and ulnar nerves, continues in the groove between the interosseus and the deep flexor tendon. Note the communication between the medial and lateral palmar nerves around the superficial flexor tendon (Figs. 10–1 and 10–2). It always runs from medial to lateral and distally. The dorsopalmar sequence of the vein, artery, and nerve is often represented by the initials VAN. Note, however, that the artery is deeper than the vein and nerve in the distal fourth of the metacarpus, where the nerve is usually blocked. Just proximal to the fetlock joint each palmar nerve gives off a dorsal branch and is continued as the medial or lateral palmar digital nerve (see Figs. 10–1 and 10–2). A second dorsal branch may arise from the palmar digital nerve.

The deep palmar branch of the ulnar nerve supplies sensation to the interosseus, part of the carpal joint, and the accessory ligament of the deep flexor. It terminates as the palmar metacarpal nerves. For a diagnostic block of the interosseus, flex the carpus and insert the needle from the palmar surface 3 cm. distal to the accessory carpal bone. The needle passes between the lateral border of the flexor tendons and the distal ligament of the accessory carpal bone. The solution is injected into the space between the accessory ligament of the deep flexor and the interosseus.[20]

Palmar metacarpal nerves. These come from the deep palmar branch of the ulnar and run down the medial and lateral borders of the interosseus on the metacarpal bones. They supply deep branches to the palmar pouch of the fetlock joint and emerge at the distal ends of the splint bones to supply the dorsal pouch of the fetlock joint and to give variable cutaneous branches to the dorsolateral and dorsomedial sides of the fetlock joint and proximal part of the pastern. They do not exchange fibers with twigs of the dorsal branches of the palmar nerves where they cross. The medial nerve may reach the coronary region.[17, 25]

The dorsal branch of the ulnar nerve (see Fig. 10–1).This descends on the lateral surface of the metacarpus but not beyond the fetlock joint.[27]

To anesthetize the digit, including the fetlock joint for surgery, block both palmar nerves below their communicating branch and both palmar metacarpal nerves. The latter may be blocked either by infiltrating the deep palmar branch of the ulnar or by superficial and deep injections at the ends of the splint bones (see Figs. 10–1 and 10–2).

For cutaneous anesthesia at the fetlock joint it may be necessary to block the dorsal branch of the ulnar nerve on the dorsolateral surface of the third metacarpal at the level of the distal end of the fourth metacarpal, and the distal termination of the medial cutaneous antebrachial nerve on the dorsomedial surface of the third metacarpal at the same level. Alternatively, the dorsal branch of the ulnar nerve can be blocked where it is palpable on the lateral surface of the ulnaris lateralis a few centimeters proximal to the accessory carpal bone, and the medial cutaneous antebrachial nerve can be blocked where it is palpable on the lacertus fibrosus at the elbow. These nerves may have to be blocked to diagnose villonodular synovitis of the fetlock joint, which primarily affects the proximal extent of the joint capsule on the dorsal surface of the third metacarpal bone.

10c. RADIOGRAPHS, METACARPUS AND FETLOCK JOINT, HORSE

Observe that the sesamoid bones articulate with the metacarpal bone, not with the proximal phalanx. The large metacarpal bone has a distal epiphysis that unites with the shaft at 6 to 12 months.[1]

On an angiogram identify the medial palmar artery and the medial and lateral digital arteries. Note the extent of the fetlock joint on an arthrogram.[2] Relate the position of the pouch to the landmarks for injection into it. Consider the relationship of soft tissue structures to the bones at the fetlock joint.

The head (distal end) of the third metacarpal is subject to fracture, most commonly in young racing Thoroughbreds.[26] These fractures are usually longitudinal and extend through the articular cartilage. Subchondral cysts occur on both the dorsal and palmar aspects of the articular surface of the head of the third metacarpal.[15, 22]

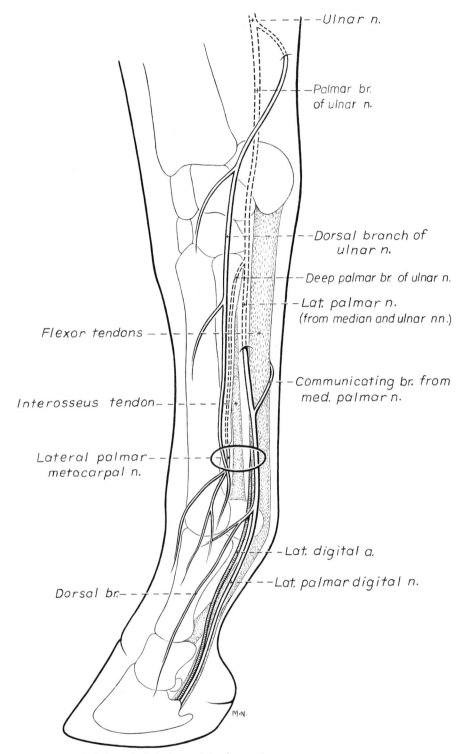

-- Ulnar n.

-- Palmar br.
of ulnar n.

-- Dorsal branch of
ulnar n.

-- Deep palmar br. of ulnar n.

-- Lat. palmar n.
(from median and ulnar nn.)

Flexor tendons -- -- -- --

-- Communicating br. from
med. palmar n.

Interosseus tendon -- -- -- --

Lateral palmar -- -- -- --
metacarpal n.

-- Lat. digital a.

-- Lat. palmar digital n.

Dorsal br. -- -- -- --

Figure 10–1. Left thoracic limb, horse, lateral aspect.

10d. LIVE HORSE

Identify the following structures:

Distal end of the great metacarpal bone. This indicates the level of the fetlock joint.

Distal ends of the small metacarpal bones. These are subject to fracture, and the distal fragment

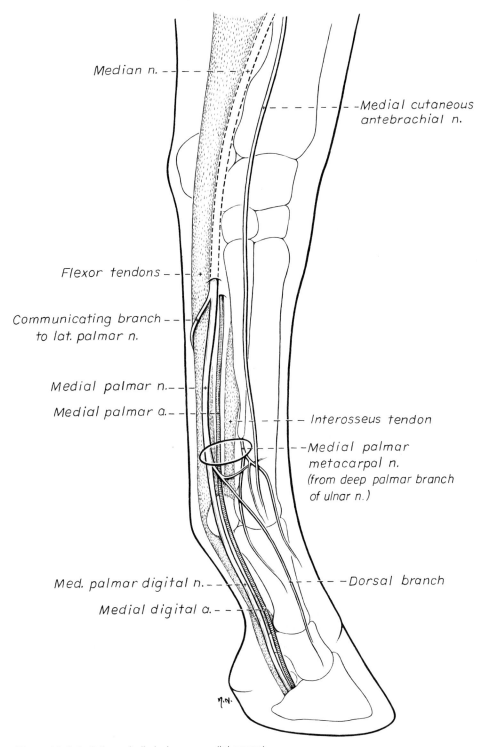

Median n.

Medial cutaneous antebrachial n.

Flexor tendons

Communicating branch to lat. palmar n.

Medial palmar n.

Medial palmar a.

Interosseus tendon

Medial palmar metacarpal n. (from deep palmar branch of ulnar n.)

Med. palmar digital n.

Dorsal branch

Medial digital a.

Figure 10–2. Left thoracic limb, horse, medial aspect.

must be removed. They are also useful landmarks for palmar metacarpal nerve blocks, but they vary in length (see Plate I).

Sesamoid bones and medial and lateral collateral sesamoid ligaments. Pick up the foot to relax the interosseus and make the sesamoid bones movable.

Interosseus. Trace the branches to the sesamoid bones and to the extensor tendon.

Superficial flexor tendon in the metacarpus. Pick up the foot to relax the tendons and separate the superficial from the deep flexor tendon.

Deep flexor tendon. The accessory ligament is not palpable in the normal state. Try to palpate it proximally between the splint bone and the deep flexor tendon (see Plate I).

The superficial flexor tendon and the interosseus are taut when the fetlock joint is in the standing position of overextension. Hold the foot up and manipulate the digit while palpating the tendons. If the fetlock joint is held in a neutral position and the dorsal part of the hoof is pulled dorsally, extending the coffin joint, only the deep flexor is tightened. Flex and extend the fetlock joint with the coffin joint in the neutral position and palpate the effect on the interosseus and superficial flexor tendons. Correlate these functions with the differential diagnosis of tendon rupture.

Proximal end of the digital sheath of the flexor tendons. Proximal to the sesamoid bone, between the interosseus and flexor tendons. It is not palpable normally (see Plate I).

Sheath-free area of metacarpus. The third quarter distally.

Proximal pouch of the fetlock joint capsule. Proximal to the sesamoid bone, distal to the end of the small metacarpal, between the large metacarpal and the interosseus (see Plate I). Injections are made into the joint at this site.

Arteries. Trace the course of the medial palmar and medial and lateral digital arteries.

Palmar nerves. Palpate them as they cross the abaxial faces of the sesamoid bones and divide into the palmar digital nerves and the dorsal branches. In the proximal three quarters of the metacarpus, the palmar nerves are covered by deep fascia and lie too deep in the groove between the interosseus and the deep flexor tendon to be palpated readily in the standing horse.

Communicating branch between the medial and lateral palmar nerves. It leaves the medial nerve about the middle of the metacarpus and runs distolaterally across the surface of the superficial flexor tendon, where it is distinctly palpable under the skin.

Locate the site of nerve blocks described in section 10b.

10e. DISSECTION, MODEL, AND LIGAMENTOUS PREPARATIONS, METACARPUS AND FETLOCK JOINTS, OX

Identify and understand the following structures on the specimens provided. The axis of the limb is between the third (medial) and fourth (lateral) digits. The terms axial and abaxial are used to refer to the sides of the digits.

Superficial flexor tendons. They form, with two bands from the interossei, the sleeves through which the deep flexor tendons pass.

Interosseus muscles. The cow has two interossei, each equivalent to that of the horse and fused along their axial borders. In the middle of the metacarpus, they give off a flat band that bifurcates and joins the branches of the superficial flexor tendon. Above the fetlock joint each interosseus muscle gives off an abaxial tendon, which terminates on the abaxial sesamoid and gives off a branch that continues obliquely across the abaxial surface of the digit to join the tendon of the medial or lateral digital extensor. The axial tendons of the interossei terminate on the axial sesamoids. Their extensor branches remain fused until they pass through the notch in the distal end of the metacarpal bone. Then they separate and join the tendons of the medial and lateral digital extensors (see Fig. 12–1).

The terminations of the interosseus of each digit are the same as in the horse, except that in the horse there is no band to the superficial flexor and the extensor branches go to the common extensor.

On the dorsolateral surface of the proximal half of the metacarpus are three palpable digital extensor tendons. The middle one is the common digital extensor. The other two are the medial and lateral digital extensors. The medial one is considered part of the common extensor.

The two branches of the common digital extensor tendon are round where they are located in the middle of the dorsal surface of the distal metacarpus. They pass between the heads of the metacarpal bone and along the dorsal axial surface of each digit, where they are palpable. They terminate on the extensor process of the corresponding third phalanx. The medial and lateral digital extensor tendons are more flat. They pass distally on the dorsal abaxial surface of each digit, are joined by the extensor branches of the interosseus, and terminate on the second and third phalanges of each digit.

Collateral ligaments of the fetlock joints.

Medial and lateral collateral sesamoid ligaments, from the abaxial sesamoid bones to the proximal end of P I.

Anesthesia of the digits of the forelimbs, including the dewclaws, requires four injections. The order of injection makes it possible to work systematically around the metacarpus (dorsal, lateral, palmar, and medial). The following description is simplified by omitting the innervation of the second and fifth digits, or dewclaws (see Figs. 10–3 to 10–6).

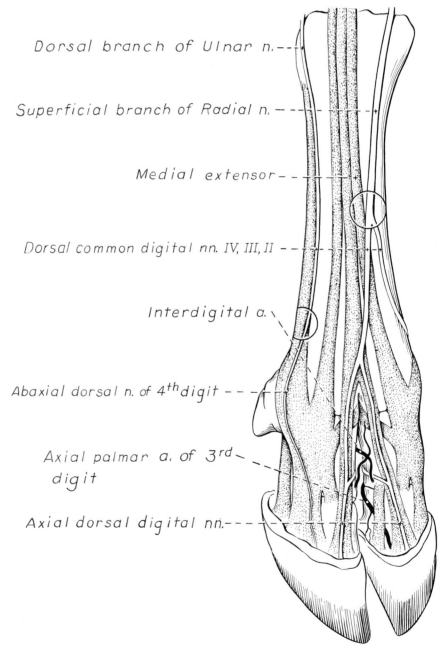

Dorsal branch of Ulnar n.

Superficial branch of Radial n.

Medial extensor

Dorsal common digital nn. IV, III, II

Interdigital a.

Abaxial dorsal n. of 4thdigit

Axial palmar a. of 3rd digit

Axial dorsal digital nn.

Figure 10–3. Right forefoot, cow, dorsolateral aspect.

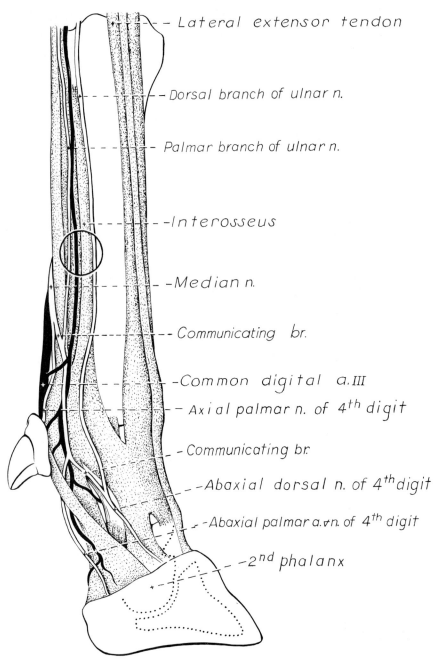

Figure 10–4. Right forefoot, cow, lateral aspect.

1. Superficial branch of the radial nerve. Palpate it on the bone medial to the tendon of the medial extensor where the latter begins to diverge from the common extensor a little below the middle of the dorsal surface of the metacarpus. Injection at this point blocks the axial dorsal nerves of both digits and the abaxial dorsal nerve of the third digit (see Fig. 10–3).

2. Dorsal common digital nerve IV from the dorsal branch of the ulnar nerve. This is continued as the abaxial dorsal digital nerve of the fourth digit. Inject in the groove between the interosseus and the metacarpal bone on the lateral side in the middle of the metacarpus. Notice that the abaxial dorsal nerves cross the fetlock joints in close association with the abaxial palmar nerves.

3. Palmar branch of the ulnar nerve. It receives the communicating branch from the median nerve and is continued as the palmar common digital nerve IV, which becomes the abaxial palmar nerve of the fourth digit. Inject in the groove between the interosseus and the deep flexor tendon on

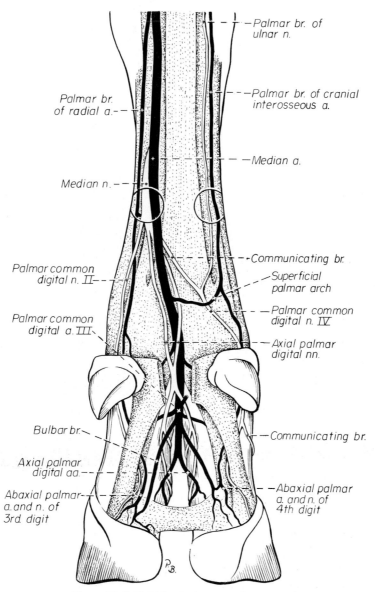

Figure 10–5. Right forefoot, cow, palmar aspect.

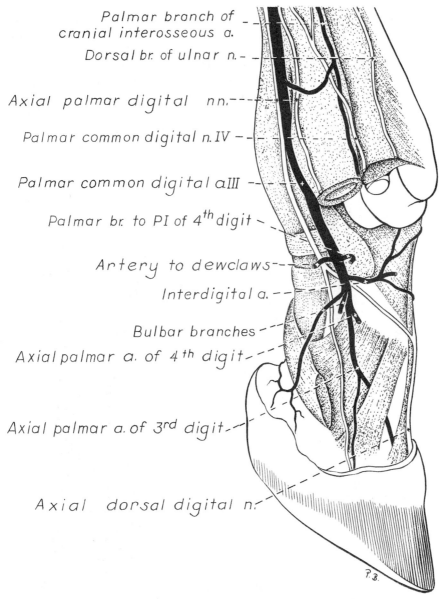

Palmar branch of cranial interosseous a.

Dorsal br. of ulnar n.

Axial palmar digital nn.

Palmar common digital n. IV

Palmar common digital a. III

Palmar br. to PI of 4th digit

Artery to dewclaws

Interdigital a.

Bulbar branches

Axial palmar a. of 4th digit

Axial palmar a. of 3rd digit

Axial dorsal digital n.

Figure 10–6. Right forefoot, cow, axial surface of the third digit.

the lateral side. Injections 2 and 3 can be made with one insertion of the needle over the interosseus.

4. Median nerve. This supplies the axial palmar digital nerves, the abaxial palmar nerve of the third digit, and a communicating branch to no. 3, the palmar branch of the ulnar nerve, in the distal third of the metacarpus. Inject in the groove between the interosseus and the deep flexor tendon on the medial side above the middle of the metacarpus. The large median artery is on the palmar surface of the nerve at the point of injection. The needle should be inserted from the medial side, close to the interosseus.

The large palmar common digital artery III is the continuation of the median artery at the superficial palmar arch; it passes obliquely across the palmar surface of the medial branch of the superficial flexor tendon and into the axial groove between the two branches of the tendon. It divides in the interdigital space into the axial palmar digital arteries (see Fig. 10–5). These are the major blood supply to each digit.

Intravenous local anesthesia of the distal metacarpus and digits has been advocated. A tourniquet applied distal to the carpus will distend three superficial veins in the distal part of the metacarpus: (1) Dorsal common digital vein III from the accessory cephalic (Fig. 10–7) on the surface of the superficial branch of the radial nerve. It courses medial to the extensor tendons in mid-metacarpus and passes into the interdigital space. This vein is recommended because the accompanying artery is so small that the danger of puncturing it and producing a hematoma is negligible.[10]

(2) Palmar common digital vein II (see Fig. 10–8) emerges from the deep distal palmar arch in the medial groove palmar to the interosseus and continues across the sesamoid bone dorsal to the dewclaw as the abaxial palmar vein of the third digit. It accompanies a small artery. (3) Palmar common digital vein IV has the same origin as palmar common digital vein II but on the lateral side. It is continued as the abaxial palmar vein of the fourth digit with a small artery.

Figure 10–7. Superficial veins of left forefoot, cow, dorsal aspect.

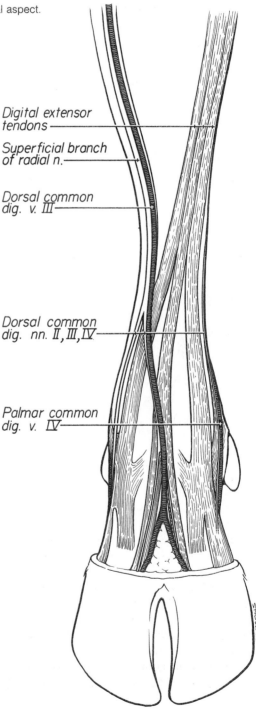

Digital extensor tendons

Superficial branch of radial n.

Dorsal common dig. v. III

Dorsal common dig. nn. II, III, IV

Palmar common dig. v. IV

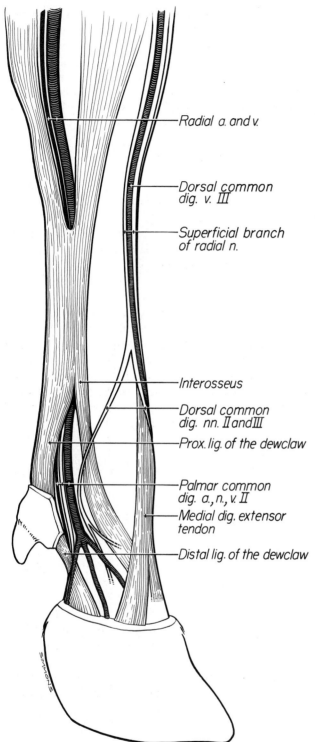

Radial a. and v.

Dorsal common dig. v. III

Superficial branch of radial n.

Interosseus

Dorsal common dig. nn. II and III

Prox. lig. of the dewclaw

Palmar common dig. a., n., v. II

Medial dig. extensor tendon

Distal lig. of the dewclaw

Figure 10–8. Superficial veins of left forefoot, cow, medial aspect.

Palmar common digital vein III, which is often double and comes from the median vein, accompanies the largest artery of the metacarpus (see Fig. 10–5) along the medial side of the flexor tendons and into the interdigital space. It is not recommended for injection because the artery may be punctured and because the vessels are covered by thick fascia.

If the tourniquet is applied above the carpus, the large radial vein (Fig. 10–8), the continuation of the cephalic, is accessible. These veins may also be used for the local administration of antibiotics.

10f. LIVE COW

Palpate all the structures given as landmarks in section 10e for anesthesia of the digits. Take the pulse from the large palmar common digital artery as it crosses over the palmar surface of the medial branch of the superficial flexor tendon. It is clearly indicated by an elongated bulge.

10g. DISSECTION, METACARPUS, DOG AND CAT

On the dorsal surface of the metacarpus in the dog and cat, the cranial superficial antebrachial artery forms the small dorsal common digital arteries. The superficial branch of the radial nerve also branches here, supplying the dorsal common digital nerves (see Fig. 9–1).

On the palmar surface in the dog, the median artery, the main supply to the digits, passes through the carpal canal in the palmar groove of the deep flexor tendon, accompanied by the median nerve. The median artery gives off a branch to the first metacarpal space and trifurcates into palmar common digital arteries II, III, and IV. Estimate the position of the metacarpal pad and consider the vulnerability of the arteries in the fossa proximal to the pad.

The palmar common digital nerves are supplied by the median and ulnar nerves.

In the cat, the main blood supply to the digits is not the median artery but a perforating artery, which comes from the dorsal carpal branch of the radial. Actually, the radial, the largest artery of the distal part of the forearm in the cat, is continued in point of size by its dorsal carpal branch, which passes deep to the tendon of the abductor pollicis longus to reach the dorsal surface. It then goes deep to the tendon of the extensor carpi radialis and perforates between the proximal ends of the second and third metacarpal bones to the palmar surface, where it supplies the palmar metacarpal arteries. There is an oblique vascular groove on the dorsal surface of the second metacarpal bone. The axial palmar artery of each digit can be traced from the palmar metacarpal to the foramen in the axial side of the distal phalanx very close to the claw.

The median artery and the palmar common digital arteries are minute in the cat. The ulnar artery is large as far down as the carpal canal.

10h. RADIOGRAPHS, METACARPUS, DOG

The largest artery is the median. It is seen on an angiogram dividing into the palmar common digitals, and the latter can be traced to the axial palmar digital arteries, which enter the distal phalanx and extend to the end of the unguicular process.

Identify the metacarpals, proximal sesamoids, and the phalanges of each digit.

Metacarpal bones 2 to 5 have only distal epiphyses. The first metacarpal bone has only a proximal epiphysis, and the first digit lacks a middle phalanx. The proximal and middle phalanges have only proximal epiphyses. All are fused at 5 to 7 months in the dog and at 4 ½ to 10 months in the cat.

The axial proximal sesamoid bones of the second and fifth digits are subject to fracture in Greyhounds. The fragments are pressed into the interosseous spaces by the flexor tendons and cause lameness until they are removed.

10i. LIVE DOG AND CAT

Palpate all of the metacarpal bones and the metacarpophalangeal articulations. Note the relationship of the joints to the metacarpal pad.

In the dog, the median artery passes through the carpal canal between the superficial and deep digital flexor tendons, where it is not palpable. Proximal to the carpal canal it courses from deep to the flexor carpi radialis to its position beween the flexor tendons in the canal. The pulse may be felt in this artery here in the distal third of the antebrachium. Place your fingers gently against the flexor carpi radialis tendon and the digital flexor tendons on the medial side of the distal antebrachium.

In the cat, the pulse may be felt in the dorsal carpal branch of the radial artery on the dorsomedial side of the carpus just before the perforating artery passes between the second and third metacarpal bones.

Use your knowledge of the terminations of the flexor tendons to determine which tendons were severed in a wound of the palmar surface of the metacarpus.

References

1. Adams, O. R.: Lameness in Horses, 3rd ed. Lea & Febiger; Philadelphia, 1974.
2. Allan, G. S.: Radiography of the equine fetlock. Equine Pract. *1* (1979):40–47.
3. Bowman, K. F., L. H. Evans, and M. E. Herring: Evaluation of surgical removal of fractured distal splint bones in the horse. Vet. Surg. *11* (1982):116–120.
4. Bramlage, L. R., A. A. Gabel, and R. P. Hackett: Avulsion fractures of the origin of the suspensory ligament in the horse. JAVMA *176* (1980):1004–1011.
5. Campbell, J. R. and R. Lee: Radiological estimation of differential growth rates of the long bones of foals. Equine Vet. J. *13* (1981):247–250.
6. Davis, P. E., C. R. Bellenger, and D. M. Turner: Fractures of the sesamoid bones in the Greyhound. Austral. Vet. J. *45* (1969):15–19.
7. Derksen, F. J.: Diagnostic local anesthesia of the equine front limb. Equine Pract. *2* (1980):41–48.
8. Fackelman, G. E.: Compression screw fixation of proximal sesamoid fractures. J. Eq. Med. Surg. *2* (1978):32–39.
9. Fackelman, G. E.: Flexure deformity of the metacarpophalangeal joints in growing horses. Comp. Cont. Ed. *1* (1979):S1–S7.
10. Fehlings, K.: Intravenöse regionale Anästhesie an der Vena digitalis dorsalis communis III bei Eingriffen an den Vorderzehen des Rindes. Deutsche tierärztl. Wschr. *87* (1980):4–7.
11. Forsell, G.: Untersuchungen über die Wirkungsweise der Beugesehnen am Vorderfuss des Pferdes. Z. Tiermed. *18* (1915):184–188.
12. Fretz, P. B. and C. W. McIlwraith: Wedge osteotomy as a treatment for angular deformity of the fetlock in horses. JAVMA *182* (1983):245–250.
13. Gray, B. W., H. N. Engel, Jr., P. F. Rumph, et al.: Clinical approach to determine the contribution of the palmar and palmar metacarpal nerves to the innervation of the equine fetlock joint. Am. J. Vet. Res. *41* (1980):940–944.
14. Habel, R. E.: Guide to the Dissection of Domestic Ruminants, 3rd ed. Ithaca, N. Y.: Habel, 1977.
15. Hornof, W. J. and T. R. O'Brien: Radiographic evaluation of the palmar aspect of the equine metacarpal condyles: a new projection. Vet. Radiol. *21* (1980):161–167.
16. Kingsbury, H. P., M.A. Qua, J. R. Rooney, et al.: A laboratory system for production of flexion rates and forces in the forelimb of the horse. Am. J. Vet. Res. *39* (1978):365–369.
17. Koch, T.: Über die Nervenversorgung an den Gliedmassenspitzen des Pferdes. Tierärztl. Rundsch. *44* (1938):333–337.
18. Lamy, E.: Anatomie pour la pratique. 5 Complément de recherches sur l'innervation de l'extrémité du membre thoracique ("main") et la construction fonctionnelle des articulations phalangiennes chez le cheval. Schweiz. Arch. Tierheilkd. *91* (1949):564–580, 652–669.
19. Leach, D. H. and A. I. Dagg: A review of research on equine locomotion and biomechanics. Equine Vet. J. *15* (1983):93–102.
20. Magda, I. I.: Mestnoe Obezbolivanie. Moscow: State Publ. Agric. Lit., 1955. Also available in Ger. transl. Lokalanästhesie. Anleitung für Tierärzte. Jena: Fischer, 1960.
21. Nilsson, S. A.: Bidrag till kännedomen om fotens innervation hos häst. Skand. Vet. Tidskr. *38* (1948):401–459.
22. O'Brien, T. R., W. J. Hornof, and D. M. Meagher: Radiographic detection and characterization of palmar lesions in the equine fetlock joint. JAVMA *178* (1981):231–237.
23. Palmer, S. E.: Radiography of the abaxial surface of the proximal sesamoid bones of the horse. JAVMA *181* (1982):264–265.
24. Pharr, J. W. and P. B. Fretz: Radiographic findings in foals with angular limb deformities. JAVMA *179* (1981):812–817.
25. Pohlmeyer, K. and R. Redecker: Die für die Klinik bedeutsamen Nerven an den Gliedmassen des Pferdes einschliesslich möglicher Varianten. Deutsche tierärztl. Wschr. *81* (1974):501–505, 537–541.
26. Rick, M. C., T. R. O'Brien, R. R. Pool, et al.: Condylar fractures of the third metacarpal bone and third metatarsal bone in 75 horses: radiographic features, treatments, and outcome. JAVMA *183* (1983):287–296.
27. Sack, W. O.: Nerve distribution in the metacarpus and front digit of the horse. JAVMA *167* (1975):298–305.
28. Spurlock, G. H. and A. A. Gabel: Apical fractures of the proximal sesamoid bones in 109 Standardbred horses. JAVMA *183* (1983):76–79.
29. Wagner, D. C., S. M. Reed, and G. A. Hegreberg: Contracted tendons (flexural deformities) in the young horse. Comp. Cont. Ed. *4* (1982):S101–S110.
30. White, K. K.: Diaphyseal angular deformities in three foals. JAVMA *182* (1983):272–279.

CHAPTER 11

DIGIT, HORSE

OBJECTIVES

1. To be able to recognize by palpation and in radiographs the bony prominences of the proximal and middle phalanges, where functionally and clinically important ligaments are attached. Swelling and pain at these points may indicate inflammation of the ligament. Identification of the bony prominences makes it possible to describe the attachments of the ligaments accurately.
2. To recognize the metacarpal and phalangeal epiphyses.
3. To recognize the radiographic features of the phalanges, the digital joints, especially the coffin joint, and the navicular bone.
4. To know the course of the digital arteries.
5. To be able to gain access to the digital sheath of the flexor tendons and to understand the digital annular ligaments, which are thickenings of the fibrous part of the sheath.
6. To understand the attachment and normal function of the cartilages of the hoof and the effect of ossification.
7. To be able to gain access to the digital joints for withdrawing fluid or injecting drugs.
8. To understand the relations of the navicular bursa to the coffin joint and to the distal end of the digital sheath of the flexor tendons.
9. To understand the anatomical and mechanical factors involved in the sequelae of laminitis.
10. To be able to estimate from the position of a nail hole on the ground surface of the hoof what structures might be penetrated and infected inside the hoof.
11. To be able to utilize diagnostic blocks to localize pain in the digit and determine the possible value of digital neurectomy in a given case of lameness.
12. To understand the surgical anatomy of operations on the digit and to be able to palpate the landmarks.
13. To understand the growth of the hoof and the effect of injuries to various parts of the dermis.

Note: The descriptions of the digit in the horse apply also to the hind limb, with the substitution of plantar for palmar.

11a. PROXIMAL AND MIDDLE PHALANGES, HORSE

In the list below, the features of the bones that can be recognized by palpation or radiography are related to the attached ligaments and tendons, so an inflammation or exostosis at a certain point on a bone can be evaluated clinically according to the function of the structure attached there. The short and cruciate sesamoid ligaments are accessible only by surgery. The ligaments are described in section 11b.

Proximal Phalanx (P I).

Triangular area on the proximal mid-dorsal surface—common or long extensor tendon. The lateral extensor in the forelimb ends lateral to this area.

Abaxial palmar margin of the proximal end—short and cruciate sesamoid ligaments.

Proximal collateral tubercles—collateral ligaments of the fetlock joint and sesamoid bones, proximal attachment of the proximal digital annular ligament.

Triangle on the palmar surface—oblique sesamoid ligaments.

Intermediate tuberosity in the middle of each border—abaxial palmar ligaments of the pastern joint.

Area between the distal part of the intermediate tuberosity and the margin of the triangle—axial palmar ligaments of the pastern joint.

Distal collateral tubercles—distal attachment of the proximal digital annular ligament and the proximal attachment of the collateral ligaments of the pastern joint (proximal interphalangeal joint).

Rough oval areas on the palmar surface behind the distal tubercles—superficial flexor.

Oblique crest on the distal half of each border, connecting the intermediate tuberosity with the distal collateral tubercle—distal digital annular ligament and ligament to the cartilage of the hoof.

Depressions on the sides of the distal end—collateral (suspensory) ligaments of the navicular bone.

Middle Phalanx (P II).

Flexor tuberosity on the palmar border of the proximal end—attachment of the fibrocartilage, which: (1) enlarges the articular surface of P II, (2) forms the bearing surface for the deep flexor tendon, and (3) serves as the attachment of the straight sesamoid ligament and the palmar ligaments of the pastern joint.

Extensor process on the mid-dorsal surface of the proximal end—extensor tendon.

Proximal collateral tubercles—collateral ligaments of the pastern joint and the superficial flexor tendon.

Depressions on the sides of the distal end—collateral ligaments of the coffin joint (distal interphalangeal joint).

Rough eminences dorsal to the depressions on the distal end—ligaments to the cartilages of the hoof.

11b. LIGAMENTOUS PREPARATIONS, DIGIT, HORSE

Cartilage of the hoof. The proximal and palmar borders can be palpated. The cartilage is attached by ligaments to all three phalanges, the navicular bone, and the digital cushion. The inner surface of the cartilage is in contact with the coffin joint capsule. The cartilage gives flexibility to the quarters (lateral and medial parts) and heels (palmar borders) of the hoof so they can expand. This expansion is the reason that the branches of the horseshoe are not nailed to the parts of the hoof behind the greatest width. The upper surface of a worn horseshoe is polished by this movement. When the digital cushion is compressed between the frog and the deep flexor tendon, it exerts pressure on the inner surface of the cartilage. Ossification of the cartilage (side bone) causes rigidity and sometimes lameness.

Proximal digital annular ligament. This is attached by its four corners to the proximal and distal collateral tubercles of P I. The distal attachments are blended with the terminations of the superficial flexor tendon on P I.

Distal digital annular ligament. It is attached to the border of P I and to the extensor tendon on each side and forms a sling around the deep flexor tendon. There are connections from the annular ligament to the digital cushion. The ligament of the ergot is attached to the annular ligament.

Extensor branches of the interosseus join the common (long) digital extensor tendon on the dorsal surface of P I.

Extensor tendon. This is very wide in the coronary region. It terminates on all three phalanges.

Superficial digital flexor tendon. This is on the palmar side of P I, covered by the proximal digital annular ligament; it divides and terminates on the palmar side of the distal collateral tubercles of P I and on the proximal collateral tubercles of P II.

Deep flexor tendon. This is seen through the gap between the annular ligaments on the palmar surface at the level of the pastern joint.

Oblique sesamoid ligaments (V ligament). One ligament comes from the base of each sesamoid bone and is attached along the border of the triangle of P I. They are visible between the flexor tendons and P I.

Straight sesamoid ligament (Y ligament). The branches of the Y come from the bases of the sesamoid bones, and the stem is attached to P II through the fibrocartilage. The ligament lies on the axis of the digit in the palmar groove between the thicker oblique ligaments.

Cruciate sesamoid ligaments. Each ligament runs from the base of the sesamoid to the other side of the palmar margin of the proximal end of P I deep to the straight ligament.

Short sesamoid ligaments. These are best seen from the inside of the joint. Each ligament runs abaxially from the base of a sesamoid bone to the abaxial palmar margin of the proximal end of P I.

It will be recalled from Chapter 10 that the sesamoid bones are also attached to the interosseus tendon and the intersesamoid and collateral sesamoid ligaments. All of these fibrous attachments make the surgical removal of fragments difficult. The oblique and straight sesamoid ligaments provide the main mechanical opposition to the interosseus in the suspensory apparatus supporting the fetlock.

When it is impossible to get a needle into the proximal pouch of the fetlock joint capsule (section 10b), the distal approach may be used.[21] There is a palpable depression bounded proximally by the sesamoid bone, dorsally by the oblique sesamoid ligament, on the palmar side by the superficial digital flexor, and distally by the proximal attachment of the proximal digital annular ligament. The digital vessels and nerves covering the depression can be palpated subcutaneously and pushed aside. The needle is directed to the axis of the digit and proximally to enter the distal palmar pouch of the joint capsule (see an arthrogram).

Abaxial palmar ligaments of the pastern joint. They originate from the intermediate tuberosities of P I and end on the flexor tuberosity of P II via the fibrocartilage. They are crossed superficially by the distal digital annular ligament and the superficial digital flexor tendon terminates deep to them.

Axial palmar ligaments of the pastern joint. These originate from the area between the distal part of the intermediate tuberosity and the border of the triangle of P I and end on the flexor tuberosity of P II via the fibrocartilage medial to the superficial digital flexor tendon.

Collateral ligaments of the pastern joint. In the standing position, they pass vertically from the collateral tubercles of P I to the collateral tubercles of P II, which are usually located at the proximal borders of the cartilages of the hoof.

Collateral (suspensory) ligaments of the navicular bone. They arise from the depressions in P I dorsal to the collateral ligaments of the pastern joint and are blended with those ligaments. They descend across the sides of P II to the ends of the navicular bone and attach to the entire proximal border, forming a continuous loop. They form, together with the navicular bone and its distal ligament (see sections 11d and 11e), a suspensory apparatus for the palmar side of the articular surface of P II. This is similar to the suspensory apparatus of the fetlock joint; it absorbs some of the thrust of P II. The navicular bone enlarges the articular surface and protects the joint from tendon pressure.

11c. RADIOGRAPHS, DIGIT, HORSE[11, 16]

Dorsopalmar View:

Sesamoid bones at the fetlock joint. Lateral one may be slightly longer (proximodistally), and it has a more concave lateral surface.

Triangular dark outline of the marrow cavity of P I. Fractures of P I are common. The fracture is usually articular and longitudinal.

Radiolucent zones representing articular cartilages. The radiolucent zone is normally widest in the coffin joint, narrower in the pastern joint, and narrowest in the fetlock joint.

Collateral tubercles of P I and P II.

Epiphyses. Unlike the epiphyses of metacarpal bones, the epiphyses present on P I and P II after birth are proximal. They fuse at 6 to 9 months.[1] The distal phalanx ossifies from a single center.

Dorsoproximal-Palmarodistal Oblique Views: These views are used to evaluate the navicular bone and P III. The navicular bone must be superimposed on P II. If the x-ray tube is directed at the dorsal surface of the coffin joint and then moved 45° proximally, an oblique view will be made that will delineate the proximal border of the navicular bone. If the angle is increased to 65° the distal border will be delineated.

Navicular Bone. Identify the proximal and distal borders and the extremities. The navicular bone receives blood vessels through its ligaments. The palmar branch to P II from the digital artery supplies the central region of the proximal border through the attachment of the collateral (suspensory) ligaments. The entire distal border is supplied by arteries that enter it perpendicularly through the distal ligament. They are fed by the palmar branches to P III from the digital arteries. In the adult, these enter through conical nutrient foramina, with the base of the cone at the border of the bone. As the horse performs more work, these cones enlarge but maintain their conical shape. Enlargement of the proximal apical portion is a radiographic sign of navicular disease and is thought to be related to vascular thrombosis and ischemia. Oval or round, pea-sized, radiolucent areas in the center of the navicular bone are most significant.[6, 10]

Medial and lateral palmar processes of P III with foramina or notches. These vary in development with age, and between individual animals. They are small in immature animals.

Medial and lateral grooves on the parietal surface for the dorsal branch of the digital artery.

Sole foramina and canal of P III. The medial and lateral digital arteries enter the foramina and anastomose in the canal. This can be demonstrated on an angiogram.

Vascular channels run distally and dorsally from the sole canal to the sole border and parietal surface of P III respectively. These are normal. A radiolucent line that reaches the coronary border is a fracture. A marginal notch may be present normally at the mid-dorsal part of the sole border.

Coffin Joint. In the 65° oblique view differentiate the head of P II from the extensor process and coronary border of P III and the palmar border of the articular surface of P III.

Paracuneal and central cuneal grooves. These features of the frog must not be mistaken for bone lesions. Usually they will be seen to extend beyond the border of the bone. If the grooves are cleaned and filled with tallow or soap, they will not show in the radiograph.

Lateromedial View:

Sesamoid bones.

Marrow cavities of phalanges.

Prominence at the distal third of the palmar surface of P I (apex of the triangle).

Relation of the pastern and coffin joints to the coronary border of the hoof.

Position of P II and P III with regard to the dorsal surface of the wall and the palmar border of the hoof.

P III. Differentiate between the medial and lateral sides of the sole border, which may be asymmetrical because of their different positions relative to the x-ray tube and film. With the x-ray tube centered on P I, the lateral side of the sole border is closer to the x-ray tube and falsely enlarged. The medial side is next to the radiograph and will appear more proximal and in sharper contrast.

Differentiate between the sole borders and the mid-dorsal part of the concave sole surface. Identify the sole canal for the terminal arch of digital arteries.

Palmar processes with notch or foramen. Notice that the normal cartilage of the hoof is not seen in the radiograph. It is visible when it is ossified in sidebone.[1]

Articulation of P II with P III and the navicular bone.

Navicular bone. Proximal and distal borders. Notice that the edge of the flexor surface normally projects from the distal border of the bone. The distal navicular ligament attaches here.

Articulation with P II and P III.

Navicular disease comprises a complex of lesions that involve the bone, its ligaments, and the bursa (bursitis podotrochlearis).[20] The cause and relative significance of each of these are uncertain. Early changes may occur on the flexor surface of the bone and the apposed surface of the digital flexor tendon. Painful lesions may be in the distal navicular ligament, which becomes shorter and thicker and ossifies at both attachments.[25] Ossification at its attachment to the distal border of the flexor surface of the navicular bone may be visible in a lateral radiograph but must not be mistaken for the normal border. Ossification of the P III attachment can only be seen at autopsy. Incongruence may occur at the articulation of P III with the navicular bone.

Fractures of P III usually involve the articular surface of the coffin joint. They are most common in racing horses, and those in the forelimb often involve the lateral side of the left P III or the medial side of the right P III.[14] These portions bear the most weight on the counterclockwise turns.

Palmar 55 to 80° Proximodistal Oblique View: In this view x-rays pass from proximal to distal along the palmar surface of the digit. Identify the flexor surface of the navicular bone with its median ridge that glides on the flexor tendon. The navicular bursa is between them.

On an angiogram identify the following:

Lateral and medial digital arteries.

Dorsal and palmar branches to P I and P II.

Branch to the digital cushion.

Dorsal branches to P III, and the terminal arch formed by the anastomosis of the medial and lateral digital arteries in the sole canal. Note the large number of arteries that pass through the third phalanx to the dermis.

11d. DISSECTION, DIGIT, HORSE

Observe the relationship of the cartilage of the hoof, the digital cushion, the termination of the deep digital flexor, and the navicular bone and its ligaments. The distal ligament of the navicular bone is in the deep wall of the navicular bursa but in the superficial wall of the coffin joint. Incision of the distal ligament opens the coffin joint on the palmar side. Observe carefully the positions of these structures in relation to the angles of the sole and the apex of the frog. The navicular bone lies across the middle of the frog, with its proximal border on a line connecting the angles of the sole. The deep flexor tendon is attached to P III deep to the apex of the frog.

On the flexor surface of the pastern, the deep flexor tendon and its synovial sheath are exposed in the gap between the proximal and distal digital annular ligaments. The sheath extends 2 cm. farther distal on the dorsal surface of the tendon than it does on the surface exposed. This is, however, the lowest accessible point of drainage.

Foals with severe flexure deformity of the distal interphalangeal joint may require tenotomy of the deep digital flexor tendon where it is superficial between the proximal and distal digital annular ligaments just proximal to the bulbs.[7] The tendon is exposed by incising its tendon sheath. After the tenotomy, the exposed tendon sheath is excised to permit fibroblastic proliferation to form a bridging scar between the cut ends of the tendon.

Distinguish the large medial or lateral palmar digital nerve from the smaller dorsal branch or branches given off near the fetlock joint. The palmar digital nerve is the direct continuation of the palmar nerve. Observe the dorsopalmar sequence of the vein, artery, and palmar digital nerve (VAN) in the middle of P I. The nerve is palpable on the border of the flexor tendons. The ligament of the ergot takes an oblique course across the superficial surface of these structures and can be palpated if it is tensed by pulling the ergot proximally. The palmar digital nerve is blocked distal to this ligament at the level of the pastern joint by injection on the palmar surface. This is just proximal to the proximal border of the lateral cartilage. It is important to block only the palmar digital nerve and not the dorsal branch if the results of palmar digital neurectomy are to be prognosticated (see Figs. 10–1 and 10–2). The accuracy of the nerve block may be tested by pinching the skin with forceps. The dorsal coronary region should remain sensitive. In one study, 56 percent of horses examined 3 years after neurectomy for uncomplicated navicular disease were still not lame.[13] It is illegal in New York to race a horse with scars of neurectomy at or above the fetlock joint. The reason for the rule is that neurectomy in the metacarpus makes a horse dangerous to ride or drive and results in hopeless atrophic damage: exungulation, rupture of the deep flexor tendon, or fractures.

Blocking the palmar nerves above the fetlock joint will anesthetize most of the digit but not the fetlock joint or the skin on the dorsolateral and dorsomedial sides of the fetlock joint and proximal pastern, which are supplied by the palmar metacarpal nerves from the deep palmar branch of the ulnar nerve. The palmar metacarpal nerves can be blocked by superficial and deep injections at the ends of the splint bones (see Figs. 10–1 and 10–2).

Note the rich blood supply to the coronary region. The terminal part of the digital artery courses in the sole groove of P III. Observe the size and number of the veins in the coronary plexus. Plexuses of large veins cover both sides of the cartilage. The plexuses are connected by veins that perforate the cartilage.

The hoof is the common integument of the end of the digit. It includes the epidermis, which is cornified except for the deepest layers; the dermis (corium); and the subcutaneous tissue. In the part of the wall covering the distal phalanx there is no subcutaneous tissue because the dermis is fused with the periosteum. Under the coronary dermis the subcutaneous tissue is thickened to form the coronary cushion. The greatest development of the subcutaneous tissue is the digital cushion, divided in the horse into a part deep to the frog (cuneal part) and a bulbar part. The bulbs are the two soft, rounded prominences situated above and behind the frog. Together with the frog they form the digital pad (torus digitalis) of the horse.

Study the six areas of the dermis. These are local differentiations of the same general connective tissue layer, which is continuous with the dermis of the skin. For histological details see reference 19.

1. The perioplic dermis is a narrow band of light-colored papillae around the proximal edge of the dermis of the hoof. It is continuous with the dermis of the bulbs.

2. The coronary dermis is an extremely important part of the hoof. The epidermis that it nourishes produces the thick middle layer of the wall. The coronary dermis is pigmented when the hoof is dark and bears papillae 4 to 6 mm. long in the natural state. A wound of the coronary dermis and its covering epidermis results in a defect in the horny wall that eventually descends to the sole border. It can be repaired only by new growth downward from the healed epidermis on the coronary dermis. The rate varies from 4 mm. to 13.6 mm. per month, with an average of 8.25 mm. It is faster in hind hoofs, unshod hoofs, and certain horses.[8]

3. The laminar dermis suspends the distal phalanx from the inside of the wall. The 600 primary laminae of the dermis of each hoof bear about 100,000 secondary laminae with a total surface area of a square meter. These interlock with the primary and secondary epidermal laminae. The tension is thus transmitted from the horny wall through its primary laminae and the living cells of the epidermal secondary laminae to the dermal laminae and to the distal phalanx by means of connective tissue fibers that penetrate the bone.

The laminar dermis is covered by living epidermis, but this area produces only enough cells under normal conditions to maintain the adhesion between living and cornified epidermal cells as the wall grows distally. The horny laminae increase somewhat in height and thickness from their coronary origin to the sole.[4]

In laminitis the attachment of the living cells of the epidermal laminae to the horny laminae is disrupted, allowing the distal phalanx to be rotated on its transverse axis by the tension on the deep digital flexor tendon (supporting the fetlock), so that the dorsal surface of P III pulls away from the wall and the tip rests on the sole. The sole cannot support the weight and it "drops" or bulges toward the ground. The space between the wall and the epidermis remaining on the dermal laminae is filled with blood and transudate, which are gradually displaced by proliferating laminar epidermis. This cornifies, filling most of the space with abnormal horn. Some cavities may remain.

The normal dermal laminae are not pigmented, but the epidermis on the terminal papillae on their distal ends produces pigmented horn, continuous with the horny sole, which fills the gaps between the ends of the white horny laminae (see section 11f).

4. The dermis of the sole is pigmented and has long papillae.
5. The dermis of the bulbs is papillated like the perioplic dermis.
6. The dermis of the frog is pigmented and has fine papillae that produce wavy horn tubules.

11e. SAGITTAL SECTION, DIGIT, HORSE

Identify the following structures:

Common digital extensor tendon.

Cavities of the fetlock, pastern, and coffin joints. Relate the proximal and distal extremities of the capsules to external landmarks.

Periople, perioplic dermis.

Coronary, laminar, sole dermis.

Digital cushion.

Phalanges.

Superficial digital flexor tendon. Ends between the middle and distal thirds of P I at its bifurcation.

Deep digital flexor tendon.

Sesamoid bone.

Straight and oblique sesamoid ligaments.

Navicular bone.

Collateral ligaments of the navicular bone. These extend from the distal end of P I across P II to attach to the proximal border of the navicular bone, where the medial and lateral ligaments are continuous. Note the T-shaped section of the junction formed by the collateral ligaments of the navicular bone and the connective tissue between the deep flexor tendon and the back of P II.

Distal ligament of the navicular bone. Passes from the distal border of the navicular bone to the flexor surface of P III between the deep digital flexor tendon and the coffin joint.

The navicular bursa is between the deep face of the deep flexor tendon and the flexor surface of the navicular bone with its ligaments. On the articular side of the navicular bone is the coffin joint. Latex injected into the bursa will not pass through the navicular ligaments into the joint, nor will it pass in the reverse direction. The proximal palmar pouch of the joint capsule is in contact with the connective tissue that extends from the deep flexor to P II, and the pouch communicates through openings in the connective tissue with a proximal diverticulum that touches the distal end of the digital synovial sheath of the flexor tendons. Latex injected into the joint passes into the digital sheath only in foals.[5] In spite of their impermeability to latex, the membranes between these three synovial structures permit the diffusion of anesthetic solutions from one to the other.

This permeability complicates the differential diagnosis of navicular disease. It is important to know the source of pain that is relieved by palmar digital nerve block. It is usually navicular disease, which is the only indication for palmar digital neurectomy, but in some cases radiographs may also implicate arthrosis of the coffin joint. It is also possible that the lesion is in the bulb, palmar border, frog, or sole, which are also innervated by the palmar digital nerve. After the effect of the nerve block has worn off, injection of anesthetic into either the navicular bursa or the coffin joint (see section 11g) will relieve pain from both of them and thus eliminate the other structures of the sole and palmar digital regions from the diagnosis, but it will not differentiate between the joint and the bursa unless the palmar digital nerve block is negative. The latter combination of results indicates that the coffin joint alone is affected and is transmitting pain through the dorsal digital branch.[3, 12, 13, 15, 23] Table 11–1 summarizes the diagnosis of navicular disease.

Table 11–1. DIAGNOSIS OF NAVICULAR DISEASE

Site of Lesion	Pain Relieved By:	
	Palmar Digital Block	*Coffin Joint Injection*
Navicular Bursa	+	+
Coffin Joint	±	+
Bulb, Palmar Border, Frog, Sole	+	−

11f. CORNIFIED HOOF, HORSE

Interior Features.

Coronary groove. Most of the middle layer (stratum medium) of the wall is pigmented, but the deep part, next to the laminae, is not. The laminae are unpigmented. The deep, unpigmented part of the middle layer, plus the distal ends of the horny laminae, are the white components of the white zone on the ground surface.

Reflection of the wall at the palmar borders, forming the bars.

Spine of the frog.

Transverse Sections and Sole.

Dermis of the distal border of P III, highly vascular.

Part of the digital cushion in the crura of the frog.

The dark horn filling the spaces between the distal ends of the horny laminae in the white zone is produced by epidermis on the terminal papillae on the ends of the dermal laminae. Horseshoe nails are driven outside the white zone through the middle layer of the wall to avoid the sensitive laminae.

11g. LIVE HORSE

Palpate the following structures:

Proximal phalanx. Proximal and distal collateral tubercles, lateral and medial borders (see Plate I).

Cartilages of the hoof. The palmar borders of the cartilages are easily palpated above the hoof (see Plate I).

Bulbar parts of the digital cushion. Palpable inside the cartilages of the hoof behind the deep flexor tendon.

Digital annular ligaments. Normally, the edges of these ligaments are too thin to palpate, except for the proximal edge of the distal digital annular ligament where it crosses the deep flexor tendon. This is the lowest point of access to the digital synovial sheath of the flexor tendons.

Extensor tendon. The borders are too thin for actual palpation, but the tendon is about 4 cm. wide at the coronary border of the hoof.

Superficial flexor tendon. The terminations are behind the distal collateral tubercles of P I and on the proximal collateral tubercles of P II.

Deep flexor tendon. The edges are palpable from the branches of the superficial flexor to the digital cushion.

Oblique sesamoid ligaments. Not normally distinguishable. To examine for exostosis of the attachments of the oblique ligaments, raise the foot and palpate with both thumbs from the borders of P I to the palmar surface, in the grooves between the bone and flexor tendon (see Plate I).

Pastern joint. The articulation may be palpated on the dorsal, medial, and lateral surfaces, but the palmar surface is covered.

Collateral ligaments of the pastern joint. They may be palpated as they run vertically from the distal collateral tubercles of P I to the proximal collateral tubercles of P II at the proximal borders of the cartilages of the hoof. The proximal end of P II is wider than the distal end of P I. The attachments of the collateral ligaments, tendons, and joint capsule are subject to exostosis (high ringbone). This may also occur around the coffin joint (low ringbone). At the fetlock joint it is called an osselet.

Abaxial palmar ligaments of the pastern joint. The origins from the middle of the borders of P I are palpable. Exostosis may occur here.

Access to the fetlock joint from the distal approach. See the description in section 11b and palpate the structures.

Access to the pastern joint capsule. Palpate dorsally from the distal collateral tubercles of P I, along the articular line, to the border of the extensor tendon (2 cm from the dorsal midline of the digit). Direct the needle dorsally and axially under the extensor tendon.

Access to the coffin joint capsule. Insert the needle 1.5 cm. proximal to the coronary border of the hoof at the border of the extensor tendon. Direct the needle obliquely distally and axially.

Origins of the collateral ligaments of the navicular bone. They are dorsal to the collateral ligaments of the pastern joint, in and above the depressions dorsal to the distal collateral tubercles of P I.

Periople.

Wall and bars of the hoof.

White zone.

Frog, composed of two crura with paracuneal and central grooves.

Estimate the position of the navicular bone and coffin joint by means of the external features of the hoof (see section 11d).

Digital arteries. Palpate the pulse on the sesamoid bones. More distally the artery may be pressed into the groove between P I and the flexor tendons. Obstruction of at least one digital artery, usually the medial one, is common. The cause is thought to be trauma.[2]

Nerve blocks in the manus and pes for the diagnosis of lameness are performed medially and laterally, from distal to proximal, in the following order:

1. Palmar/plantar digital nerve block. This is done at the level of the pastern joint distal to the point where the nerve passes deep to the ligament of the ergot with the digital vessels. The nerve is palpable at the level of the middle of P I beside the flexor tendons. The ligament of the ergot is palpable if it is tensed by pulling on the ergot. The site is just proximal to the proximal border of the lateral cartilage. Only a small amount of anesthetic (1.5 to 2.5 ml.) should be injected to prevent diffusion dorsally to other nerve branches. An accurate injection will anesthetize the palmar/plantar and distal parts of the hoof and most of its contents, including the bulbs, digital cushion, frog, sole, palmar/plantar border, most of the laminar dermis, navicular bone and bursa, termination of the deep flexor tendon, P III, and most or all of the coffin joint. The region anesthetized is smaller in the hind limb because of the presence of the dorsal metatarsal nerves (Chapter 16), which innervate the dorsal parts of the pastern and coffin joints and the dorsal parts of the coronary and laminar dermis.

2. Nerve block at sesamoids. This block is useful only on the forelimb, where the metacarpal nerves do not reach the coffin joint. Block the palmar digital nerve and the dorsal branches where they are still coursing together on the abaxial surface of the proximal sesamoid. They can be palpated subcutaneously and are blocked at the level of the base of the sesamoid. This will anesthetize the entire digit distal to the fetlock joint, with the exception of an area of skin on the proximal dorsal surface of the pastern. If the palmar digital nerve block is negative and the nerve block at the sesamoids is positive, navicular disease is eliminated. Arthrosis of the coffin joint or pastern joint can be differentiated by the signs of pain remaining after the palmar digital nerve block and before the block at the sesamoids. Coffin joint pain comes from the level of the hoof, whereas pastern joint pain is elicited by direct palpation and manipulation. Radiographs or injection of anesthetic into the coffin joint with elimination of the lameness provide confirmation.

3. Distal metapodial (metacarpal/metatarsal) block. In the forelimb (see section 10b) at the level of the distal ends of the small metacarpal bones, block the palmar nerves between the interosseus and the deep digital flexor tendons. Block the palmar metacarpal nerves subcutaneously at the distal ends of the splint bones and deeply between the interosseus and large metacarpal bone. Medial and

lateral injections should meet in the middle of the palmar surface of the bone. This will anesthetize the entire digit including the fetlock joint, sesamoids, and sesamoid ligaments. An exception may be the proximal extension of the dorsal portion of the fetlock joint capsule.

In the hind limb, the plantar nerves and the plantar metatarsal nerves are blocked at the same site (see section 16c). In addition, the dorsal metatarsal nerves must be blocked on the medial and lateral surfaces of the large metatarsal bone just dorsal to the distal ends of the small metatarsals. This can be done from the same injection site used for the plantar metatarsals. This will anesthetize the entire digit as described for the forelimb.

4. Proximal metapodial (metacarpal/metatarsal) block. This block is done at the proximal end of the metapodium between the base of the small metapodial bones and the interosseus and digital flexor tendons. The nerves are covered by thick fascia and are not palpable. In the forelimb on the lateral side, this site is medial to the distal ligament of the accessory carpal bone. This will block the palmar/plantar nerves and the deep branch of the palmar branch of the ulnar nerve in the forelimb (see section 10b) and the deep branch of the lateral plantar nerve from the tibial nerve in the hind limb (see section 16c). These deep branches give rise to the palmar/plantar metapodial nerves. This block will anesthetize the entire digit in the forelimb and almost all of the structures on the palmar/plantar surface of the large metapodial bone. The accessory ligament of the deep digital flexor may be spared if it receives innervation from the carpus/tarsus where it arises. This will not anesthetize the dorsal surface of the metapodium and the anesthesia of the sides will result from concomitant infiltration of the overlying cutaneous nerves. The dorsal surface of the hind digit will not be anesthetized.

References

1. Adams, O. R.: Lameness in Horses, 3rd ed. Philadelphia; Lea & Febiger, 1974.
2. Bibrack, B.: Uber die formale und kausale Genese der Zehenarterienobliteration beim Pferd. Zbl. Vet. Med. A10 (1963):67–84.
3. Bolz, W.: Neurektomie der Volarnervenäste bei chronischer Podotrochlitis und anderen Hufkrankheiten. Tierärztl. Rundsch. 44 (1938):797–801, 813–816.
4. Budras, K. D. and F. Preuss: E/M Untersuchungen zur Hornbildung im Hyponychium des Pferdehufes. Prakt. Tierärzt. 60 (1979):729–731.
5. Calislar, T. and L. E. St. Clair: Observations on the navicular bursa and the distal interphalangeal joint cavity of the horse. JAVMA 154 (1969):410–412.
6. Colles, C. M. and J. Hickman: The arterial supply of the navicular bone and its variations in navicular disease. Equine Vet. J. 9 (1977):150–154.
7. Fackelman, G. E., J. A. Auer, J. Orsini, and B. von Salis: Surgical treatment of severe flexural deformity of the distal interphalangeal joint in young horses. JAVMA 182 (1983):949–952.
8. Lungwitz, A.: Über das Wachsthum und die Abreibung der Hornwand des Pferdehufes. Deutsche Zschr. f. Thiermed. 7 (1881):75–107.
9. Milne, F. J.: Clinical examination and diagnosis of the diseased equine foot. JAVMA 151 (1967):1599–1608.
10. Pohlmeyer, K.: Die arteriellen Versorgungsgefässe und deren intraossearer Verlauf in den Extremitätenknochen beim Pferdefohlen. IV Ossa digitorum manus. Deutsche tierärztl. Wschr. 86 (1979):113–119.
11. Rendano, V. T. and B. Grant: The equine third phalanx: its radiographic appearance. J. Am. Vet. Radiol. Soc. 14 (1978):125–136.
12. Sack, W. O.: Nerve distribution in the metacarpus and front digit of the horse. JAVMA 167 (1975):298–305.
13. Schebitz, H.: On navicular disease. Cornell Vet. 55 (1965):518–520.
14. Scott, E. A., M. McDole and M. H. Shires: A review of third phalanx fractures in the horse: sixty-five cases. JAVMA 174 (1979):1337–1343.
15. Seiferle, E.: Peripheres Nervensystem. In Nickel, A., A. Schummer, and E. Seiferle (eds.): Lehrbuch der Anatomie der Haustiere. Vol. 4. Berlin: Paul Parey, 1975, p. 214.
16. Shively, M. J.: Normal radiographic anatomy of the equine digit. J. Eq. Med. Surg. 2 (1978):77–84.
17. Stump, J. E.: Anatomy of the normal equine foot, including microscopic features of the laminar region. JAVMA 151 (1967):1588–1598.
18. Taylor, T. S. and J. T. Vaughan: Effects of denervation of the digit of the horse. JAVMA 177 (1980):1033–1039.
19. Trautmann, A. and J. Fiebiger: Fundamentals of the Histology of Domestic Animals. Habel, R. E. and E. L. Biberstein (trans.), Ithaca, N.Y.: Comstock, 1957.
20. Turner, T. A. and J. F. Fessler: The anatomic, pathologic, and radiographic aspects of navicular disease. Comp. Cont. Ed. 4 (1982):S350–S356.
21. Van Pelt, R. W.: Intra-articular injection of the equine carpus and fetlock. JAVMA 140 (1962):1181–1190.
22. Vukelic, E. and J. Marolt: Beitrag zur Kenntnis der aseptischen Podotrochlitis. Tierärztl. Umsch. 10 (1961):294–299.
23. Westhues, M.: Über das Wesen, die Diagnostik, und die Therapie der Podotrochlitis chronica des Pferdes. Berl. Münch. tierärztl. Wschr. (1938):781–785, 797–802.
24. Wintzer, H. J., and K. Dämmrich: Zur Bewertung des Röntgenbildes vom Strahlbein des Pferdes in der Lahmheitsdiagnostik. Schweiz. Arch. Tierheilkd. 112 (1970):471–479.
25. Wintzer, H. J. and K. Dämmrich: Untersuchungen zur Pathogenese der sog. Strahlbeinlahmheit des Pferdes. Berl. Münch. tierärztl. Wschr. 84 (1971):221–225.
26. Zietzschmann, O. and O. Krölling: Lehrbuch der Entwicklungsgeschichte der Haustiere, 2nd ed. Berlin: Paul Parey, 1955.

CHAPTER 12

DIGIT, OX, DOG, AND CAT

OBJECTIVES

A. Surgical anatomy of the bovine digit
   1. To be able to palpate the landmarks of the pastern joint. The recommended site of amputation is through the middle of P I.
   2. To know the tendons and ligaments cut in amputation.
   3. To be able to palpate the distal interdigital ligament in the standing cow and to avoid it in minor surgery of the interdigital space.
   4. To understand the relations of the synovial structures of the digits in connection with purulent infections.
   5. To know the course of the main artery of the digit and where it is cut in amputation.
B. Anatomy of hoof trimming in cattle
   1. To understand the characteristic structure of the horn of the parts of the bovine hoof and the difference between bulb and sole.
   2. To understand the differences between the horse and cow in the laminar dermis and in hoof adhesion.
   3. To understand the pathology of the deep structures of the digit caused by overgrowth of the hoof.
   4. To be able to judge the amount of horn to remove in order to restore the normal angle of the hoof at the toe and the normal thickness of the ground surface.
C. Surgical anatomy of the digit in the cat and dog
   1. To be able to locate the joints and phalanges by palpation.
   2. To be able to avoid the main artery of the digit in removal of a broken phalanx.
   3. To be able to remove the claws of the cat effectively.
D. Anatomy of claw trimming in the dog
   1. To know the extent of the sensitive tissue inside the claw.
   2. To understand the regional characteristics of the claw dermis and their effect on claw growth.
   3. To be able to use the claw trimmer painlessly by correct application of the shearing force.

12a. SKELETON AND RADIOGRAPHS OF DIGIT, OX

Study the bones with the ligamentous preparations (Fig. 12–1).

Proximal Phalanx

Axial proximal collateral tubercles. The interdigital phalangosesamoid ligaments pass from the sesamoid bones of one digit to the axial tubercle of P I of the other digit.

Rough area in the proximal half of the axial surface for attachment of the proximal interdigital ligament.

Depression on the distal end of the axial surface for the common collateral ligament of the pastern and coffin joints.

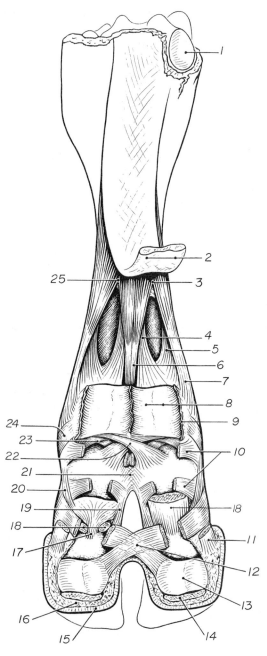

Figure 12–1. Palmar aspect of right forefoot, cow. *1*, ulnar carpal bone; *2*, bands from interossei to branches of superficial flexor tendon; *3*, interosseus IV; *4*, axial tendon, *5*, abaxial tendon, *6*, axial extensor branch, *7*, abaxial extensor branch, of interosseus IV; *8*, proximal sesamoid bones; *9*, palmar annular ligament; *10*, annular ligaments of digit; *11*, ligament of dewclaw; *12*, distal interdigital ligament; *13*, distal sesamoid (navicular) bone; *14*, termination of deep flexor muscle; *15*, dermis of hoof; *16*, digital cushion; *17*, central palmar ligament of pastern joint; *18*, terminations of superficial flexor, stump remains on fourth digit; *19*, axial palmar ligament of pastern joint; *20*, abaxial palmar ligament of pastern joint; *21*, proximal interdigital ligament; *22*, interdigital phalangosesamoid ligaments; *23*, cruciate sesamoid ligaments; *24*, collateral sesamoid ligament; *25*, interosseus III.

Middle Phalanx

Large abaxial collateral tubercle of the proximal end of P II. The superficial part of the distal interdigital ligament originates here.

Flexor tuberosity on proximal end of palmar surface for attachment of palmar ligaments of pastern joint and termination of superficial digital flexor.

Deep depression on the axial surface at the distal end for the axial collateral ligament of the coffin joint, which is especially strong. It may cause difficulty in amputation through the coffin joint.

Distal Phalanx

Depression distal to the articular margin on the axial surface, for attachment of the axial collateral ligament of the coffin joint and the axial common collateral ligament of the pastern and coffin joints.

Large foramen on the axial side of the extensor process. The axial foramen receives the axial palmar digital artery.

Navicular bone, where fibers of the distal interdigital ligament are attached, as well as collateral and distal ligaments of the navicular bone.

Radiographs

Identify the distal end of the metacarpal bone, phalanges, sesamoids, and the articulations in the dorsopalmar and lateromedial views.[13] On the dorsopalmar view, identify:

Sagittal ridge of each head of the metacarpal bone, articulating with the groove in the base of P I.

Proximal abaxial collateral tubercle of P I and P II.

Sagittal ridge of the base of P II, articulating with the groove in the head of P I.

Flexor tubercle of P III.

Distal sesamoid superimposed over distal P II.

Vascular channels and foramina in P III.

Rudimentary phalanges may be evident in the dewclaws at the level of the fetlock joint.

12b. LIGAMENTOUS PREPARATIONS, DIGITS, OX

Cruciate sesamoid ligaments. They attach the distal ends of the sesamoid bones to the proximal end of P I of the same digit.

Interdigital phalangosesamoid ligaments. They pass from the distal ends of the sesamoid bones of one digit to the axial tubercle of P I of the other digit.

Proximal interdigital ligament. This short, thick ligament connects the proximal halves of the proximal phalanges (Fig. 12–1).

Ligaments of the dewclaws. These are parts of the digital fascia. They attach the second and fifth digits in lieu of any skeletal connections. The proximal ones come from the deep metacarpal fascia, and the distal ones (palpable) are attached to the abaxial side of P III and to the navicular bone (see Fig. 10–5).

Collateral ligaments of the pastern joint. They are difficult to distinguish from overlying tendons.

Palmar ligaments of the pastern joint include an abaxial, an axial, and a central ligament.

The common collateral ligament is clearly seen on the axial side of the digit. It extends from the depression on the distal end of P I, receives fibers from P II, and ends distal to the articular margin of P III (see Fig. 10–6). The corresponding abaxial ligament is weak.

The elastic dorsal ligament, from the axial surface of the proximal end of P II, passes deep to the common collateral ligament and is attached to the extensor process of P III. This is a homologue of the dorsal ligaments that keep the claws of Carnivora raised.

The distal interdigital ligament (see Figs. 10–5, 10–6, and 12–1). The deep part goes directly across the interdigital space from the axial side of the distal end of P II to the opposite P III and navicular bone. The superficial part extends from the abaxial tubercle on the proximal end of P II, around the back of the deep flexor tendon, to the navicular bone of the other digit. The superficial part is analogous to the distal digital annular ligament of the horse.

Common or long extensor tendon. The branches go to the extensor process of P III of each large digit (see Fig. 10–3).

Medial and lateral (proper) digital extensor tendons. These terminate primarily on the proximal end,of P II, partially on P III. The proper extensors receive the extensor branches of the interossei (see Fig. 10–4).

Superficial flexor tendon. Each branch terminates on the flexor tuberosity on the palmar surface of the proximal end of P II.

Deep flexor tendon. Surrounded by the superficial digital flexor tendon at the fetlock joint, passes over the flexor surface of the navicular bone at the coffin joint, and terminates on the thick proximal end of the sole surface of P III, the flexor tubercle. A navicular bursa is located between the tendon and the navicular bone.

The digital flexor tendons are supported by the palmar annular ligament at the fetlock joint and digital annular ligaments on the palmar aspect of P I. The deep digital flexor is also supported by the superficial part of the distal interdigital ligament.

Interdigital communication occurs between the fetlock joint capsules and sometimes between the digital synovial sheaths of the flexor tendons.[14]

The digital flexor tendons function in preventing overextension of the fetlock and interphalangeal joints. In addition, overextension of the fetlock joint is prevented by the interosseus muscle and its terminations on the sesamoid bones and the proper digital extensor tendon and by the distal sesamoid ligaments that attach to P I. Overextension of the pastern joint is resisted by the palmar ligaments. At the coffin joint, the navicular bone and its ligamentous attachments resist overextension. Separation of the digits is prevented by the interdigital ligaments—distal, proximal, and phalangosesamoid. Within each digit the larger collateral ligaments on the axial side resist abaxial movement of the distal bone at the pastern and coffin joints. These axial and interdigital ligaments also protect the joints from penetrating objects.

12c. DISSECTION, DIGITS, OX

Observe the position of the distal interphalangeal articulation with respect to the coronary border of the hoof (see Fig. 10–4). When the hoof is amputated by sawing in a straight line through the coffin joint, the extensor process of P III or the navicular bone or both may be left in the stump and should be dissected out. This method of amputation has fallen into disfavor because it leaves a large blocky stump close to the ground, where it is constantly injured.

The perioplic dermis is a narrow band at the proximal border of the hoof. The coronary dermis is relatively wider than that of the horse, extending about halfway down the wall (see Fig. 10–5). The laminae are correspondingly short in comparison with those in the horse and have no secondary laminae. Therefore, the surface area for adhesion of the horny hoof is smaller than that in the horse, and less of the weight is born by suspension of the distal phalanx. A larger share of the weight is born by the bulb. Nevertheless, in bovine chronic laminitis the laminae separate, and the distal phalanx is rotated or "dropped."

Nerves

Observe the course of the nerves in the digits (see Figures 10–3 to 10–6). Anesthesia of the digits is discussed in Chapter 10. There is no indication for injection of the nerves distal to the fetlock joints in the ox.

1. Axial dorsal digital nerves. These result from the bifurcation of the small dorsal common digital nerve III lying on the common or long extensor tendon. These nerves are joined by communicating branches from the axial palmar digital nerves at the level of the pastern joints.

In the pelvic limb the dorsal metatarsal nerve joins the dorsal common digital nerve III in the interdigital space before the latter divides into axial dorsal digital nerves.

2. Abaxial dorsal nerve of digit IV crosses the sesamoid bone dorsal to the abaxial palmar digital vein.

3. Abaxial palmar nerve of digit IV crosses the sesamoid bone behind the vein and superficial to the abaxial palmar digital artery; it supplies the deep structures of the bulb and the abaxial dermis.

4. Axial palmar digital nerves run on both sides of the palmar common digital artery III between the dewclaws. These nerves give off the interdigital communicating branches to the axial dorsal nerves and continue to the axial dermis.

5. Abaxial palmar nerve of digit III. This nerve has the same course as the abaxial palmar nerve of digit IV. It passes deep to the distal ligament of the medial dewclaw and goes to the abaxial surface of the third phalanx. Note that the four palmar nerves are much larger and are distributed to a greater area than the dorsal nerves.

6. Abaxial dorsal nerve of digit III has the same course as the abaxial dorsal nerve of digit IV.

Arteries

Examine the arteries of the digits (see Figs. 10–3 to 10–6).

1. The dorsal metacarpal artery III is very small and of no surgical significance. It lies in the groove on the dorsal surface of the metacarpal bone, covered by tendons and deep fascia. In the interdigital space it joins the palmar common digital artery III, which is the major source of blood to the digits.

2. The abaxial palmar artery of digit IV runs across the sesamoid bone deep to the nerve and continues on the abaxial palmar border of the digit to the bulb. It enters the foramen on the abaxial side of the palmar process of P III. The anastomosis with the palmar common digital artery is easily broken.

3. The abaxial palmar artery of digit III occupies the corresponding position.

4. The palmar common digital artery III is the main supply to both digits. It arises from the median artery, which passes distally on the medial surface of the digital flexor tendons. The palmar common digital artery III passes superficially over the palmar surface of the medial branches of the digital flexor tendons at the fetlock joints and runs into the space between the branches of the flexor tendons, deep to the nerves. A palmar branch emerges between the nerves and supplies the dewclaws. At this level, palmar branches to P I of digits III and IV originate from the sides of the palmar common digital artery and pass deep to the flexor tendons, between the annular ligaments, to join the abaxial palmar digital arteries. The common digital artery bifurcates proximal to the pastern joint, forming the axial palmar arteries of digits III and IV. The palmar common digital artery is vulnerable to injury during amputation at the middle of P I. It is important to keep the cutting instrument close to the digit being amputated to avoid the axial palmar digital artery of the opposite digit. Near the bifurcation, each artery gives off a bulbar branch, which passes backward, supplying the bulb and anastomosing with the abaxial palmar digital artery. The axial palmar digital artery continues forward in the interdigital space, gives a branch to the dermis, passes deep to the common collateral ligament, and enters the foramen on the axial side of the extensor process of P III. It forms the terminal arch in the sole canal, where it anastomoses with the abaxial palmar digital artery and supplies the dermis on P III.

The axial palmar digital artery appears to be the only large artery cut in amputation at the level of the coffin joint. It will be observed, however, that a great many small vessels are exposed in the cut edge of the dermis.

How many ligations of large arteries would be necessary in amputating through the middle of P I? This is the preferred site for amputation of a digit. The bone is beveled by pulling a wire saw proximally and abaxially, leaving a smooth surface that can be entirely covered by skin flaps.

Substantial veins accompany each of the arteries just discussed.

Pelvic Limb. The arteries of the digits in the pelvic limb are similiar to those of the thoracic limb except that the main source of arterial blood is the dorsal metatarsal artery from the dorsal pedal and cranial tibial arteries. The dorsal metatarsal artery courses distally in the groove on the dorsal surface of the metatarsal bone into the interdigital space, receives a communication from the small plantar common digital artery III, and bifurcates into the axial plantar arteries of digits III and IV (see Fig. 16–5) that have a distribution similiar to the axial palmar digital arteries in the forelimb.

12d. SAGITTAL SECTION, DIGIT, COW

Identify the phalanges and observe that the sole surface of P III is normally parallel to the ground and the pastern joint is. slightly flexed. Identify the coffin joint cavity, navicular bone, navicular bursa, and the pastern joint cavity (Fig. 12–2). Note the relationship of the coffin joint to the proximal border of the hoof wall.

Identify the termination of the deep flexor tendon on the prominent flexor tubercle of P III and the termination of the superficial flexor on the flexor tuberosity of P II.

The digital cushion is thickest in the base of the bulb. It extends between the bulbar dermis and the bone to the middle of the sole surface of P III, marking the apex of the bulb. The rest of P III is surrounded by very vascular sole dermis, laminar dermis, and coronary dermis.

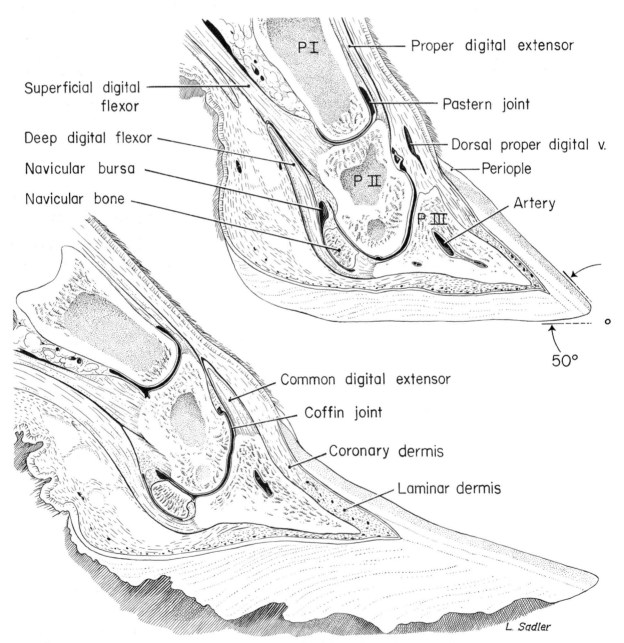

Figure 12–2. Sagittal sections of the digit of the thoracic limb, cow. Normal digit in standing position, cut abaxial to extensor process of P III. Overgrown hoof, digit slightly flexed and cut through extensor process of P III.

The large vessel inside P III is the terminal arch of the axial palmar digital artery. It supplies the dermis by branches that pass out through the bone.

The wall of the hoof grows distally at the rate of 4.7 mm. per month in adults and 5.9 mm. in calves.[11] Normal growth and wear maintain an angle of about 50° between the dorsal border of the wall and the ground in the forelimb and 45° in the hind limb. If the animal is stabled on manure, wear is prevented, the wall grows long, the angle becomes more acute, and the toe turns up. The elevation of the toe overextends the coffin joint, raising the tip of P III so that its sole surface is at an angle of 8 to 28° from the ground. This places great tension on the deep digital flexor. The change in position of P III causes inflammation of the dermis by tension and pressure. The weight is rocked back on the bulbs, putting pressure on the navicular bones and the soft tissue of the bulbs. The cow adopts a sickle-hocked stance, which is bad for her conformation rating if she is purebred; lies down as much as possible; consumes less feed; and produces less milk. In some animals the abaxial border of the wall is pried away from the sole by the overgrowth, causing a separation at the white zone and infection of the dermis.

The growth of horn on the sole surface also builds up. Bulbar horn is softer, has more inter-tubular cells than the wall, and tends to be separated in layers by the action of the alkaline fluids of manure. The resulting fissures often penetrate obliquely upward to the bulbar dermis, causing infections.

The shape of P III is changed by the pressure of the coronary border of the wall, sometimes causing atrophy of the extensor process. Exostosis occurs at the termination of the deep flexor. Many other changes in the bones, joints, ligaments, and tendons result from overgrowth of the hoofs.[10]

12e. CORNIFIED HOOF, OX

Observe the following structures:

The junction of the wall with the periople (see Fig. 12–3). Some of the periople may have been destroyed in removing the hoof.

The width of the coronary groove. It is really too shallow to be called a groove. The holes formed by the papillae are minute. As in the horse, the wall is composed of hard, mostly tubular horn.

The small laminae.

The periople is continuous with the bulbar horn. The base of the bulb is demarcated from the wall by a deep oblique axial groove and a less distinct abaxial groove. The horn is thinnest along the axial groove. Observe the relationship of the proximal end of the axial groove to the navicular bursa and coffin joint.

The apex of the bulb extends forward about two thirds of the length of the ground surface of the hoof, but if the surface is worn smooth, the apex of the bulb is not distinguishable from the sole on the outside. The bulb varies greatly in thickness with the amount of wear. When overgrown, it is stratified, fissured, and undermined by disintegration of the horn. The true sole is the harder smooth horn between the apex of the bulb and the white zone. It consists of a body and axial and abaxial crura, embracing the apex of the bulb. The crura terminate as the angles of the sole at the axial and abaxial grooves. The white zone is marked by the distal ends of the laminae.

12f. DIGIT, LIVE COW

Palpate the following structures:

Proximal collateral tubercle of P I (see Plate II).

Distal ligament of the dewclaw.

Distal interdigital ligament.

Flexor tendons. These are best palpated on the axial border of the digit.

Common extensor tendon.

Proper extensor tendon. The foot must be raised and flexed and extended. The termination of the tendon on the mid-dorsal extensor process of P II can be palpated about 3 cm. above the coronary border of the hoof.

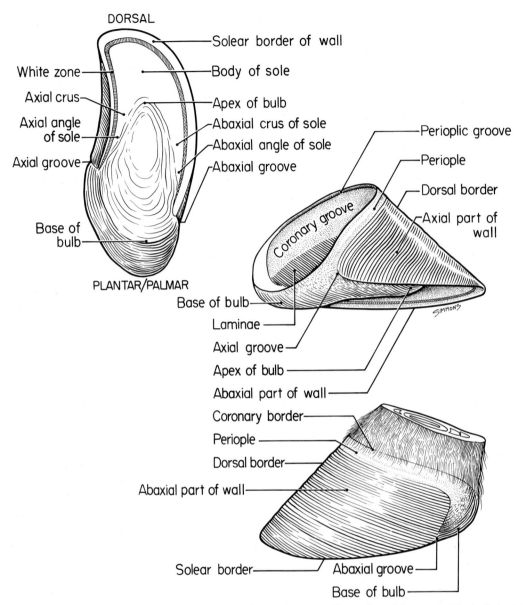

Figure 12–3. Three views of the lateral hoof of the left hind foot, cow. The outline of the apex of the bulb is determined by the extent of the digital cushion inside the hoof and by the amount of wear. It may not be visible on the surface.

Pastern joint. Marked by the extensor process and the prominent abaxial collateral tubercle of P II. These are important landmarks for amputation through P I (see Plate II).

Estimate the position of the coffin joint. The extensor process of P III extends proximally as far as the coronary border of the hoof. The most distal part of the curve of the head of P II is about 2 cm. distal to the coronary border of the hoof.

Trace the periople to the bulb and to the interdigital space, where it is continuous with the periople of the other hoof.

Estimate the position of the apex and the abaxial margin of P III. How much of the toe and abaxial part of the wall can be removed in trimming without endangering the dermis? The normal angle between the dorsal border of the wall and the sole is about 50° in the forelimb and 45° in the hind limb. The normal ratio of the length of the dorsal border to the height of the hoof at the bulb is 2:1. When the hoof is overgrown, the angle is decreased. Cattle stabled continuously on soft moist bedding or manure should have 2 to 5 cm. of wall trimmed off twice a year. The sole surface should be shaved down until it is smooth and the horn yields slightly to thumb pressure (see Fig. 12–2).

Lameness due to hoof lesions is more common in the hind limb. These lesions are more common in the medial hoof of the forelimb and in the lateral hoof of the hind limb.[12]

Consider the posture assumed by the cow in painful conditions of one digit. Fractures of the distal phalanx occur more often in the forelimb. If the fracture is in the third (medial) digit, the affected foot is placed before the other. If bilateral fractures of the third digits are present, the feet are crossed. If the fourth digit is affected, the limb is abducted.[16] The same mechanism operates in laminitis. Usually the third digits of the forefeet and the fourth digits of the hind feet are more painful.[9]

In a sheep, observe the opening of the interdigital sinus between the proximal phalanges. It is the opening of a bent cutaneous tube lined by glands that secrete into its lumen.

12g. BONES OF THE DIGIT AND DISSECTION OF THE PAW, DOG AND CAT

Note the location of the largest artery that supplies the digit. It lies on the axial side of the palmar surface. The other three digital arteries are minute. The position of the main artery of the digit is the same in the cat, although it has a different origin, as described in section 10g. When it is necessary to amputate a digit, the pad should be preserved, if possible, by removing the bones from an incision on the dorsal surface.

Observe the position of the digital pads. They support the distal interphalangeal joints. At rest, the digital axis is broken by flexion at the proximal interphalangeal joint and by overextension at the distal joint. The digital pad is homologous to the bulb and frog in the horse.

The elastic dorsal ligaments are of little clinical importance, but they are interesting in that they oppose the action of the deep digital flexor, keeping the claws raised off the ground in ordinary walking. In the dog, the ligaments are attached to the tubercles on the proximal end of the middle phalanx and inserted mid-dorsally on the unguicular crest of P III.

In the cat, the elastic ligaments are more complex.[17] A short thick dorsal ligament extends from the lateral side of the distal end of P II to the dorsal part of the unguicular crest of P III. Long thin dorsal ligaments run from the proximal interphalangeal joint to the sides of the base of the unguicular process. There are also palmar (plantar) elastic ligaments from the deep surface of the deep flexor tendon to the distal end of P II. These ligaments pull the deep flexor tendon distally when the muscle is relaxed so that the terminal part of the tendon pushes P III into overextension, aiding the dorsal ligaments in retraction of the claw. The articular surface of the distal end of P II is oblique and beveled and extends laterally so that the dorsal ligaments pull P III to the lateral side of P II, "sheathing the claw." Examine the skeleton to see the relation of each P III to P II. The digital extensor tendons have their primary insertion on P II and do not act to overextend the distal interphalangeal joint in the cat. The resistance of the elastic ligaments permits flexion of the carpal, metacarpophalangeal, and proximal interphalangeal joints without protrusion of the claw. Co-contraction of both flexor and extensor muscles is necessary for protrusion of the claws.[6] The extensors fix the metacarpophalangeal and proximal interphalangeal joints, permitting flexion at the distal interphalangeal joint, which protrudes the claw.

The main part of the horny claw corresponds to the wall of the equine hoof. It grows in a curve because more horn is produced on the dorsal surface than on the sides. This mechanism also keeps the claw sharp as it wears. The soft horn in the cavity between the thin margins of the wall is the sole. Note the unguicular crest of P III. This shelf of bone overlaps the proximal margin of the claw. Note the length of the unguicular process of P III. The dermis of the tip of this process is often injured in clipping the claws. This is painful and an unnecessary exposure to infection. Although the resulting hemorrhage can be stopped in the office, it may recur in the home. Damage to the dermis can be avoided with a minimal knowledge of anatomy. If unpigmented claws are transilluminated, the vascular dermis and the artery in the unguicular process color the danger zone pink. In cutting pigmented claws, the unguicular process can be avoided by keeping the cutting blade parallel to the palmar surface of the base of the claw or parallel to the ground surface. The curvature of the horny

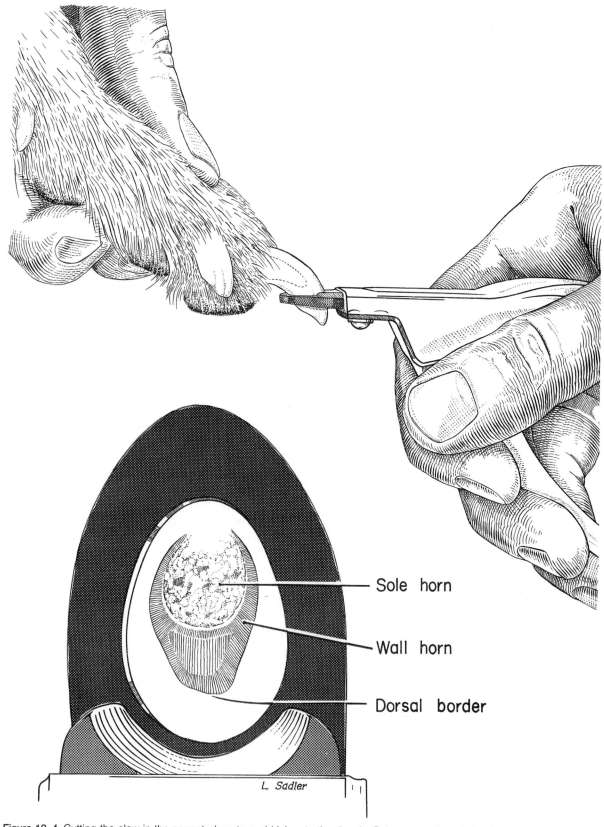

Sole horn

Wall horn

Dorsal border

L. Sadler

Figure 12–4. Cutting the claw in the correct plane to avoid injury to the dermis. Below: a section of claw in the instrument.

claw is much greater than the curvature of the unguicular process because of the faster growth of horn on the dorsal surface. Much pain can be avoided if the cutting edge of the guillotine claw clipper moves through the claw in the dorsopalmar direction rather than from side to side. When the claw is cut from side to side the soft sole horn presents no resistance to the sides of the wall when they are pinched together. The pressure is transmitted to the sensitive dermis between the wall and the unguicular process (Fig. 12–4).

In the operation for declawing the cat it is necessary to remove all of the unguicular crest to prevent regrowth of the claw.[8] This is usually done with the guillotine type of claw clipper. The joint is flexed by the operator to expose the claw. Some operators prefer to place the clipper so that the base of the distal phalanx is preserved with the collateral ligaments of the joint and the insertion of the deep flexor. This also preserves the digital pad. Others prefer to remove all of P III to avoid a possible sequestrum.[4]

12h. ANGIOGRAM

The axial palmar digital artery enters the distal phalanx and extends to the end of the unguicular process. Observe the relation of the end of the unguicular process to the end of the claw and the difference in curvature between them. Epiphyseal fusion in the phalanges is discussed in section 10h.

12i. DIGIT, LIVE DOG, CAT

Palpate the relationship between the digital pad and the distal interphalangeal joint. Define the extremities of the first and second phalanges (see Plate III).

Find the demarcation between the wall and the sole of the claw. Estimate the extent of the sensitive tissues into the tip of the claw. This is easily determined in unpigmented claws by transillumination and in pigmented claws by projection of the plane of the palmar/plantar surface of the base of the claw. In the cat, flex the distal interphalangeal joint to expose the claw. This must be done to position P III for removal in the declawing procedure.

References

1. Burns, J. and J. Cornell: Angiography of the caprine digit. Vet. Radiol. *22*(1981):174–176.
2. Estill, C. T.: Intravenous local analgesia of the bovine lower leg. Vet. Med.—Small Anim. Clin. *72* (1977):1499–1502.
3. Fowler, M. E.: Hoof, claw, and nail problems in nondomestic animals. JAVMA *177*(1980):885–893.
4. Fowler, M. E. and S. E. McDonald: Untoward effects of onychectomy in wild felids and ursids. JAVMA *181*(1982):1242–1245.
5. Gogi, S. N., J. M. Nigam, and A. P. Singh: Angiographic evaluation of bovine foot abnormalities. Vet. Radiol. *23*(1982):171–174.
6. Gonyea, W. and R. Ashworth: The form and function of retractile claws in the felidae and other representative carnivorans. J. Morphol. *145*(1975):229–238.
7. Greenough, P. R., F. J. MacCallum, and A. D. Weaver: Lameness in Cattle, 2nd ed. Philadelphia: Lippincott, 1981.
8. Herron, M. R.: Declawing the cat. Mod. Vet. Pract. *48* No. 10 (1967):40–43.
9. Maclean, C. W.: Observations on acute laminitis in cattle. Vet. Rec. *77*(1965):662–672.
10. Pohly, W.: Die Stallklauen der Rinder. Arch Tierheilk. *44*(1918):39–66.
11. Prentice, D. E.: Growth and wear rates of hoof horn in Ayrshire cattle. Res. Vet. Sci. *14*(1973):285–290.
12. Rebhun, W. C. and E. G. Pearson: Clinical management of bovine foot problems. JAVMA *181*(1982):572–577.
13. Shively, M. J. and J. E. Smallwood: Normal radiographic and xeroradiographic anatomy of the bovine manus. Bovine Pract. *14*(1979):74–82.
14. Sisson, S. and J. D. Grossman: The Anatomy of the Domestic Animals. Philadelphia: W. B. Saunders, 1955.
15. West, D. M.: Anatomical considerations of the distal interphalangeal joint of sheep. New Zeal. Vet. J. *31*(1983):58–60.
16. Wintzer, H. J.: Bedekte klauwbeenfracturen bij het rund. Tijdsch. diergeneesk. *86*(1961):455–461.
17. Wünsche, A. and F. Preuss: Zur Mechanik des Krallengelenks der Katze. Zool. Beitr. *18*(1972):91–100.

CHAPTER 13

HIP AND THIGH

OBJECTIVES

1. To be able to palpate the tuber coxae, tuber sacrale, tuber ischiadicum, and trochanter major in the horse. These landmarks are useful in the diagnosis of dislocations and fractures.
2. To be able to diagnose trochanteric bursitis in the horse by observation of the stance, gait, and response to palpation and manipulation.
3. To be able to palpate the medial saphenous vein in the horse or cow. The vein is a landmark for the saphenous nerve. The saphenous artery is convenient for taking the pulse in the cow.
4. To be able to recognize the caudal thigh muscles and their fascial sheaths in connection with the drainage of abscesses. To appreciate the extensor function of these muscles and the strain it places on sutures in them.
5. To understand the clinical signs associated with fibrotic ossifying myopathy.
6. To be able to palpate the subiliac (prefemoral) lymph nodes in the horse and cow.
7. To be able to insert a needle into the hip joint in the horse and dog.
8. To be able to find the sciatic lymph node in the split bovine carcass without mutilating the quarter.
9. To be able to avoid the sciatic nerve in operations on the hip joint and in injections into the caudal thigh muscles in small animals, calves, young pigs, and small ruminants.
10. To know the centers of ossification in the pelvis and femur of the dog.
11. To understand the mechanical effect of the origin of the gastrocnemius on the displacement of the fragments of the femur in the dog.
12. To be able to make a prognosis for the viability of the head of the femur in fractures of the proximal end of the femur.
13. To be able to determine the direction of luxation of the head of the femur of the dog and cat by manipulation.
14. To be able to gain surgical access to the canine hip joint from the dorsal, cranial, caudal, or ventral approach.
15. To be able to insert a needle into the femoral vein in the dog.
16. To be able to diagnose paralyses and sensory deficits caused by injury to the four main nerves of the hind limb.
17. To understand the cause of peroneal paralysis associated with calving.
18. To be able to recognize hip laxity by palpation.

Nerves of the Pelvic Limb

A general knowledge of the origin and distribution of the four clinically important nerves of the hind limb is necessary for the diagnosis of injuries to the spinal cord and nerves.[19, 23, 27] There is

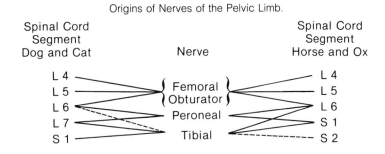

Origins of Nerves of the Pelvic Limb.

considerable variation between individuals, and the lines drawn in the diagram are only indications of the major spinal nerve contributions.

The following clinical signs are associated with loss of function of the nerves listed.[45, 48]

Femoral Nerve. Section of this nerve paralyzes the quadriceps femoris, resulting in collapse of the stifle and therefore in total lack of support of the limb. No compensation occurs. The sartorius is also paralyzed. There is a sensory deficit in the field of the saphenous nerve on the medial surface of the limb, extending to the paw or fetlock. In the dog, the contribution of the ventral branch of the fifth lumbar nerve is the most important for preservation of the patellar reflex.[47]

The femoral nerve courses through the psoas major muscle to enter the quadriceps and is protected from fragments of fractured bones. Femoral nerve paralysis occurs in beef calves that require assistance at birth because of a hip or stifle lock.[44] Excessive extension of the hips causes contusion or tearing of the femoral nerve, usually where it enters the quadriceps muscle.

Obturator Nerve. The muscles supplied comprise the adductor group: external obturator, pectineus, adductors, and gracilis. Section in the dog results in a marked inability to prevent the paw from slipping laterally on a smooth surface. Bilateral section causes the animal to go down in a split. The effect is not noticeable on a nonskid surface. Adult cattle are usually able to stand and walk after avulsion of both obturator nerves if they have good footing. On slippery concrete they will go down, with the hind limbs abducted and flexed.[13]

Peroneal Nerve. Transection of this branch of the sciatic nerve results in some extension of the hock and an inability to extend the digits. The foot often rests on the dorsal surface of the flexed digits. If the foot is placed on the plantar surface, the limb supports weight, as in distal radial nerve paralysis. In peroneal nerve paralysis, the animal learns to compensate by flipping the foot forward so that it lands properly, but only if the tibial nerve is intact. Apparently the tibial nerve conducts the necessary proprioceptive impulses.[5] There is a sensory deficit on the craniolateral surface of the crus and the dorsal surface of the metatarsus and digits (see Fig. 13–1).

Peroneal paralysis is fairly common in the cow after difficult parturition.[13, 14, 16] At least half of the peroneal nerve is derived from the sixth lumbar nerve, which emerges between the last lumbar and the first sacral vertebrae and must pass through the pelvic inlet to reach the sacral plexus. Compression of the nerve against the wing of the sacrum during parturition will cause this paralysis. Avulsion of the obturator and sixth lumbar nerves bilaterally produces signs similar to calving paralysis with flexed fetlock joints.[15]

The peroneal nerve crosses the proximal end of the fibula, where it can also be compressed if that limb is down in lateral recumbency and pressed against the edge of the gutter or other hard surface.

Tibial Nerve. Section of this branch of the sciatic nerve causes a marked change in gait by paralyzing the extensors of the hock and the flexors of the digits. The hock flexes in a sickle-hocked posture when bearing weight. In the dog, the tuber calcis will be closer to the ground when the limb is bearing weight. In the cat, the entire plantar surface of the paw will be on the ground. The claws are elevated in the dog. In the cow, the flexion of the hock with the foot on the ground produces a

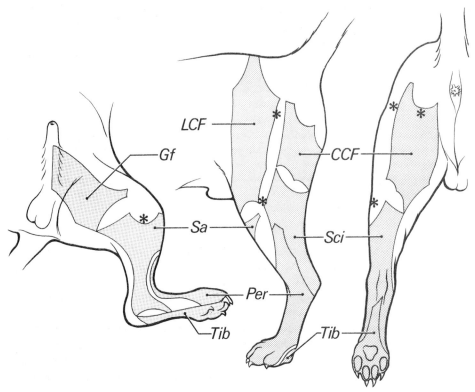

Figure 13–1. Autonomous zones of the cutaneous innervation of the canine pelvic limb. Caudal cutaneous femoral *(CCF)*, genitofemoral *(Gf)*, lateral cutaneous femoral *(LCF)*, peroneal *(Per)*, saphenous *(Sa)*, sciatic *(Sci)*, tibial *(Tib)*. Asterisks indicate palpable bony landmarks—medial and lateral tibial condyles, greater trochanter, and lateral end of tuber ischiadicum.[30] The sciatic nerve autonomous zone is for lesions proximal to the greater trochanter and includes the zones for the peroneal and tibial nerves. For sciatic nerve lesions caudal to the femur, the autonomous zone varies depending on how many of its cutaneous branches are affected.

peculiar flexion of the fetlock; this joint buckles forward and the pastern becomes vertical. The sensory deficit is on the plantar surface of the metatarsus and digits (Fig. 13–1).

Sciatic Nerve. Transection at the greater sciatic foramen causes paralysis of the caudal thigh muscles and all the muscles of the joints below the stifle. The limb does not collapse when weight is borne on it because the stifle is fixed by the quadriceps, but the limb is very unstable. The hock passively flexes and extends, and the animal stands on the dorsal surface of the flexed digits. There is no sensation below the stifle, except on the medial surface. Noxious stimulation of the fifth digit of the dog or cat will not elicit a reflex or pain perception because of the interference with sensory neurons. Stimulation of the medial side of the metatarsus will elicit a pain response and flexion of the hip but not the stifle, tarsus, or digits. This is mediated through the saphenous nerve, lumbar spinal cord segments and lumbar nerves to the psoas major and rectus femoris muscles that flex the hip. Do not confuse hip flexion with a normal flexor response of the pelvic limb. Injury to the sciatic nerve in the caudal thigh distal to its innervation of the caudal thigh muscles will not abolish flexion of the stifle.

Common sites and causes of injury to the sciatic nerve or the spinal nerves that form it include: fracture of the seventh lumbar vertebra, sacroiliac luxation, sacral fracture, fracture of the body of the ilium at the greater sciatic notch, misdirected gluteal muscle injection, misdirected intramedullary pin proximal to the femur, femoral fracture, and misdirected caudal thigh muscle injection. The last can be avoided by pressing one's thumb between the biceps femoris and semitendinosus proximal to the stifle and injecting medial or lateral to it.

Occasionally the sciatic nerve becomes entrapped in the fibrosis and callus of healing that follow fracture or surgery in the area of the pelvis and hip. This usually results in persistent pain and reluctance to use the limb. Other signs may include neurogenic atrophy, loss of sensation in the autonomous zone of the nerve, and standing on the dorsum of the paw if the limb is used.

Cranial Gluteal Nerve. In the dog, injury to this nerve will cause a lateral rotation of the thigh during the support phase of the gait. This will be most obvious at the stifle when the limb is extended just prior to the next protraction.

13a. PELVIS AND FEMUR, HORSE

The iliac crest includes the tuber sacrale and tuber coxae. In large animals the tuber coxae includes the cranial ventral iliac spine plus a thickened portion of the iliac crest. Locate the following structures:

Tuber coxae. It is normally about 5 cm. ventral to the summits of the tuber sacrale and the sacral spinous processes. It is an important landmark in the diagnosis of fractures of the pelvis (see Plate I), and for obtaining CSF from the lumbosacral space.

Tuber ischiadicum.

Trochanter major. Note especially the cranial part, over which the tendon of the gluteus accessorius (part of the gluteus medius) passes to its termination on the crest below. The trochanteric bursa is between the tendon and the cranial part of the trochanter.

Trochanter tertius. It is the termination of the gluteus superficialis, and it is sometimes fractured.

Groove on the ventral surface of the cranial branch of the pubis. The ligament of the head of the femur originates here and in the fossa acetabuli. It is covered by the accessory ligament.

Fovea of the head of the femur. Palpate the great depth of the fovea as compared with that of the ox. In the horse, it is the point of attachment of two ligaments, the ligament of the head and the accessory ligament.

Trochanter minor. This is the termination of the iliopsoas.

13b. HIP JOINT, HORSE

The accessory ligament passes from the prepubic tendon through the acetabular notch to the head of the femur. The notch is bridged by the transverse ligament, a part of the circular labrum acetabulare. The ligament of the head is deep to the accessory ligament and mostly intra-articular, except for the part that is attached in the groove on the pubis.

Occasionally rupture of the ligament of the femoral head occurs alone without luxation.[1] This permits lateral rotation of the femur, and the stifle will appear more lateral than normal. Associated with this, the tarsus will be positioned medial to the stifle and the hoof will be directed laterally (stifle out—hock in—toe out). The limbs will be of equal length. With craniodorsal luxation of the hip the horse must extend the limb to rest the hoof on the ground. This will cause the tuber calcis of the affected limb to be proximal to that in the normal limb. The displaced greater trochanter may be palpable and the tuber coxae may be lower on the affected side.

13c. DISSECTION, CROUP AND THIGH, HORSE

Tensor fasciae latae. It is separated from the superficial and middle gluteal muscles by a fascial septum.

Subiliac (prefemoral) lymph nodes. They form a chain 7 cm. long and lie about halfway between the tuber coxae and the patella.

Trace the intermuscular septa between:

Superficial gluteal and the biceps femoris.
The three divisions of the distal part of the biceps (see Plate I).
Biceps femoris and semitendinosus.
Semitendinosus and semimembranosus. This septum is strongly curved.
Semimembranosus and gracilis.

Reflection of the superficial gluteal and the two parts of the middle gluteal at their terminations demonstrates the trochanteric bursa. When the bursa is inflamed, the limb is abducted so that the weight is placed on the medial side of the hoof. At the end of the supporting phase, the hoof breaks over the medial side of the dorsal part and this causes more wear at that point. The stride is shortened, and the hoof of the affected limb swings in a medially convex arc as it is advanced. The spine is bent laterally in the caudal lumbar region, so that the hindquarters deviate toward the sound side and the horse trots "dog-fashion." The region of the cranial part of the major trochanter is sensitive to pressure. In chronic bursitis the gluteal muscles are atrophied, but this sign is also seen in tarsitis.

Severe atrophy of the middle gluteal and tensor fasciae latae occurs with denervation from lesions of the cranial gluteal nerve or the cell bodies of its motor neurons in the L 5, L 6, and S 1 spinal cord segments. The latter has been observed with focal lesions in the ventral gray column that are related to a protozoal infection.

On the medial side of the thigh the saphenous nerve, artery, and medial saphenous vein emerge between the sartorius and pectineus. The deep inguinal lymph nodes are in the femoral triangle.

13d. RADIOGRAPHS, PELVIS AND HIPS, HORSE

Identify the bones of the pelvis, sacrum, acetabulum, femoral head, and greater trochanter. Look for the sacroiliac articulation and the articulation between the body and transverse processes of L 6 with the sacrum. There are separate ossification centers for the ilium, ischium, and pubis, which unite between 10 and 24 months. Additional ossification centers for the iliac crest, tuber coxae, tuber ischiadicum, caudal border of ischium, and acetabular fossa unite with the adjacent bones by 4 to 5 years. In the proximal femur, the major trochanter, femoral head, and the third trochanter are all separate centers of ossification. The major trochanter and head unite with each other and the diaphysis between 18 and 36 months.

13e. LIVE HORSE

Fractures of the pelvis occur more commonly in the wing of the ilium of older horses from jumping injuries and in the body of the ischium, pubis, or acetabulum of young horses that fall and severely abduct their limbs.[26] Hip lameness may produce a head-nod on the forelimb that strikes the ground simultaneously with the lame hind limb, an elevation of the gluteal area and tail head when the affected hind limb strikes the ground, pain on manipulation of the affected coxofemoral joint, and gluteal muscle atrophy in chronic cases. No abnormal deviation of the swing phase of the gait occurs. Some fractures can be palpated on rectal examination.

Tuber coxae. Palpate the dorsal and ventral extremities and observe their normal relationship to the tuber sacrale. Fracture of the tuber coxae may not be readily recognized in the lateral view because the tuber becomes less prominent. The symmetry of the pelvis should be checked from the rear.

The tubera sacralia project above the sacrum and may become more prominent in chronic partial sacroiliac luxation. This is referred to as "hunter's bumps." In other horses a lowered tuber coxae may be evident plus mild disuse atrophy of the gluteal muscles.

Tuber ischiadicum. See Plate I.

Tensor fasciae latae. It extends distally from the tuber coxae on the craniolateral surface of the thigh.

Subiliac (prefemoral) lymph nodes. This is a chain of small nodes on the cranial surface of the tensor fasciae latae, halfway between the tuber coxae and the patella. Place the fingertips in the groove between the tensor fasciae latae and the abdominal wall and draw forward. The lymph nodes will slip caudally out from under the fingertips.

Quadriceps femoris. Palpate the muscle in the distal third of the cranial part of the thigh. This muscle is essential to the supporting function of the whole limb. If the stifle is not fixed, the hock and hip also collapse. Exertional rhabdomyolysis sometimes affects the quadriceps, causing collapse and subsequent atrophy.

Trochanter major. Palpate it through the superficial gluteal. The trochanter is divided by a notch into cranial and caudal parts. The cranial part is palpated for tenderness in the diagnosis of trochanteric bursitis. The notch is the landmark for insertion of a needle into the joint. The summit of the caudal part is normally on the line connecting the tuber coxae and tuber ischiadicum.

Biceps femoris. Palpate the septum between the biceps and the semitendinosus near the caudal border of the lateral surface of the thigh.

Semitendinosus. This muscle is on the caudolateral border of the thigh, but the termination is on the medial surface of the leg. The septum separating this muscle from the semimembranosus extends distally from the tuber ischiadicum, curving cranially under the gracilis near the stifle.

Semimembranosus. It is palpable on the caudomedial border of the thigh.

The three powerful caudal thigh muscles are frequently injured with large L-shaped flap wounds. The intermuscular septa are therefore important in surgical repair and in drainage. The caudal thigh muscles are powerful extensors of the stifle when the limb has been advanced and the foot planted. A sutured wound in these muscles is placed under a severe strain by the animal's efforts to rise if it is allowed to lie down.

Acute or chronic injury to the caudal thigh muscles (semimembranosus, semitendinosus, and less often the biceps femoris and gracilis) may result in fibrosis and even ossification of the injured area and shortening of these muscles. This prevents full extension of the limb during the cranial part of the swing phase of the gait and abruptly shortens the stride when the foot is 6 to 10 cm. above the ground, causing it to be suddenly slapped to the ground. This fibrotic-ossifying myopathy occurs in horses that constantly back against the restraining chain on a trailer or as a result of an acute injury in working rodeo horses.

Palpate the pulse in the saphenous artery.

13f. ACETABULUM AND FEMUR, OX

The depression on the head of the femur for the attachment of the ligament of the head is very small. If the head of the femur is articulated with the acetabulum, the course of the ligament may be traced from the ventral border of the ischium at the margin of the obturator foramen through the acetabular notch to the fovea capitis. The weakness of this ligament is cited as a factor in luxation in the ox. There is no accessory ligament. Another factor may be the notch in the dorsocranial margin of the acetabulum. This is most apparent in the dorsal view.

13g. SUPERFICIAL DISSECTION, CROUP AND THIGH, CALF

Lateral surface:

The muscle of the cranial border of the proximal part of the thigh is the tensor fasciae latae. When its point of origin, the tuber coxae, is fractured, the animal will not advance the thigh during the acute stage. On the abdominal wall cranial to the muscle is the large and important subiliac lymph node (see Plate II).

The largest muscle on the lateral surface of the thigh is the biceps femoris. Its principal action, together with the semitendinosus and semimembranosus, is to extend the limb when the foot is advanced and fixed. The caudal thigh muscles also raise the hock in the last phase of the stride and deliver the power behind the kick. It has been reported that a violent fall can cause the cranial border of the biceps to be torn from the fascia and to be caught behind the trochanter major. The resulting forced extension of the stifle and hock resembles proximal fixation of the patella. It is relieved by an incision in the cranial border of the muscle.[40]

In the triangle between the tensor fasciae latae and biceps is the gluteus medius. There is no gluteus superficialis and no trochanter tertius in the cow.

Reflection of the origin of the biceps from the lesser sciatic foramen shows the caudal gluteal vessels and the sciatic lymph node. The latter receives lymph from the hip joint and the muscles of the gluteal region and caudal thigh. It is therefore one of the important lymph nodes of the carcass.

In meat inspection, it is more easily reached from the inside of the split carcass by an incision through the sacrosciatic ligament dorsal to the lesser sciatic foramen. It may be in the foramen.

The sciatic nerve passes through the greater sciatic foramen and distally, dorsal then caudal to the hip joint.

Note on the Nomenclature. The dog has a sacrotuberous ligament. The ungulates have a sacrosciatic ligament (ligamentum sacrotuberale latum), which incorporates the sacrotuberous ligament in its caudal border. The cat has neither. The English term sciatic is the usual translation of the Latin ischiadicus.

Medial surface:

From cranial to caudal in the distal part of the thigh the muscles are: the tensor fasciae latae, the vastus medialis, the sartorius, and the gracilis. The femoral vessels are deep to the sartorius, and the saphenous vessels and nerve emerge from its caudal border.

Not all adductor paralysis is caused by intrapelvic injury to the obturator nerve during parturition (see Fig. 25–6). Recovery in many cases is too rapid for a nerve injury. Necropsy of cows that do not get up after treatment of parturient paresis usually reveals traumatic hemorrhagic injury or ischemic degeneration of the adductor, gracilis, and pectineus muscles.[28] This myopathy probably results from local ischemia associated with compression of muscles within their osteofascial compartments.[16] After 6 hours of anesthesia-induced recumbency on one pelvic limb, muscle and nerve damage may be extensive enough to prevent the animal from rising on that limb.[16] Ischemic muscle necrosis is evident, especially in the semitendinosus, as well as neuropathy of the sciatic nerve in the thigh. Other possibilities include the tearing of medial thigh muscles under the pelvis when the cow goes down from parturient paresis with both hind limbs in extreme flexion and abduction, or ischemia from compression of the deep femoral artery.[20, 37]

13h. LIVE COW

Trochanter major femoris. The summit and the cranial border may be palpated easily through the biceps. Note that the trochanter is normally below a line connecting the tuber coxae and tuber ischiadicum. Visualize the position of the trochanter in dorsal and ventral displacement of the head of the femur (see Plate II).

Tuber coxae. In dorsal luxation of the hip the tuber coxae is lower on the affected side in the standing animal because the weight of the viscera pulls the pelvis down and the dislocated femur does not support it. The symmetry of the tubera coxarum is also destroyed in fracture of one tuber coxae.

Tuber sacrale. Note that the tuber sacrale does not project dorsal to the crest of the sacrum. In luxation of the sacroiliac articulation, the tuber sacrale is prominent and the crest of the sacrum is sunken.

Subiliac (prefemoral) lymph node. It is located on the abdominal wall cranial to the tensor fasciae latae, a short distance above the level of the patella. The node is 8 to 12 cm. long. It should not be confused with a small superficial lymph node that may be palpable on the surface of the tensor fasciae latae.

Saphenous artery. It is large and easily palpable as it emerges around the caudal border of the sartorius muscle. This is a convenient place to feel the pulse.

13i. PELVIS AND FEMUR, RADIOGRAPHS, DOG

The pelvis is second only to the femur in number of fractures sustained. Most pelvic fractures are in the ilium.[31] In dogs, the ilium, ischium, pubis, and os acetabuli are fused together at 4 to 6 months.[12, 22] Secondary ossification centers for the tuber ischiadicum and the margin of the ischial arch fuse with the ischium at about 1 year.[22] The crest of the ilium may remain separate radiologically for 2 1/2 years or more. The union of the pelvic symphysis begins at the caudal end and may not be complete until the sixth year.

The femur is the most frequently fractured bone in the dog.[31] About one-fifth of femoral fractures are in the head and neck, and the rest are in the shaft and distal end.

The proximal end of the femur ossifies from three centers—head, major trochanter, and minor trochanter.The ossification centers for the head and major trochanter fuse together prior to their fusion with the shaft.[38] All three are fused with the shaft at 6 to 13 months in dogs[12, 22] and 7 to 11 months in cats.[42] Epiphyseal separation of the head of the trochanter major may occur in young animals.

The distal epiphysis is mortised to receive the four points on the distal end of the shaft. Epiphyseal separation may also occur here. Fusion occurs at 6 to 12 months in dogs and 13 to 19 months in cats.

In mid-shaft fractures, the distal fragment is usually displaced caudally by the caudal thigh muscles and the gastrocnemius. The end of the proximal fragment forms a prominence on the front of the thigh. There is marked overriding of the fragments.

Supracondylar fractures usually result in flexion of the distal fragment at the stifle because of the spasm of the gastrocnemius, but if the break is distal to the origin of the gastrocnemius, as in epiphyseal separation, the distal fragment may be tilted forward and may lie in front of the distal end of the shaft.

The evaluation of radiographs for the early detection of hip dysplasia in susceptible breeds is an exacting task. The prognosis may mean serious financial loss to the dog breeder. It is essential to begin with proper positioning of the animal according to a fixed standard such as that established by a panel of the American Veterinary Medical Association.[50] The dog is placed on its back with the hind limbs extended. The pelvis must be level from side to side and craniocaudally. The limbs are rotated medially so that the divergent rays will cast the shadow of the patella in the middle of the femoral trochlea. This is done to get the head of the femur in the standard position. The radiograph must meet the following criteria or it will not yield a reliable diagnosis: the obturator foramina should have the same shape and equal size, the wings of the ilia should be equal, the radiolucent zones of the sacroiliac joints should be of equal thickness, and the head of the femur should show a central flat spot—the fovea.[51] Dysplasia is evidenced by a change in the normal congruence of the acetabulum to the hemispherical head. Note, however, that only the facies lunata is in contact with the head—the acetabular fossa, opposite the fovea, is not. In hip dysplasia the acetabulum becomes shallow, and there is a loss of the cranial rim. The head becomes flattened and distorted by exostosis.

Sometimes the standard view is supplemented by one with the limbs fully flexed and abducted to rotate the femoral head to a different profile.

Examine the head of the femur on the bone specimens and note the foramina around the margin of the articular surface. The arteries of the canine hip joint are supplied mainly from the medial and lateral circumflex femoral arteries, with a smaller contribution from the caudal gluteal.[29, 39] These branches form an extracapsular vascular ring at the attachment of the joint capsule to the femoral neck. Ascending branches from this ring penetrate the capsule and ascend the neck between the bone and the synovial membrane. These intracapsular arteries are best developed on the cranial and dorsal surface of the femoral neck. At the epiphysis these vessels anastomose to form a subsynovial intracapsular ring from which epiphyseal arteries enter the foramina to supply the femoral head. The arteries in the ligament of the femoral head have not been observed to supply the femoral head. Rupture of this ligament in hip luxation does not compromise the vascular supply to the femoral head. It is important that surgical approaches do not disrupt the cranial and dorsal aspects of the extracapsular vascular ring or their source, especially the ascending branch of the lateral circumflex femoral artery. Intracapsular fractures or epiphyseal separation may deprive the proximal fragment of its blood supply and cause necrosis. However, accurate reduction and rigid internal fixation in small animals apparently permit adequate revascularization because subsequent vascular necrosis is uncommon.

Necrosis of the capitular epiphysis occurs without separation in young dogs of small breeds. Ischemia of the head is produced by some unknown cause; the bone dies, then is demineralized. The absence of this condition in adults may be due to the free anastomosis between intraosseous metaphyseal and epiphyseal arteries that follows the disappearance of the epiphyseal cartilage barrier.

Using the bones, produce the common dorsocranial luxation with lateral rotation and the dorsocaudal luxation with medial rotation. Determine the effect that these would have on the length of the limbs in various positions. Abduct the femur and note that luxation in that position is very difficult. In extreme adduction, however, the head is pried out of the acetabulum. Forced abduction when the limb is extended may cause the less common caudoventral luxation. Affected dogs carry their limb slightly abducted and rotated medially. The femoral head is displaced medially into the obturator foramen, making it difficult to palpate the greater trochanter.[49]

A surgical method to repair dorsolateral hip luxations is to pass a metal pin cranially, starting just ventral to the tuber ischiadicum.[17] The pin passes lateral to the dorsal rim of the acetabulum and is inserted into the wing of the ilium. This acts as an extension of the acetabular rim to prevent luxation. It is important to stay lateral to the sciatic nerve. This method cannot be used in cats because the wing of the ilium does not curve laterally and the pin cannot be inserted in it. The ilium of the cat is straight compared with those in other species.

To avoid injury to the sciatic nerve when passing an intramedullary pin through the trochanteric fossa, or a needle to obtain bone marrow, the femur should be adducted and not rotated laterally.

13j. DISSECTION, HIP JOINT, DOG

The direction of pull of the largest muscles attached to the proximal end of the femur is dorsocranial. Associated with this is the predominance of dorsocranial luxations.

There are four main approaches to the hip joint: dorsal, cranial, caudal, and ventral.[36] The most used one is dorsal. The skin is incised over the greater trochanter, and the cranial border of the biceps is separated from the tensor fasciae latae. The flat tendon of the superficial gluteal is transected over the greater trochanter.Then the middle gluteal and the underlying piriformis are separated from the deep gluteal by blunt probing, and the sciatic nerve is located and protected. Now the middle and deep gluteals can be reflected either by tenotomy near the greater trochanter or by osteotomy of the greater trochanter. Reflection of these muscles exposes the joint capsule and the small articularis coxae muscle that crosses the joint capsule to the neck of the femur. This muscle is used as a guide for opening the joint capsule. The capsule is incised just caudal and parallel to the articularis coxae. This spares the blood vessels that enter the capsule at the neck of the femur. If the tendons are cut, they are reattached by sutures; if the trochanter is removed, it is reattached by pins or a screw.[46]

A cranial approach gives access to the cranial surface of the hip joint by separation and retraction without transection of muscles.[11] A long incision is made in the skin and fascia lata from the mid-dorsal line along the cranial border of the biceps femoris to the stifle. The tensor fasciae latae and the cranial border of the biceps are separated and reflected. The vastus lateralis is separated from the rectus femoris by blunt dissection, preserving the branches of the lateral circumflex femoral artery and femoral nerve that cross the upper part of the vastus intermedius to the vastus lateralis.

The caudal approach is useful for open reduction of craniodorsal luxation.[35] A curved proximodistal incision is made around the caudal surface of the greater trochanter. The fascia lata is incised along the cranial border of the biceps and the muscle is retracted caudally with precautions to identify and protect the underlying sciatic nerve. The gluteal muscles are retracted craniodorsally. The gemelli and the tendon of the internal obturator are isolated and transected to expose the caudal surface of the joint.

The ventral approach is difficult, but it is recommended to preserve the gluteal muscles in excision of the femoral head. A T-shaped incision is made with the stem of the T along the pectineus and the bar of the T in the inguinal groove. The pectineus is transected and reflected, sparing the femoral, deep femoral, and caudal femoral vessels. The iliopsoas muscle, running caudodistally to reach its termination on the lesser trochanter, covers the joint. It is retracted cranially and the adductor is retracted caudally to expose the rim of the acetabulum.

Observe the position of the femoral vein caudal to the femoral artery in the femoral triangle. Note that the pectineus muscle is prominent enough to palpate and that the vein lies between the muscle and the artery, which is easily located by its pulsation. The pectineus has been the subject of much investigation since it was discovered that transection of the muscle relieved the pain of hip dysplasia.[8] Contraction of this muscle elevates the femoral head against the dorsal rim of the acetabulum. Section of the pectineus in puppies does not effect the incidence of hip dysplasia as they grow older.[34]

The sciatic nerve in the thigh has the same position in all domestic animals. It lies between the biceps femoris laterally and the semitendinosus and semimembranosus medially. It may be reached for diagnostic stimulation by inserting a needle between the biceps and semitendinosus, 2.5 cm. distal to the tuber ischiadicum, to a depth of 5 cm. (see Plate III).

Tendon transfers have occasionally been used to correct the deficits associated with permanent peripheral nerve lesions.[7, 32] The procedures involve joining the tendon of a normally innervated muscle to the tendon of one of the denervated muscles. For sciatic nerve deficits the tendon of the vastus lateralis can be sutured to the long digital extensor tendon at the stifle. This is combined with talocrural arthrodesis. For peroneal nerve deficits the tendon of the long digital flexor can be sutured to the long digital extensor tendon in the proximal metatarsus.

13k. DISSECTION OF THE THIGH, DOG

The shaft of the femur is exposed for repair of fractures by a lateral approach through a skin incision from the major trochanter to the patella. The fascia lata is incised just cranial to the muscle fibers of the biceps femoris. Retraction of the biceps femoris caudally and the vastus lateralis cranially exposes the femur. The sciatic nerve will be observed coursing distally caudal to the femur on the adductor, which terminates on the caudal side of the femur.

13l. LIVE DOG

Palpate the tuber coxae and the tuber ischiadicum and compare the positions of the right and left greater trochanters. Hip luxation is usually dorsocranial and occurs when a dog is hit on the side opposite to the limb that is extended and supporting weight.[2] The pelvis is forced laterally over the femur of the supporting limb, which acts like a lever and is adducted. The head is forced out of the acetabulum as the ligament of the femoral head ruptures and the joint capsule tears. The gluteals pull the proximal femur dorsocranially. In most cases of luxation, the limb is rotated laterally and is shorter in caudal extension, indicating dorsocranial displacement. Place the thumb in the depression between the tuber ischiadicum and the greater trochanter and rotate the femur laterally, so that the trochanter forces the thumb out of the space. The failure of this test is partial evidence for luxation because the head is no longer fixed as a fulcrum. A fracture of the neck or separation of the capital epiphysis would also give this sign (see Plate III). To replace a femur that is luxated dorsocranially, the hip should be extended and the femur drawn caudally and then rotated medially.

Dogs with hip dysplasia have joint laxity.[34] This can be determined best by manipulation of the joint in the anesthetized dog. With the dog in lateral recumbency and the hip and stifle flexed at 90° place one hand on the pelvis and lift the femur directly lateral to determine how far the head can be lifted out of the acetabulum. It is normal to lift it out a few millimeters. This distance will be greater in puppies, even up to 1 cm. Then determine if the joint can be luxated by adducting the femur and slowly pushing it toward the dorsal rim of the acetabulum. If luxation occurs, abduction of the limb will suddenly replace the head in the acetabulum, often accompanied by a snapping sound.

To insert a needle into the hip joint, penetrate the skin just cranial to the summit of the greater trochanter and direct it medially, keeping it perpendicular to the median plane, until synovia is obtained.

Palpate the crest of the ilium. In most medium- and large-sized dogs, bone marrow can be obtained here with local anesthesia. In most small dogs and cats, this bone is too thin, and the femoral bone marrow is aspirated under general anesthesia. Palpate the greater trochanter and pass the needle down its medial side into the trochanteric fossa. Keep the femur perpendicular to the sacrum, or adducted slightly to avoid the sciatic nerve.

Palpate, on the medial surface of the thigh, the femoral artery in the femoral triangle. The latter is bounded cranially by the sartorius, caudally by the pectineus, and deeply by the iliopsoas and vastus medialis. The femoral vein, caudal to the artery and cranial to the pectineus, is a possibility for intravenous injection. Palpate the pectineus muscle and abduct the limb to determine the amount of tension placed on this muscle. Dogs with pectineal myopathy associated with hip dysplasia have a shortened pectineus muscle, which limits abduction of the limb.[10]

Palpate the caudal thigh muscles. Athletic dogs, especially Greyhounds, injure their caudomedial thigh muscles and develop a fibrosis and contracture that limits the swing phase of the gait similar to that which occurs in the horse. Find the depression beween the biceps femoris and semitendinosus where the thumb should be placed to avoid injections into the sciatic nerve.

Note that the dog and cat do not have a subiliac (prefemoral) lymph node.

The cutaneous innervation of the thigh involves the overlapping of numerous peripheral nerves.[30, 43] The autonomous zones listed can be tested for specific nerves (see Fig. 13–1).

Lateral surface—middle of cranial part: lateral cutaneous femoral nerve (L 3, L 4, L 5).

Lateral surface—middle of caudal part: caudal cutaneous femoral (L 7, sacral segments).

Caudal surface—middle part: caudal cutaneous femoral.

Medial surface—middle proximal part: genitofemoral nerve (L 3, L 4).

Medial surface—middle distal part: saphenous nerve (L 4, L 5, L 6).

References

1. Adams, O. R.: Lameness in Horses, 3rd ed. Philadelphia: Lea & Febiger, 1974.
2. Alexander, J. W.: Coxofemoral luxations in the dog. Comp. Cont. Ed. *4* (1982):575–583.
3. Allam, M. W., F. E. Nulsen, and F. H. Lewey: Electrical intraneural bipolar stimulation of peripheral nerves in the dog. JAVMA *114* (1949):87–89.
4. Bardet, J. F., and R. B. Hohn: Quadriceps contracture in dogs. JAVMA *183* (1983):680–685.
5. Bego, U., M. Pajtl, and K. Cermak: Beitrag zu den peripheren Nervenlähmungen am Hinterbein beim Hund, mit besonderer Berücksichtigung des N. fibularis. Deutsche tierärztl. Wschr. *70* (1963):120–123.
6. Bennett, D.: An anatomical and histological study of the sciatic nerve, relating to peripheral nerve injuries in the dog and cat. J. Small Anim. Pract. *17* (1976):379–386.
7. Bennett, D. and L. C. Vaughan: Peroneal nerve paralysis in the cat and dog: an experimental study. J. Small Anim. Pract. *17* (1976):499–506.
8. Bowen, J. M., R. E. Lewis, S. K. Kneller, et al.: Progression of hip dysplasia in German shepherd dogs after unilateral pectineal myotomy. JAVMA *161* (1972):899–904.
9. Budras, K. D.: Zur Homologisierung der Mm. adductores und des M. pectineus der Haussäugetiere. Zbl. Vet. Med. (C) *1* (1972):73–91.
10. Cardinet, G. H., L. J. Wallace, M. R. Fedde, et al.: Developmental myopathy in the canine with type II muscle fiber hypotrophy. Arch. Neurol. *21* (1969):620–630.
11. Cawley, A. J., J. Archibald, and W. J. B. Ditchfield: Fractures of the neck of the femur in the dog. I. A technique for repair of fractures of the femoral neck. JAVMA *129* (1956):354–358.
12. Chapman, W. L.: Appearance of ossification centers and epiphyseal closures as determined by radiographic techniques. JAVMA *147* (1965):138–141.
13. Cox, V. S., J. E. Breazile, and T. R. Hoover: Surgical and anatomic study of calving paralysis. Am. J. Vet. Res. *36* (1975):427–430.
14. Cox, V. S.: Understanding the downer cow syndrome. Comp. Cont. Ed. *3* (1981):S472–S478.
15. Cox, V. S.: Pathogenesis of the downer cow syndrome. Vet. Rec. *111* (1982):76–79.
16. Cox, V. S., C. J. McGrath, and S. E. Jorgensen. The role of pressure damage in pathogenesis of the downer cow syndrome. Am. J. Vet. Res. *43* (1982):26–31.
17. Duff, S. R. I. and D. Bennett: Hip luxation in small animals: an evaluation of some methods of treatment. Vet. Rec. *111* (1982):140–143.
18. Fitzgerald, T. C.: Blood supply of the head of the canine femur. Vet. Med. *56* (1961):389–394.
19. Fletcher, T. F.:Lumbosacral plexus and pelvic limb myotomes of the dog. Am. J. Vet. Res. *31* (1970):35–41.
20. Gräub, E.: Ischämische Nekrose der Oberschenkelmuskulatur infolge der Geburt bei der Kuh. Arch. Wiss. u. Prakt. Tierhlk. *34* (1908):645–665.
21. Ham, A. W.: Histology, 7th ed. Philadelphia: J. B. Lippincott, 1974, p. 425.
22. Hare, W. C. D.: Radiographic anatomy of the canine pelvic limb. Part II. Developing limb. JAVMA *136* (1960):603–611.
23. Huddleston, O. L. and C. S. White: Segmental motor innervation of the tibialis anterior and gastrocnemius-plantaris muscles in the dog. Am. J. Physiol. *138* (1943):772–775.
24. Hulth, A., I. Norbergh, and S. E. Olsson: Coxa plana in the dog. J. Bone and Joint Surg. *44A* (1962):918.
25. Ihlemelander, E. C., G. H. Cardinet, M. M. Guffy, et al.: Canine hip dysplasia: differences in pectineal muscles of healthy and dysplastic German shepherd dogs when two months old. Am. J. Vet. Res. *44* (1983):411–416.
26. Jeffcott, L. B.: Pelvic lameness in the horse. Equine Pract. *4* (1982):21–47.
27. Jefferson, A.: Aspects of the segmental innervation of the cat's hind limb. J. Comp. Neurol. *100* (1954):569–596.
28. Jönsson, G. and B. Pehrson: Studies on the downer syndrome in dairy cows. Zbl. Vet. Med. (A) *16* (1969):757–784.
29. Kaderly, R. E., B. G. Anderson, and W. D. Anderson: Intracapsular and intraosseous vascular supply to the mature dog's coxofemoral joint. Am. J. Vet. Res. *44* (1983):1805–1812.
30. Kitchell, R. L.: Personal Communication, 1983.
31. Leonard, E. P.: Orthopedic Surgery of the Dog and Cat. Philadelphia: W. B. Saunders, 1960.
32. Lesser, A. S. and S. S. Soliman: Experimental evaluation of tendon transfer for the treatment of sciatic nerve paralysis in the dog. Vet. Surg. *9* (1980):72–73.
33. Lust, G., P. H. Craig, G. E. Ross, Jr., et al.: Studies on pectineus muscles in canine hip dysplasia. Cornell Vet. *62* (1972):628–645.

34. Lust, G., W. T. Beilman, and V. T. Rendano: A relationship between degree of laxity and synovial fluid volume in coxofemoral joints of dogs predisposed for hip dysplasia. Am. J. Vet. Res. *41* (1980):55–60.

35. Piermattei, D. L.: Surgical approaches to the joints. Am. Anim. Hosp. Assoc. Proc. 38th Mtg. (1971):368–378.

36. Piermattei, D. L. and R. G. Greeley: An Atlas of Surgical Approaches to the Bones of the Dog and Cat, 2nd ed. Philadelphia: W. B. Saunders, 1980.

37. Prather, E. K.: Observations on downer cow syndrome. JAVMA *155* (1969):1794.

38. Rendano, V. T., C. B. Quick, G. S. Allan, and G. D. Ryan: Radiographic evaluation of femoral head and neck fractures: the value of the flexed ventrodorsal and oblique projections in diagnosis. J. Am. Anim. Hosp. Assoc. *16* (1980):485–491.

39. Rivera, L. A., Y. Z. Abdelbaki, C. W. Titkemeyer, et al.: Arterial supply to the canine hip joint. J. Vet. Orthop. *1* (1979):20–33.

40. Silbersiepe, E., E. Berge, and H. Muller: Lehrbuch der speziellen Chirurgie für Tierärzte und Studierende, 14th ed. Stuttgart: Enke, 1965.

41. Smith, R. N.: The normal and radiological anatomy of the hip joint of the dog. J. Small Anim. Pract. *4* (1963):1–9.

42. Smith, R. N.: Fusion of ossification centers in the cat. J. Small Anim. Pract. *10* (1969):523–530.

43. Spurgeon, T. L. and R. L. Kitchell: Electrophysiological studies of the cutaneous innervation of the external genitalia of the male dog. Zbl. Vet. Med. (C) *11* (1982):289–306.

44. Tryphonas, L., G. F. Hamilton, and C. S. Rhodes: Perinatal femoral nerve degeneration and neurogenic atrophy of quadriceps femoris muscle in calves. JAVMA *164* (1974):801–807.

45. Vaughan, L. C.: Peripheral nerve injuries: an experimental study in cattle. Vet. Rec. *76* (1964):1293–1300.

46. Wheaton, L. G., R. B. Hohn, and J. W. Harrison: Surgical treatment of acetabular fractures in the dog. JAVMA *162* (1973):385–392.

47. Wilson, J. W.: Relationship of the patellar tendon reflex to the ventral branch of the fifth lumbar spinal nerve in the dog. Am. J. Vet. Res. *39* (1978):1774–1777.

48. Worthman, R. P.: Demonstration of specific nerve paralysis in the dog. JAVMA *131* (1957):174–178.

49. Thatcher, C., and S. C. Schrader: Caudal ventral hip luxation in the dog: a review of 14 cases. J. Am. Anim. Hosp. Assoc. *21* (1985): 167–172.

50. Whittington, K., W. C. Banks, W. D. Carlson, et al.: AVMA Council on Veterinary Services. Report of panel on canine hip dysplasia. JAVMA *139* (1961): 791–806.

51. Rendano V. T., and G. Ryan: Canine hip dysplasia evaluation: a positioning and labeling guide for radiographs to be submitted to the Orthopedic Foundation for Animals. Vet. Radiol. In press, 1985.

CHAPTER 14

STIFLE AND LEG, HORSE AND OX

OBJECTIVES

1. To be able to identify the bony prominences at the stifle, the patella, and the collateral and patellar ligaments by palpation.
2. To be able to insert a needle into the femoropatellar joint capsule or either sac of the femorotibial capsule.
3. To be able to differentiate between proximal fixation and dislocation of the patella in the horse.
4. To be able to perform medial patellar desmotomy in the horse.
5. To be able to diagnose rupture of the peroneus tertius.
6. To be able to work on the hind foot of a horse without fighting the reciprocal mechanism of the stifle and hock.
7. If embryotomy is indicated in a breech presentation, to be able to disconnect the stifle and hock by simple tenotomy.
8. To avoid the mistake of attributing lameness to a congenital defect in the ossification of the fibula seen in a radiograph.
9. To be able to anesthetize the hock, metatarsus, and digit by nerve blocks in the crus.
10. To be able to anesthetize the digit or digits by nerve blocks in the crus.
11. To be able to identify the muscles of the crus and the medial saphenous vein by palpation. They are landmarks as well as sites of injury and inflammation.
12. To be able to recognize and understand the cause of the gait abnormality in calves with spastic paresis.
13. To be able to denervate the gastrocnemius for the treatment of spastic paresis in calves.
14. To be able to locate the bicipital bursa at the stifle in the ox.
15. To be able to find the popliteal lymph node of food animals with minimum damage to the round.
16. To be able to palpate the common peroneal nerve in the proximal crus.

Table 14–1. DEEP DIGITAL FLEXOR MUSCLES*

Nomina Anatomica Veterinaria, 2nd ed.	Nomina Anatomica Veterinaria, 3rd ed.
M. flexor digitorum [digitalis] profundus	Mm. flexores digitorum [digitales] profundi
M. flexor digiti I [hallucis] longus	M. flexor digitorum [digitalis] lateralis
M. flexor digitorum [digitalis] longus	M. flexor digitorum [digitalis] medialis
M. tibialis caudalis	M. tibialis caudalis
	Tendo communis

*Data from Nomina Anatomica Veterinaria. Vienna: International Committee on Veterinary Anatomical Nomenclature, 2nd ed., 1973, and 3rd ed., 1983.

Notes on the Nomenclature. The crus is the anatomical leg or gaskin; it is the part of the pelvic limb between the stifle and the hock. The anatomist recognizes no four-legged animals.

It is well to keep in mind that the carpus and hock flex in opposite directions. On the hind limb the flexors of the digit are extensors of the hock, and the extensors of the digit are flexors of the hock. The analogue of the common digital extensor is the long digital extensor. It is so named because there is also a short digital extensor on the hind limb. The most cranial and superficial muscle in the crus is the long digital extensor in the horse, the peroneus tertius in the ox, and the cranial tibial in the dog.

The names of the deep digital flexor muscles have been adapted to quadrupeds as shown in the column on the right of Table 14–1.

14a. RADIOGRAPHS, BONES, HORSE

The medial and lateral condyles of the femur ossify from one center, the distal epiphysis. This unites with the femoral diaphysis at 21 to 30 months. The tibial tuberosity is a separate ossification center that joins the proximal articular epiphysis of the tibia at 8 to 14 months. These fused centers unite with the shaft of the tibia at 23 to 38 months. The proximal tibial epiphysis forms the tibial condyles. Examine the fibula on a skeleton. It ossifies from three or more centers. The shaft usually does not ossify in the distal third. This leaves the distal epiphysis isolated and it unites with the distal tibia 3 to 6 months after birth, forming the lateral malleolus. The ossification of the head does not begin until after birth, and it unites with the shaft slowly and irregularly so that about 50 percent of adult horses have a congenital defect between the head and the shaft, which should not be mistaken for a fracture.[3]

Identify the skeletal structures comprising the femoropatellar and femorotibial joints.[9] Note the relationship of the patella to the medial ridge of the trochlea on both the lateromedial and caudocranial views. Osteochondrosis is most common in the stifle as a subchondral cyst in the medial femoral condyle and as a dissecting lesion in the lateral ridge of the trochlea.[6, 13]

14b. LIGAMENTOUS PREPARATION, HOCK AND STIFLE, HORSE

Flex and extend the stifle and note the identical action of the hock, produced mechanically in the horse by the tendinous peroneus tertius and superfical digital flexor. The bones, joints, and tendons involved are often called the reciprocal mechanism. Rupture of the peroneus tertius is diagnosed by observing that the hock can be extended with the stifle flexed. On initiation of the swing phase of the stride the stifle flexes normally, but the hock flexes poorly and appears loose. The horse supports weight normally, but a small depression (dimple) may be evident in the common calcanean tendon. This is more evident when the limb is picked up. Rupture of the peroneus tertius occurs when horses get a pelvic limb caught and struggle to free it or it may be associated with excessive extension of the pelvic limb at the start of a race.

This simultaneous action of the hock and stifle creates an obstetrical problem when the fetal foal or calf presents flexed hocks at the pelvic inlet. Simple traction on the flexed hocks after they have entered the birth canal will lock the stifles in flexion and prevent delivery. If the hocks have not entered the pelvis, traction will cause some extension of the stifle and this in turn will open the hock angle and jam the crus and metatarsus in the pelvic inlet. The fetus should be repelled and the feet raised into the maternal pelvis as the hocks, stifles, and hips are extended. If this is impossible and embryotomy is indicated, the common calcanean (Achilles) tendons may be severed, permitting delivery with the hocks in complete flexion and the stifles extended. This is easier than amputation at the hocks.

Another application of the reciprocal mechanism is encountered in raising the hind limb to work on the hoof. After the hind foot has been picked up, all the joints are flexed. To see the sole of the hoof it is necessary to carry the foot a step to the rear to get some extension of the stifle and hock.

Observe the course of the gastrocnemius tendon. It winds around the lateral side of the superficial digital flexor tendon (see Plate I).

14c. DISSECTIONS, STIFLE, HORSE

The stifle joint consists of three subsidiary joints: the femorotibial, femoropatellar, and proximal tibiofibular. The articular surfaces of the femur and tibia are separated by medial and lateral menisci, which glide caudally on the tibia when the joint is flexed. Each horn of each meniscus is attached to the tibia. In addition, the caudal horn of the lateral meniscus is attached to the back of the femur between the condyles by the meniscofemoral ligament, and the cranial horns of the menisci are connected by the transverse ligament in carnivores and the ox.

The femorotibial joint has medial and lateral collateral ligaments and cranial and caudal cruciate ligaments. The cruciate ligaments are intercondylar and named from their attachments to the tibia. The cranial one is lateral to the caudal one where they cross near their femoral origin.

The femoropatellar joint has three patellar ligaments in the horse and ox, the medial, intermediate, and lateral. In the carnivores, sheep, goats, and man, there is only one patellar ligament. The medial and lateral femoropatellar ligaments are thin bands in the retinacula (see section 15b). There is fat between the patellar ligaments and the stifle joint.

Examine the two sacs of the femorotibial joint capsule. Although the femoropatellar capsule usually communicates with the medial femorotibial sac by a narrow slit at the distal end of the medial trochlear ridge, it communicates with the lateral sac in only one fourth of the animals examined. Communication between the two femorotibial sacs is rare in the horse. Therefore, practical considerations require that if the femoropatellar joint or either sac of the femorotibial joint is infected, all three should be considered infected, but that each must be treated separately for therapeutic purposes. Several points of access are available for each sac. The following are recommended:

Lateral femorotibial, between the lateral collateral ligament and the tendon of origin of the long digital extensor. Note the distal prolongation of the lateral sac under the tendon of origin of the long digital extensor.

Medial femorotibial, between the medial collateral and medial patellar ligaments.

Femoropatellar, caudal to the lateral patellar ligament near the patella, or between the medial and intermediate patellar ligaments. For the latter site insert the needle proximal to the tibial tuberosity one-third of the distance to the patellar attachments and direct the needle proximally toward the gliding surface of the patella.

The femoropatellar joint is best studied on a specimen in which the cartilage is preserved. Examine the trochlea of the femur. The medial ridge is thickened by a smooth tubercle on the proximal end of the medial surface. This tubercle of the femoral trochlea, although it does not articulate with the patella, is covered with articular cartilage because it provides a friction catch for the patellar fibrocartilage and medial ligament. The patellar articular surface of the trochlea presents an abrupt change of direction at the proximal end, so that the upper portion, a transverse zone about 1.5 cm. wide, faces dorsocranially in the standing horse. It may be termed the resting surface of the trochlea, and the remainder, which is much larger, may be called the gliding surface.[10, 12]

Examine the patella. The medial angle to which the fibrocartilage is attached is more prominent than the lateral. The articular surface is divided into a resting part and a gliding part. The resting part is a zone about 1.5 cm. wide along the distal border. Between the apex and the medial angle of the patella the resting part forms an angle of about 130° with the medial part of the gliding surface. The resting part also extends about 2 cm. lateral to the apex. The gliding surface conforms to the corresponding surface of the trochlea. The function of these parts of the joint can be studied by palpation of the live horse (see section 14e).

14d. DISSECTION, CRUS, HORSE

Peroneal nerves. The superficial and deep peroneal nerves are seen emerging from the distal end of the biceps femoris on the proximal end of the lateral digital extensor. They run close together slightly distal to the head of the fibula, which can be palpated in the dissection or in the live animal at the origin of the lateral digital extensor. The nerves are subject to injury here, resulting in paralysis of the extensors of the digit and the flexors of the hock. The nerves may be blocked at this point in any animal to produce, with blocks of the tibial, caudal cutaneous sural, and saphenous nerves, surgical anesthesia of the hock, metatarsus, and digit. However, the peroneal nerves should not be blocked at this level for diagnostic purposes because the anesthetic affects the muscular branches and causes knuckling. This makes it impossible to see whether the anesthetic has eliminated the lameness (see Plate I and Figs. 16–1 and 16–2).

The caudal nerve is the superficial peroneal. It supplies the lateral digital extensor and the skin of the craniolateral surface of the limb down to the fetlock. It courses subcutaneously in the groove between the long and lateral digital extensor muscles.

The cranial nerve is the deep peroneal. It runs obliquely craniodistally into the space between the long and lateral digital extensors, where it gives branches to the long digital extensor and the tibialis cranialis and descends on the cranial surface of the lateral edge of the tibialis cranialis. The deep peroneal nerve supplies a sensory branch to the interior of the hock joint and continues to the dorsal surface of the metatarsus and digit. The usual site for blocking is 10 cm. proximal to the tibiotarsal articulation, cranial to the septum between the long and lateral digital extensors. The superficial peroneal nerve is easily blocked with the same insertion of the needle.

The tibial nerve. This is seen on the medial surface of the leg, on the caudomedial surface of the deep digital flexors. The relations of the accompanying caudal branches of the saphenous artery and medial saphenous vein vary slightly. The artery may be double. The motor branches to the extensors of the hock and flexors of the digit are given off proximal to the site for nerve block, which is 10 cm. proximal to the tuber calcanei. The tibial nerve supplies the plantar nerves. Tibial and deep peroneal nerve blocks will anesthetize the digit (see Plate I and Fig. 16–2).

If anesthesia of the hock and metatarsus is desired, one must also block three cutaneous nerves:

1. The superficial peroneal.

2. The saphenous nerve may be traced down the medial surface of the limb. Its branches run on both sides of the medial saphenous vein.

3. The caudal cutaneous sural nerve becomes subcutaneous laterally at the beginning of the gastrocnemius tendon, accompanies the lateral saphenous vein across the surface of the hock, and continues to the fetlock on the lateroplantar aspect of the metatarsus (see Fig. 16–1).

14e. LIVE HORSE

Palpation of this large and complex joint should begin with an easily recognized feature—the tibial tuberosity. By passing the fingers proximally, two soft depressions can be felt between the intermediate patellar ligament and the medial and lateral patellar ligaments. Continuing proximally between the intermediate and medial ligaments, one can feel the smooth, rounded prominence of the medial ridge of the trochlea. Palpation of this surface is blocked proximally by the distal border of the patella and its fibrocartilage. Palpate the cranial surface of the patella, its base (proximal), and the continuity of the fibrocartilage with the medial patellar ligament. The lateral patellar ligament should be traced to the patella. The femoropatellar joint capsule is injected caudal to the lateral patellar ligament near the patella (see Plate I).

Beginning with the tibial tuberosity again, palpate caudally across the extensor groove, occupied by the common tendon of origin of the long digital extensor and peroneus tertius, and a diverticulum of the joint capsule. Caudal to the extensor groove is the lateral tibial condyle and the head of the fibula. The lateral collateral ligament can be palpated from the lateral epicondyle of the femur to the head of the fibula. The lateral sac of the femorotibial joint is injected here between the lateral collateral ligament and the tendon of origin of the long digital extensor.

Return to the tibial attachment of the medial patellar ligament and palpate caudally to the medial collateral ligament. This extends vertically from the medial epicondyle of the femur to the tibia below the medial condyle. The medial sac of the femorotibial joint is injected between these ligaments.

Determine by palpation the resting and gliding positions of the patella.[10]

When the horse is standing squarely on both hind limbs, the patella is at the proximal end of the trochlea, the resting articular surfaces are in contact, and the cranial border of the medial patellar ligament can be palpated one finger-breadth behind the cranial surface of the medial ridge of the trochlea. When the patella is on the resting surface of the trochlea, little force is required to prevent the patella from slipping off to the gliding surface. Palpation of the quadriceps femoris will show that it is relaxed when the horse is standing. However, the biceps femoris and tensor fasciae latae are attached to the lateral patellar ligament, and the sartorius and gracilis are attached to the medial patellar ligament. They may help to hold the patella in the resting position.

When the horse rests one hind limb on the toe of the hoof, the supporting limb undergoes slight flexion with the added weight, and the hindquarters sink about 4 cm. The pelvis is tilted, with the supporting side higher. In the supporting limb, the fibrocartilage and medial patellar ligament slide farther around the tubercle of the trochlea so that the cranial border of the ligament is two finger-breadths behind the cranial surface of the medial ridge of the trochlea. The latter is readily palpated between the intermediate and medial ligaments, which, with the patella and the fibrocartilage, form a loop over the top of the medial ridge. This mechanism prevents flexion of the stifle and enables the horse to stand with little muscular effort. Some effort must be required, however, because the horse soon tires and shifts his weight to the other hind limb.

If the patella of the weight-bearing limb is palpated, the apex will be felt in close contact with the trochlea. There is a marked depression between the relaxed quadriceps and the cranial surface of the patella. As the horse begins to flex the stifle, the release of the patella can be felt as a distinct snap. The patella rotates laterally about 15° as the gliding surfaces engage and a notch becomes palpable between the apex and the trochlea. Proximally the quadriceps is now tense, eliminating the dimple at the base of the patella. Whether or not the patella goes into the resting position in the weight-bearing phase of each stride at gaits faster than the walk is unknown.

The pathological condition of proximal fixation of the patella is probably a disorder of the neuromuscular mechanism that normally releases the patella from its resting position. Spasm of the medial muscles of the thigh is a possible cause. When this occurs the affected limb is held with the stifle and hock fully extended and the fetlock and interphalangeal joints flexed so that the hoof rests on its dorsal surface. The positions of the hock and digit are related to the reciprocal mechanism and the attachments of the superficial digital flexor. The horse is unable to flex the stifle and hock and drags the limb behind. This is not a luxation because the patella is fixed in one of its normal positions. Temporary relief from proximal fixation of the patella can be obtained by pushing the medial patellar ligament and fibrocartilage off the medial ridge manually. The horse can sometimes be startled with a whip so that he jumps and unlocks the patella. A more lasting palliative measure is medial patellar desmotomy. After the medial patellar ligament is cut, a small dimple will be apparent. The taut termination of the sartorius on the distal end of the medial patellar ligament should not be confused with an uncut ligament. If the operation is done bilaterally, the animal cannot sleep standing for some time, but the ligament soon regenerates and becomes palpable again.[15] True lateral luxation, traumatic or congenital, occurs occasionally in the horse. Medial luxation is more rare.

Injury to the ligaments of the stifle can be determined by movements to displace the tibia from the femur. With the pelvic limb held off the ground, move the leg medially and laterally at the stifle. Excess abduction of the tibia indicates a rupture of the medial collateral ligament. Excessive adduction is diagnostic of a lateral collateral ligament injury. To test joint stability that is due to the cruciate ligaments, rock the supporting leg cranially and caudally. If the horse is cooperative, stand behind the limb, brace your knee against the tarsus, grasp the proximal tibia with both hands, and rock it cranially and caudally. There is no movement in the normal horse. Excessive cranial motion occurs with cranial cruciate ligament injury, and excessive caudal motion occurs with caudal cruciate ligament injury.

Palpate on the medial surface of the leg (crus) from cranial to caudal:

Tibialis cranialis.

Tibia.

Cranial branch of medial saphenous vein with branches of saphenous nerve. (See section 16c.)

Deep digital flexors. (See section 16b).

Tibial nerve. It can be palpated caudally on the medial surface of the deep digital flexors by placing the fingertips medial to the common calcanean tendon. (see Plate I).

Superficial digital flexor tendon.

Palpate on the lateral surface of the leg, from cranial to caudal:

Long digital extensor.

Point of injection for the peroneal nerves. The superficial and deep peroneal nerves can be palpated between the biceps femoris and lateral digital extensor before they enter the muscles on the craniolateral surface of the tibia. These can be blocked here or where the peroneal nerves are in the groove between the long and lateral digital extensors, 10 cm. proximal to the tibiotarsal joint. The superficial peroneal nerve is subcutaneous. The deep peroneal nerve is about 2 cm. deep and cranial to the intermuscular septum.

Lateral digital extensor.

Deep digital flexors.

Gastrocnemius tendon. It winds around the lateral surface of the superficial digital flexor tendon from the superficial to the deep position. The groove between the tendons can be palpated.

Caudal cutaneous sural nerve. This nerve can be injected subcutaneously on the craniolateral surface of the gastrocnemius tendon, near the origin of the tendon from the lateral head of the muscle.

14f. DISSECTION, STIFLE AND CRUS, OX

Locate the patellar ligaments. The cranial part of the biceps terminates by a strong tendon on the patella and lateral patellar ligament. The large bursa between this tendon and the lateral epicondyle of the femur is subject to inflammation. It may communicate with the femorotibial joint. The femoropatellar and femorotibial joints usually communicate, as do the medial and lateral femorotibial sacs. Two puncture sites are recommended for the bovine stifle: the femoropatellar joint between the intermediate and medial patellar ligaments and the lateral femorotibial sac in the muscular groove of the tibia, cranial to the tendon of the peroneus tertius.

Identify the tendon of the gastrocnemius as it winds around the lateral surface of the superficial flexor from the superficial to the deep position. These muscles are affected in calves that have a neuromuscular abnormality called spastic paresis. The hock is rigidly extended. This is exacerbated when the calf walks and the affected limb is thrust caudally in extension. This usually occurs before 6 months, and the disability limits their rate of weight gain for meat production. The cause involves an overactivity of the gamma efferent neurons to neuromuscular spindles in the gastrocnemius muscles.[4, 5] No microscopic lesions have been found. The function can be improved by denervation of the gastrocnemius muscles.[2] Inheritance has been proposed but not proven. An incision is made between the cranial and caudal parts of the biceps femoris to expose the lateral head of the gastrocnemius. The common peroneal nerve, running obliquely across the lateral surface of the lateral head, is preserved. In the fat caudal to the origins of the gastrocnemius, the tibial nerve can be isolated just before it disappears between the heads of the muscle. The muscular branch to the medial head comes from the caudal border of the tibial nerve at this point. The branch to the lateral head arises from the lateral surface near the middle of its width. These branches can be identified by electrical stimulation and cut, sparing the plantar nerves and the branches to the digital flexors. This operation should not be done bilaterally at the same time; it should not be done in adults. Affected animals should not be used for breeding.

Find the peroneus tertius, peroneus longus, and the medial, long, and lateral digital extensors. The peroneus tertius, unlike that of the horse, is broad, fleshy, and superficial. The medial digital extensor is a part of the long digital extensor.

The digits can be anesthetized by two injections in the crus. The tibial nerve is palpated on the medial side at the proximal end of the space between the common calcanean tendon and the deep digital flexors. This is about 10 cm. above the tuber calcanei. The common peroneal nerve is injected by inserting the needle caudal to the palpable proximal part of the fibula and directing it craniodistally. Part of the injection is subfascial and the rest is 4 cm. deep between the peroneus longus and the lateral digital extensor.[11]

The metatarsus is not anesthetized by this method because the saphenous and caudal cutaneous sural nerves are not blocked.

The popliteal lymph node is in the fat between the biceps and semitendinosus, just behind the proximal end of the gastrocnemius. It is reached for final inspection by an incision between the biceps femoris and semitendinosus at the level of the patella. In swine, the node is subcutaneous.

A condition of fixation of the patella occurs in the ox. The limb is extended moderately and resists flexion. Some authors consider this a proximal fixation like that of the horse; others believe it is a proximolateral luxation. A true lateral luxation also occurs occasionally in the ox. The limb is flexed and will not bear weight.[8]

14g. LIVE COW

Lameness due to lesions in the stifle will cause the animal to avoid flexing the stifle. On walking, the stifle and hock will be fixed in extension. The fetlock will be slightly flexed and only the tip of the toe will be in contact with the ground. Ligamentous injuries can be diagnosed by the same manipulations as described for the horse. Palpate the following structures (see Plate II):

> Patella.
> Medial ridge of femoral trochlea.
> Medial, intermediate, and lateral patellar ligaments.
> Medial and lateral collateral ligaments.
> Medial meniscus between the medial patellar ligament and medial collateral ligament.
> Lateral femoral epicondyle (bicipital bursa).
> Superficial digital flexor and gastrocnemius tendons.
> The muscle group formed by the peroneus tertius and the medial and long digital extensors. All three have a common origin from the extensor fossa of the femur. They lie on the craniolateral surface of the crus. Caudal to this group, palpate the peroneus longus and the lateral extensor, both of which originate from the lateral tibial condyle. Palpate the nerve block sites (see section 14f).
> Tibial nerve. It is craniomedial to the common calcanean tendon.
> Peroneal nerve. It is located on the lateral surface of the proximal fibula.

References

1. Adams, O. R.: Lameness in Horses, 3rd ed. Philadelphia: Lea & Febiger, 1974.
2. Bouckaert, J. H. and A. De Moor: Treatment of spastic paralysis in cattle: improved denervation technique of gastrocnemius muscle and postoperative course. Vet Rec. 79 (1966):226–229.
3. Delahanty, D. D.: Defects—not fractures—of the fibulae in the horse. JAVMA 133 (1958):258–260.
4. De Ley, G. and A. De Moor: Bovine spastic paralysis: results of surgical desafferentation of the gastrocnemius muscle by means of spinal dorsal root section. Am. J. Vet. Res. 38 (1977):1899–1900.
5. De Ley, G. and A. De Moor: Bovine spastic paralysis: results of selective gamma efferent suppression with dilute procaine. Vet. Sci. Comm. 3 (1979/1980):289–298.

6. McIllwraith, C. W.: Subchondral cystic lesions (osteochondrosis) in the horse. Comp. Cont. Ed. *4* (1982): S394–S404.

7. Nelson, D. R. and D. B. Koch: Surgical stabilization of the stifle in cranial cruciate ligament injury in cattle. Vet. Rec. *111* (1982):259–262.

8. Nelson, D. R.: Surgery of the stifle joint in cattle. Comp. Cont. Ed. *5* (1983):S300–S305.

9. Nichels, F. A. and R. Sande: Radiographic and arthroscopic findings in the equine stifle. JAVMA *181* (1982):918–924.

10. Preuss, F. and E. Henschel: Über die reitende Patella des Pferdes. Berl. Münch. Tierärztl. Wochenschr. *82* (1969):409–413.

11. Schreiber, J.: Die anatomischen Grundlagen der Leitungsanästhesie beim Rind. IV. Teil. Die Leitungsanästhesie der Nerven der Hinterextremität. Wiener Tierärztl. Mschr. *43* (1956):673–705.

12. Sisson, S. and J. D. Grossman: The Anatomy of the Domestic Animals. Philadelphia: W. B. Saunders, 1955, p. 118.

13. Trotter, G. W. and C. W. McIllwraith: Osteochondritis dissecans and subchondral cystic lesions in their relationship to osteochondrosis in the horse. J. Equine Vet. Sci. *1* (1981):157–163.

14. Trout, D. R., and C. L. Lohse: Anatomy and therapeutic resection of the peroneus tertius muscle in a foal. JAVMA *179* (1981):247–251.

15. Vaughan, L. C.: Upward displacement of the patella and its treatment by desmotomy. Br. Eq. Vet. Assoc. Proc. *1* (1962):28–29.

CHAPTER 15

STIFLE AND LEG, CARNIVORES

OBJECTIVES

1. To be able to identify by palpation the skeletal prominences of the distal end of the femur and both ends of the tibia and fibula.
2. To recognize the ossification centers of the tibia and fibula. To be able to distinguish between avulsion of the tibial tuberosity and the normal epiphysis in a radiograph.
3. To be able to recognize the normal sesamoids of the stifle joint by their position in a radiograph.
4. To be able to recognize the normal radiolucent menisci and articular cartilages of the femorotibial joint in craniocaudal views and to interpret asymmetry.
5. To be able to palpate the collateral and patellar ligaments, the patella, and the gastrocnemius sesamoids.
6. To be able to manipulate the stifle to diagnose the instability due to injury of the cruciate and collateral ligaments.
7. To be able to palpate a patellar luxation and understand the effect a chronic luxation has on the shape of the limb.
8. To understand the surgical anatomy necessary for correction of patellar dislocation, rupture of the cruciate ligaments, and meniscal lesions.
9. To be able to insert a needle into the stifle joint.
10. To be able to palpate the popliteal lymph node.
11. To be able to palpate the landmarks for nerve blocks in the crus.

15a. TIBIA, FIBULA, AND RADIOGRAPHS, DOG AND CAT

Orient the tibia. The lateral side of the proximal third is concave. The medial malleolus projects from the distal end. In the dog, the thin flat distal half of the shaft of the fibula is applied to the flattened lateral surface of the distal half of the tibia. In the cat, the shafts of the bones are not flattened or adherent but present opposing borders for the attachment of the interosseous membrane. The head of the fibula articulates with the caudolateral angle of the lateral tibial condyle. The lateral malleolus (distal end of the fibula) projects distally to correspond with the medial malleolus.

Table 15–1 and Table 2 of the Appendix show the approximate age of radiological union of the epiphyses with the shafts of the tibia and fibula.

Identify the following in radiographs:

In the lateral radiograph of the stifle, note the high position of the patella on the trochlea. The three sesamoid bones on the caudal surface of the joint should not be mistaken for fragments. Two are in contact with the caudal surface of the femur proximal to the condyles, at the origin of the gastrocnemius. The third is in the tendon of origin of the popliteus, where it crosses the lateral condyle of the tibia.

In the craniocaudal view, find the patella and the two gastrocnemius sesamoids. The medial sesamoid may be displaced medially and distally in some normal dogs. Excessive distal displacement in a dog that walks with overflexion of the tarsus indicates an avulsion of the origin of that head of the gastrocnemius muscle. The popliteus sesamoid may be obscured. Compare the intervals between the femoral and tibial condyles on the medial and lateral sides. The lateral one is usually slightly wider. The radiolucent zone is occupied by the menisci and articular cartilages. If the femoral and tibial condyles appear to be in contact, there is a meniscal injury.

Epiphysis of the tibial tuberosity. Notice in the lateral view of the normal stifle of the pup that there is a thick, radiolucent epiphyseal cartilage between the tibial tuberosity and the rest of the tibia. This should not be diagnosed as epiphyseal separation because the epiphysis has not been rotated outward and upward by the tension of the patellar ligament (avulsion). Note also the smooth contour of the cranial border of the tibia distal to the epiphysis. This area has a frayed appearance in avulsion. Avulsion occurs more commonly in Greyhounds, usually before they are 8 months old; it is caused by the stress of race training.[27]

Proximal articular epiphyses of the tibia and fibula. Note again the normal thickness of the epiphyseal cartilage in the pup.

The shafts of the tibia and fibula are usually fractured in the middle.

Distal epiphyses of the tibia and fibula.

Medial (tibial) malleolus and lateral (fibular) malleolus. These may be fractured in the adult.

On the arthrogram note the large extent of the cavity for the common capsule of the three joints. It extends proximal to the patella and trochlea on the shaft of the femur and lateral on the epicondyles. It surrounds both femoral condyles and the articulation of the gastrocnemius sesamoids and passes around the thin axial border of each meniscus to surround the tibial condyles. It extends around the articulation of the head of the fibula with the lateral tibial condyle and passes distally around the tendon of origin of the long digital extensor and a short distance under the tendon of the popliteus. All parts are in communication. A large fat body separates the cranial synovial part of the capsule from the fibrous part, which blends with the patellar ligament.

Note the irregular appearance of the growth plate for the distal femoral epiphysis. In the young pup, the distance between the femoral and tibial condyles appears to be large because of the carti-

Table 15–1. EPIPHYSEAL FUSION IN THE CRUS (AGE IN MONTHS)[9, 17, 35, 36]

	Dogs	Cats
Tibial tuberosity to proximal epiphysis	6–9	8–10
Tibial tuberosity and proximal epiphysis to shaft	6–15	12–18
Proximal fibula	6–12	13–18
Distal tibia	5–11	10–13
Distal fibula	5–13	10–14

lage in the condyles that has not yet ossified. The ossification center for the patella first appears at 6 to 9 weeks. Occasionally there are two ossification centers, a proximal and a distal. The sesamoids first appear radiographically at 3 months in the gastrocnemius and popliteus muscles in the dog and at 2.5 to 5 months in the cat.

15b. DISSECTIONS, PATELLAR LUXATION, DOG

Place the limb on the table with the cranial surface up. The superficial medial muscle is the sartorius, with one insertion on the patella and one on the tibia. The superficial lateral muscle is the biceps femoris, with its aponeurotic insertion on the patella and patellar ligament. Find the patella by palpation and trace the patellar ligament to the tibial tuberosity.

Traumatic luxation of the patella in a normal limb can occur in the dog, but recurrent luxation occurs medially in the toy breeds of dogs.[5, 38] The primary malformation that causes this is unknown. Classifications exist for describing the degree of medial patellar luxation.[33, 38] In severe malformation, the luxation is permanent and cannot be corrected manually. The femur deviates laterally distal to the hip and is curved with a lateral convexity. The femur may be rotated laterally or there may be torsion of the distal third. The lateral femoral condyle is larger and extends farther distally than the medial. The trochlea is shallow or absent. The proximal tibia is deviated medially at the stifle (genu varum) and is rotated medially. Most commonly what appears to be a medial displacement of the tibial tuberosity is the result of medial rotation of the tibia. This can be corrected manually when the normal position of the patella is reestablished.[38] Occasionally, a torsion of the proximal tibia contributes to this medial position of the tibial tuberosity. The proximal third of the tibia may be curved with a medial convexity, and the distal tibia may be bowed with a lateral convexity. The paw may deviate medially (varus deformity).[11, 30] When displaced medially, the quadriceps muscle, patella, and patellar ligament act like a taut bow string on the medial side of the femur between the ilium and proximal femur and the tibial tuberosity, which causes or exacerbates these deformities.[38]

Numerous surgical procedures have been described to correct this deformity in its various degrees.[5, 20, 38] A basic understanding of the femoropatellar ligaments is necessary.[30]

Each femoropatellar ligament forms a part of a retinaculum. The following is from *Nomina Anatomica Veterinaria*.

Patellar lig. (man, dog, cat, pig, sheep, goat)
Intermediate patellar lig. (ox, horse)
Medial patellar retinaculum (all spp.)
  Medial femoropatellar lig. (all spp.)
  Medial patellar lig. (ox, horse)
Lateral patellar retinaculum (all spp.)
  Lateral femoropatellar lig. (all spp.)
  Lateral patellar lig. (ox, horse)

The retinacula are derived from the deep fascia and aponeuroses on the sides of the patella and patellar ligament. Each consists of two or more layers of fibers running in two directions: (1) proximodistal fibers attached to the patella, but running mainly from the thigh muscles to the tibia; these fibers are concentrated in the medial and lateral patellar ligaments in the horse and ox; (2) deep transverse fibers, running from the proximal end of the patella to the femoral epicondyles in the horse and ox and to the gastrocnemius sesamoids in the dog—the femoropatellar ligaments.

The aponeurosis of the biceps (the part of the retinaculum directed distally) covers the thin, lateral femoropatellar ligament; the latter extends from the proximal end of the patella across the tendon of the vastus lateralis, with which it is blended in the joint capsule, and across the femur to the lateral sesamoid.

The medial femoropatellar ligament is difficult to see. The caudal belly of the sartorius covers the termination of the cranial belly of the semimembranosus on the medial sesamoid. The aponeurosis of the cranial belly of the sartorius can be drawn forward to expose the aponeurosis of the caudal part of the vastus medialis. These two aponeuroses are blended to form the part of the medial retinaculum directed distally. The medial femoropatellar ligament consists of a thin layer of transverse fibers attached to the medial border of the patella through the aponeurosis of the vastus medialis and extending to the medial gastrocnemius sesamoid and the tendon of the semimembranosus. It forms part of the fibrous joint capsule, then runs across the femur proximal to the epicondyle and deep to the descending genicular artery.

Some surgical procedures use the fascia lata to augment a weak lateral femoropatellar ligament by dissecting a strip off the vastus lateralis.[24] This is left attached distally to the patella, and the free end is drawn through the tendon of the lateral head of the gastrocnemius just over its sesamoid and sutured. Many suture materials have been used as a substitute for the fascia lata. Imbrication is often used to provide lateral support for the patella.

In most dogs when the trochlea is deepened surgically and the patella is replaced, the tibia can be derotated by passing a suture around the lateral collateral ligament and through the tibial tuberosity and tightening it.[38]

More heroic measures are employed when the bones are deformed. The tibial tuberosity can be transplanted laterally to compensate for torsion or medial rotation of the tibia as follows. The cranial edge of the origin of the tibialis cranialis is elevated from the lateral surface of the tibia and reflected. The bone here must be scraped free of muscle. The extension of the patellar ligament distal to the tibial tuberosity along the cranial border of the tibia is elevated from the bone but left attached distally. A thin slice of the tibial tuberosity 3 mm. thick is cut off with the patellar ligament attached, turned 90° laterally, and pinned to the lateral surface of the tibia. The tibialis cranialis is sutured back in place over the transplant.[11] Wedge osteotomy may be performed to correct the curvature of the bones.[30]

A pelvic limb deformity, in which the patella luxates laterally, occurs occasionally in young dogs of giant breeds.[29] The stifles are bowed medially, with the tibia deviated laterally (genu valgum). The lateral femoral condyle is smaller than the medial one. The angle between the neck and the shaft of the femur is increased, but the head of the femur is subluxated, allowing medial deviation of the femur at the hip. This condition is thought to be related to overnutrition and too rapid bone growth. Osteochondrosis results with delayed endochondral ossification on the lateral sides of the distal femur and proximal tibia.

15c. DISSECTIONS, CRUCIATE LIGAMENTS

The cranial cruciate ligament is attached caudally to the axial surface of the lateral femoral condyle. Near its origin it crosses lateral to the caudal ligament and runs craniodistally and somewhat medially to attach to the cranial intercondylar area of the tibia. This area is medial to the axis of the bone and caudal to the transverse ligament. The caudal cruciate ligament runs from the axial surface of the medial femoral condyle caudodistally to the medial border of the popliteal notch of the tibia.

Each cruciate ligament has cranial and caudal components that function independently of each other in flexion and extension.[2, 4] In general, the bulk of the cranial cruciate ligament is taut on extension and loose on flexion, whereas the caudal cruciate ligament is loose on extension and taut on flexion. These cruciate ligaments provide craniocaudal stability to the stifle. The cranial ligament limits cranial movement of the tibia on the femur and the caudal ligament limits movement of the tibia caudally. If the cranial cruciate ligament is cut, there will be a significant increase in cranial movement of the tibia (cranial drawer sign), which is a larger movement when the stifle is flexed. Section of the caudal cruciate ligament causes the opposite effect, increased caudal movement of the tibia, especially with the stifle flexed.

The cruciate ligaments also provide rotational stability to the stifle. This is primarily a function of the cranial ligament, which limits medial rotation of the tibia on the femur when the stifle is flexed. There is a considerable amount of normal medial rotation of the tibia, especially with the stifle flexed, but with rupture of the cranial cruciate ligament this is significantly increased. The cranial cruciate ligament also limits stifle hyperextension.

The cranial cruciate ligament is the one most commonly ruptured in stifle injuries in the dog. This occurs in athletic dogs that are hunting or playing vigorously and suddenly turn sharply to one side, so that the body turns toward the side of the supporting pelvic limb.[31] This forces extreme medial rotation of the tibia on the femur, and if the rotation exceeds the strength of the cranial cruciate ligament, it will tear, usually at its insertion on the tibia. Similarly if such a dog steps in a hole and overextends the stifle, the cranial cruciate ligament may tear. Older, less active dogs of any size breed are thought to have a degeneration of these ligaments, which makes them more susceptible to tearing with only mild stress applied to the joint. Surgical repair is usually necessary for rupture of the cranial cruciate ligament because it may be very painful in the acute stage, and if it is not corrected, the chronic instability will result in an incapacitating degenerative osteoarthropathy. Many surgical procedures have been described to repair these ligaments; they vary with the size of the dog and the surgeon's preference.

The classic method is to replace the ruptured ligament with a strip of fascia lata passed through holes drilled in both the femur and tibia.[26] The first step is to dissect a strip of fascia lata free along the cranial border of the biceps from the lateral condyle of the tibia to the tensor fasciae latae. The proximal end is cut off, and the distal end remains attached. The joint capsule is opened along the lateral side of the patella and patellar ligament; the patella is luxated medially, and the joint is debrided. If the menisci are damaged, they are removed. A hole is drilled through the femur from a point proximal to the end of the lateral collateral ligament to the attachment of the cranial cruciate ligament laterally in the intercondylar fossa. The hole in the tibia is drilled from the tibial attachment of the cranial cruciate ligament to the medial surface of the bone slightly distal to the medial condyle. The fascial strip is threaded through the holes and anchored to the cranial border of the tibia with wire sutures. The two holes in the bones are not in line, but the course of the fascial strip through the joint should be the same as that of the ligament; therefore, it is important to understand the points of attachment. The initial part of the fascial strip serves as a reinforcement of the lateral collateral ligament.

A modification of this classic method is to use a strip of fascia lata attached distally to the tibia, lateral to the tibial tuberosity.[13] A hole is drilled through the lateral femoral condyle as before, and the strip of fascia lata is passed caudally into the intercondylar fossa and threaded through the hole from distal to proximal. It is then pulled distally across the lateral femoral condyle, stifle, and distal attachment of the strip of fascia lata, where it is sutured.

Another modification is to isolate a strip of fascia lata from the craniolateral surface of the quadriceps. Continue this to the medial side of the patella, where a portion of the craniomedial aspect of the patella is cut off with an osteotome. The patellar ligament attached to this piece of bone is separated from the remainder but is left attached to the tibial tuberosity. The replacement ligament will consist of a strip of fascia lata, a portion of the patella, and a portion of the patellar ligament. This is passed caudally into the intercondylar fossa of the femur and threaded distal to proximal through a hole drilled in the lateral condyle. The strip of fascia lata is pulled distally and sutured to the periosteum of the lateral surface of the femoral condyle.

No drill holes are required when the same strip of fascia lata, and portions of patella, and patellar ligament are dissected and passed completely through the intercondylar fossa of the femur to the caudal side. There the fascia lata is pulled directly lateral over the lateral femoral condyle through an incision in the tendinous origin of the gastrocnemius. This is pulled taut with the limb in extension and sutured to the periosteum on the lateral side of the femoral condyle.[3, 4]

All of these procedures provide a substitute ligament that is anatomically aligned similar to the normal ligament. It is important to open the joint capsule and inspect the joint for further injury, especially of the menisci, and to remove any injured tissue .

In smaller breeds, some surgeons use various imbrication procedures to tighten the joint and reduce the instability.[4, 8, 10, 25] One of these involves passing a suture on each side from the patellar ligament at its termination or from holes drilled in the tibial tuberosity to the connective tissue around each gastrocnemius sesamoid and drawing these tight.[10]

15d. DISSECTIONS, MENISCI AND COLLATERAL LIGAMENTS, DOG

Find the medial and lateral collateral ligaments and the external edges of the menisci. Note the attachments of the collateral ligaments on the femoral epicondyles, which are caudal to the long axis of the shaft but at the axis of rotation. The medial ligament attaches to the medial border of the tibia distal to the condyle. The lateral ligament attaches to the head of the fibula. The medial collateral ligament is closely attached to its meniscus by the deep short part of the ligament that ends in the meniscus, while the lateral ligament is separated from its meniscus by the tendon of the popliteus.[6]

The collateral ligaments prevent adduction and abduction of the tibia on the femur (mediolateral hinge motion). The medial ligament is taut in all ranges of motion but especially on extension.[39] The lateral ligament is taut on extension of the stifle but is loose on flexion, which permits the normal medial rotation of the tibia that occurs on flexion. Both ligaments limit lateral and medial rotation of the tibia with the stifle extended. In flexion the medial ligament limits lateral rotation.

Injuries of these ligaments can be diagnosed with the limb in extension by the ability to open the medial side of the stifle on abduction of the tibia if the medial collateral ligament is damaged or the lateral side of the stifle on adducting the tibia if the lateral collateral ligament is injured. With rupture of either ligament, there will be excessive lateral and medial rotation of the tibia that can be palpated with the stifle extended. Rupture of the medial ligament will permit excessive lateral rotation with the joint flexed. The medial ligament is more commonly injured, and this is often associated with the stress that tears the cranial cruciate ligament. The same injury may damage the medial meniscus.[6]

The menisci are curved pieces of fibrocartilage that are thicker toward the outside of the joint. They are like washers inserted between the femoral and tibial condyles to decrease the incongruity and increase the stability of the stifle and act as shock absorbers.[22] The cranial and caudal extremity of each meniscus is attached to the tibia. The caudal attachment of the lateral meniscus is at the lateral edge of the popliteal notch. A transverse ligament attaches the two cranial extremities of the menisci, and the caudal extremity of the lateral meniscus is also attached dorsally to the intercondylar fossa of the femur by the meniscofemoral ligament. The medial meniscus is also firmly attached to the medial collateral ligament and a large portion of the joint capsule. During stifle flexion both menisci move but the lateral one is free to move farther and in extreme flexion may protrude over the caudal edge of the lateral tibial condyle.[6] This disparity in movement of the menisci is due to the firm attachment of the medial meniscus to the medial collateral ligament, joint capsule, and the tibia. The lateral meniscus is attached to the femur, which pulls it caudally as the lateral femoral condyle moves caudally over the tibia. This is enhanced by the lack of attachment to the lateral collateral ligament, less extensive joint capsule attachment, and the caudal position of its caudal tibial attachment.

As the stifle flexes, the lateral collateral ligament loosens, and the tibia rotates medially as the lateral femoral condyle and the lateral meniscus slide caudally on the tibia.

The menisci are injured when the stifle is severely stressed.[6, 16] Injury of the medial meniscus is more commonly associated with tearing of the cranial cruciate ligament and excessive medial tibial rotation. Most commonly, the inner and caudal aspect of the meniscus tears longitudinally or a portion of it folds.[16] The injured meniscus may cause a clicking sound, which is heard when the animal is walking or when the stifle is manipulated.

Medial meniscus injuries occur in 50 percent or more of dogs with cranial cruciate injuries.[21] If it is not damaged at the initial stress and injury, it may be damaged as the dog regains the ability to walk with its unstable joint. During weight bearing, the tibia glides cranially and the medial meniscus is drawn cranially with the tibia so that its caudal part moves under the medial femoral condyle, where it can be crushed.

The injured portion of the meniscus should be removed to prevent degenerative joint disease.[6] Some prefer to remove the entire meniscus when it is injured.[15] The joint capsule, which normally supplies blood to the meniscus, should be preserved. It will be the source of regeneration of granulation tissue that will ultimately change into fibrocartilage to replace the meniscus.[12] The meniscus may be removed from a cranial arthrotomy incision by pulling it forward, severing the attachments of the extremities, and dissecting the periphery from the capsule. Be careful to avoid the popliteal vessels that course just caudal to the caudal attachment of the meniscus.

15e. DISSECTION OF NERVE BLOCKS OF LEG, DOG

The paw can be anesthetized by blocking the following nerves (see Fig. 15–1):

Peroneal Nerves. Palpate the groove between the long digital extensor and the tendon of the

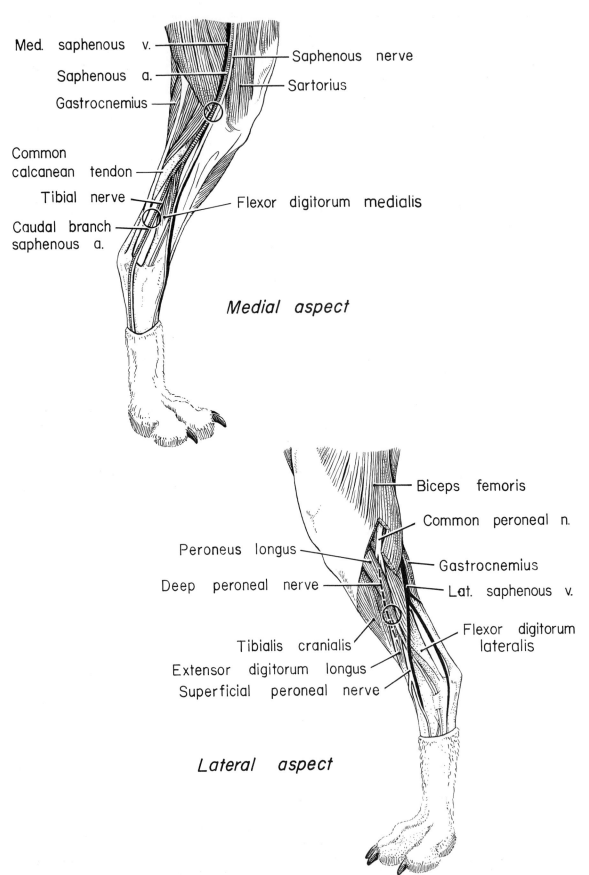

Med. saphenous v.

Saphenous a.

Gastrocnemius

Common calcanean tendon

Tibial nerve

Caudal branch saphenous a.

Saphenous nerve

Sartorius

Flexor digitorum medialis

Medial aspect

Biceps femoris

Common peroneal n.

Peroneus longus

Gastrocnemius

Deep peroneal nerve

Lat. saphenous v.

Tibialis cranialis

Flexor digitorum lateralis

Extensor digitorum longus

Superficial peroneal nerve

Lateral aspect

Figure 15–1. Nerve blocks (circled) to anesthetize the hind paw of the dog.

peroneus longus. Insert the needle in the groove, halfway between the stifle and the hock and proximal to the cranial branch of the lateral saphenous vein, and direct it distally. Make a deposit for the superficial peroneal nerve; then advance the needle medially to block the deep peroneal nerve on the craniolateral surface of the tibia. It lies lateral to the cranial tibial artery. The peroneal nerves can also be blocked where the common peroneal nerve is palpable as it crosses the head of the fibula. This will also paralyze the flexors of the hock and the extensors of the digit.

Tibial Nerve. Palpate the nerve by rolling it on the caudomedial surface of the deep digital flexors, in the webbed space in front of the common calcanean tendon. The nerve is accompanied by the caudal branch of the saphenous artery.

Saphenous Nerve. Inject in front of the medial saphenous vein behind the proximal end of the tibia.

The tibia is subcutaneous medially and is best approached from that side for open reduction of fractures. The cranial branches of the saphenous vessels, and the saphenous nerve cross the tibia obliquely and should be spared.

15f. LIVE DOG

Palpate the stifle (see Plate III).

Cranially:
> Ridges of the femoral trochlea.
> Patella.
> Tibial tuberosity, the proximal end of the cranial border of the tibia.
> Patellar ligament. With the joint in the standing position, the plane of femorotibial contact is halfway between the patella and the tibial tuberosity.
> The joint capsule is accessible on either side of the ligament caudal to the fat pad. All of the synovial sacs of the joint capsule communicate freely. Normally there is a slight depression on the medial side of the patellar ligament.

Laterally:
> Proximal end of the fibula. Articulates with the caudolateral angle of the lateral condyle of the tibia. This is the insertion of the lateral collateral ligament. Palpate the common peroneal nerve where it crosses the proximal fibula.
> Try to find the lateral sesamoid of the gastrocnemius. It is deep to the biceps and may be impossible to palpate in muscular dogs.

Medially:
> Distal margin of the medial femoral condyle.
> Medial collateral ligament.
> The medial sesamoid is easily palpated.

Caudally:
> Popliteal lymph node. Between the distal ends of the biceps femoris and semitendinosus, on the heads of the gastrocnemius.

Palpate the points of injection of the peroneal, tibial, and saphenous nerves described in section 15e.

The diagnosis of internal lesions of the stifle requires an understanding of the normal range of movement. Complete extension of the stifle to 180° is impossible in the normal joint. Extension is limited to about 150° by the cruciate, collateral, and meniscofemoral ligaments and the menisci. In maximum extension the stifle is rigid and little rotation is possible. In flexion the menisci glide backward on the tibia especially the lateral meniscus. The lateral collateral ligament is slack, and the tibia can be rotated medially until limited by the cranial cruciate ligament. The collateral ligaments prevent lateral rotation as well as mediolateral hinge motion at the stifle.

Dogs with stifle disease that causes excessive pain will not bear weight on the limb, and they carry it flexed. If they walk on the limb, the stride will be short and the weight will be carried on the forelimbs. The dog will nod on the forelimb when the lame hind limb is placed on the ground.

In examining the stifle for ligamentous injuries, the following procedure should be used:[23] Palpate the patellar ligament and the patella in the femoral trochlea. If the patellar ligament is ruptured, the limb cannot support weight. Palpate for distention of the joint capsule and crepitus on gentle flexion and extension. Determine the range of motion in the stifle. Gently adduct and abduct the tibia in a mediolateral hinge motion to assess the integrity of the collateral ligaments.

With the limb extended, rotate the tibia laterally and medially to test for collateral ligament strength. With the stifle in moderate flexion, rotate the tibia medially to test for cranial cruciate ligament integrity and laterally to test for medial collateral ligament integrity. To determine craniocaudal stability of the stifle, hold the femur from behind with the thumb on the lateral condyle and the stifle in moderate flexion. Grasp the tibia with the other hand and with the thumb on the lateral condyle, push the tibia cranially and pull it caudally. Excessive cranial movement diagnoses a cranial cruciate ligament rupture. Excessive caudal movement diagnoses rupture of the caudal cruciate ligament. In heavily muscled dogs, anesthesia may be necessary to detect excessive cranial movement of the tibia.

Another method to determine excessive cranial movement of the tibia is the tibial compression maneuver.[18, 34] Hold the limb with the stifle and hock flexed at 90°. Support the femur in this position with one hand, with the first finger over the stifle and on the tibial tuberosity. With the other hand flex the hock forcefully. This will pull on the common calcanean tendon and compress the tibia between the stifle and hock. If the cranial cruciate ligament is ruptured, the tibia will glide cranially at the stifle.

Palpate the cranial and caudal muscles in the crus. The cranial tibial muscle is the most superficial on the craniolateral aspect of the crus. It covers the long digital extensor. Palpate the two heads of the gastrocnemius muscle and the deep digital flexors on the caudal side of the crus. Identify the common calcanean tendon and its component parts.

The common calcanean tendon consists of the tendons of the gastrocnemius and superficial digital flexor muscles along with contributions from the biceps femoris laterally and the gracilis and semitendinosus medially. Through their attachment to the tuber calcis they extend the hock. Injury to one or more components results in varying degrees of overflexion of the hock when the dog bears weight on the limb.[7, 28] The stifle will overextend to compensate for this functional abnormality. All components must be damaged before a plantigrade posture results. Rupture of the origins of the gastrocnemius muscles can be diagnosed radiographically by the distal displacement of the sesamoids. If the lateral sesamoid is displaced, the origin of the superficial digital flexor is also damaged. This should be compared to a radiograph of the normal limb because of the normal variation in the radiographic position of these sesamoids. Occasionally, injury to the common calcanean tendon will spare the superficial digital flexor. The hock will be moderately overflexed (dropped) and the digits will be overflexed because of the increased tension on the superficial digital flexor tendon. The superficial digital flexor may become detached from the tuber calcanei and cause intermittent tarsal overflexion and stifle overextension. This slippage can be palpated. Fractures of the calcaneus occasionally occur in Greyhounds along with fractures of the central tarsal bone.

References

1. Alexander, J. W.: Tibial fractures and their management. Comp. Cont. Ed. *4* (1982):78–87.
2. Arnoczky, S. P. and J. L. Marshall: The cruciate ligaments of the canine stifle: an anatomical and functional analysis. Am. J. Vet. Res. *38* (1977):1807–1814.
3. Arnoczky, S. P., G. B. Tarvin, L. Marshall, et al.: The over-the-top procedure: a technique for anterior cruciate ligament substitution in the dog. J. Am. Anim. Hosp. Assoc. *15* (1979):283–291.
4. Arnoczky, S. P.: Surgery of the stifle—the cruciate ligaments (Part I). Comp. Cont. Ed. *2* (1980):106–117.
5. Arnoczky, S. P. and G. B. Tarvin: Surgery of the stifle—the patella (Part II). Comp. Cont. Ed. *2* (1980):200–208.
6. Arnoczky, S. P., G. B. Tarvin, and P. B. Vasseur: Surgery of the stifle—the menisci and collateral ligaments (Part III), Comp. Cont. Ed. *2* (1980):394–400.
7. Bonneau, N. H., M. Olivieri, and L. Breton: Avulsion of the gastrocnemius tendon in the dog causing flexion of the hock and digits. J. Am. Anim. Hosp. Assoc. *19* (1983):717–722.
8. Gambardella, P. C., L. J. Wallace, and F. Cassidy: Lateral suture technique for management of anterior cruciate ligament rupture in dogs: a retrospective study. J. Am. Anim. Hosp. Assoc. *17* (1981):33–38.
9. Chapman, W. L.: Appearance of ossification centers and epiphyseal closures as determined by radiographic techniques. JAVMA *147* (1965):138–141.
10. DeAngelis, M. and R. E. Lau: A lateral retinacular imbrication technique for the surgical correction of anterior cruciate ligament rupture in the dog. JAVMA *157* (1970):79–84.
11. DeAngelis, M.: Patellar luxation in dogs. Vet. Clin. North Am. *1* (1971):403–415.
12. De Young, D. J., G. L. Flo and H. Tvedten: Experimental medial meniscectomy in dogs undergoing cranial cruciate repair. J. Am. Anim. Hosp. Assoc. *16* (1980):639–645.

13. Dickinson, C. R. and D. N. Nunamaker: Repair of ruptured anterior cruciate ligament in the dog: experience of 101 cases using a modified fascia strip technique. JAVMA *170* (1977):827–830.
14. Dyce, K. M., R. H. A. Merlen, and F. J. Wadsworth: The clinical anatomy of the stifle of the dog. Br. Vet. J. *108* (1952):346–354.
15. Flo, G. L. and D. De Young: Meniscal injuries and medial meniscectomy in the canine stifle. J. Am. Anim. Hosp. Assoc. *14* (1978):683–689.
16. Flo, G., D. De Young, H. Tvedten, et al.: Classification of meniscal injuries in the canine stifle based upon gross pathological appearance. J. Am. Anim. Hosp. Assoc. *19* (1983):325–334.
17. Hare, W. C. D.: Radiographic anatomy of the canine pelvic limb. Part II. Developing limb. JAVMA *136* (1960):603–611.
18. Henderson, R. A. and J. L. Milton: The tibial compression mechanism: a diagnostic aid in stifle injuries. J. Am. Anim. Hosp. Assoc. *14* (1978):474–479.
19. Hohn, R. B., and J. M. Miller: Surgical correction of rupture of the anterior cruciate ligament in the dog. JAVMA *150* (1967):1133–1141.
20. Horne, R. D.: Transplantation of the cranial head of the sartorius muscle for correction of medial patellar luxations. J. Am. Anim. Hosp. Assoc. *15* (1979):561–565.
21. Hulse, D. A. and P. K. Shires: Observation of the posteromedial compartment of the stifle joint. J. Am. Anim. Hosp. Assoc. *17* (1981):575–578.
22. Hulse, D. A. and P. K. Shires: The meniscus: anatomy, function and treatment. J. Am. Anim. Hosp. Assoc. *5* (1983):765–774.
23. Keller, W. F.: Diagnosing stifle lameness in dogs. JAVMA *146* (1965):1069–1072.
24. Leonard, E. P.: Orthopedic Surgery of the Dog and Cat. Philadelphia: W. B. Saunders, 1960.
25. McCurnin, D. M., P. T. Pearson, and W. M. Wass: Clinical and pathologic evaluation of ruptured cranial cruciate ligament repair in the dog. Am. J. Vet. Res. *32* (1971):1517–1524.
26. Paatsama, S.: Ligament Injuries in the Canine Stifle Joint. Helsinki: Veterinary College, 1952.
27. Power, J. W.: Avulsion of the tibial tuberosity in the Greyhound. Aust. Vet. J. *52* (1976):491–495.
28. Reinke, J. D. and S. P. Kus: Achilles mechanism injury in the dog. Comp. Cont. Ed. *4* (1982):639–645.
29. Riser, W. H., L. J. Parkes, W. H. Rhodes, et al.: Genu valgum: a stifle deformity of giant dogs, J. Am. Vet. Radiol. Soc. *10* (1969):28–38.
30. Rudy, R. L.: Stifle joint. *In* Archibald, J. (ed.): Canine Surgery, 2nd ed. Wheaton, Ill. Am. Vet. Public., 1974.
31. Singleton, W. B.: Differential diagnosis of stifle injuries in the dog. J. Small Anim. Pract. *1* (1960):182–191.
32. Singleton, W. B.: Stifle joint surgery in the dog. Can. Vet. J. *4* (1963):142–150.
33. Singleton, W. B.: The surgical correction of stifle deformities in the dog. J. Small Anim. Pract. *10* (1969):59–69.
34. Slocum, B. and T. Devine: Cranial tibial thrust: a primary force in the canine stifle. JAVMA *183* (1983):456–459.
35. Smith, R. N. and J. Allcock: Epiphyseal fusion in the Greyhound. Vet. Rec. *72* (1960):75–79.
36. Smith, R. N.: Fusion of ossification centers in the cat. J. Small Anim. Pract. *10* (1969):523–530.
37. Sumner-Smith, G.: Observations on epiphyseal fusion of the canine appendicular skeleton. J. Small Anim. Pract. *7* (1966):303–311.
38. Trotter, E. J.: Medial patellar luxation in the dog. Comp. Cont. Ed. *2* (1980):58–68.
39. Vasseur, P. B. and S. P. Arnoczky: Collateral ligaments of the canine stifle joint: anatomic and functional analysis. Am. J. Vet. Res. *42* (1981):1133–1137.

CHAPTER 16

HOCK AND METATARSUS

OBJECTIVES

1. To be able to identify in radiographs the tarsal bones of the horse, ruminant, and carnivore, and to know which bones are normally fused in certain species.
2. To be able to palpate the bony prominences of the hock joint and its collateral ligaments.
3. To know which bones are fractured and luxated in the Greyhound.
4. To be able to palpate the primary site of bone spavin and the medial tendon of the cranial tibial muscle in the horse.
5. To know the origin and course of the nerve that supplies the interior of the tarsal joint in the horse. To be able to anesthetize the tarsal joint.
6. To know the attachments of the long plantar ligament in the horse and the effect of a swelling of the ligament.
7. To be able to palpate the pouches of the tarsocrural joint sac and to distinguish between the plantar pouches and a distention of the sheath of the deep digital flexor tendon.
8. To be able to make an injection into the tarsocrural joint sac in the horse and dog and into the distal intertarsal and tarsometatarsal joints in the horse, and to know which joint cavities of the tarsus communicate.
9. To be able to block the three nerves on each side of the distal end of the metatarsus that supply the equine digit.
10. To be able to palpate the lateral digital extensor tendon proximal and distal to the hock and the large dorsal metatarsal artery that crosses deep to the tendon.
11. To be able to trace the largest artery of the hind foot in all species and to appreciate its points of vulnerability.
12. To be able to trace the cranial branch of the medial saphenous vein across the hock in the horse and the cranial branch of the lateral saphenous vein in the ox.
13. To be able to block the nerves of the metatarsus in the ox to anesthetize the digits.
14. To know what veins can be used for intravenous local anesthesia of the distal metatarsus and digit in the ox.
15. To know the course of the lateral saphenous vein in the dog and to be able to distend it and fix it for venipuncture. To be able to distend the medial saphenous vein in the cat.

Note on the Nomenclature. The tarsal canal is not analogous to the carpal canal. The former is a channel between the third and fourth tarsal bones. In herbivores it transmits the perforating tarsal vessels, which are absent in man and carnivores. It has received special attention in the horse, where it is large, and because it also transmits a nerve to the distal intertarsal joints primarily involved in tarsitis.

The tarsal tunnel corresponding to the carpal canal is represented in the nomenclature only by the groove on the medial side of the calcaneus, where the tendon of the lateral digital flexor passes over the sustentaculum tali: sulcus tendinis musculi flexoris digitalis lateralis. The groove is converted to a tunnel by the flexor retinaculum.

16a. BONES AND RADIOGRAPHS, HOCK, HORSE

The distal epiphysis of the tibia fuses at 16 to 25 months. The lateral malleolus, distal extremity of the fibula, fuses to the distal epiphysis between 3 and 6 months.

Tibia. Identify the medial and lateral malleoli. Note groove for the tendon of the lateral digital extensor in the lateral malleolus. The two grooves and the intermediate ridge of the cochlea are oblique from caudomedial to craniolateral. In foals, fractures occur in the cranial part of this ridge and in the lateral ridge of the trochlea of the talus. Osteochondrosis commonly occurs on the cranial part of the intermediate ridge of the cochlea in young Standardbreds.[3]

Talus. Observe the relationship of the ridges of the trochlea to the cochlea and malleoli of the tibia. The tubercle on the distal part of the medial surface of the talus is a landmark for the long medial collateral ligament.

Calcaneus. The tuber calcanei extends about 5 cm. above the talus and the tarsocrural joint. The plantar surface of the sustentaculum tali forms a smooth surface for the passage of the lateral digital flexor tendon. At the distal end of the lateral surface is a rough prominence for the attachment of the long lateral collateral ligament.

The primary site of arthritis of the intertarsal and tarsometatarsal joints (bone spavin) is on the medial side between the central and third tarsal bones and between the third tarsal and the third metatarsal bones. The process may spread to the other intertarsal joints. The medial tendon of the tibialis cranialis terminates on the first tarsal bone (fused with the second). It was called the cunean tendon because the first, second, and third tarsal bones are the cuneiform bones of human anatomy.

The tarsal canal is formed by the apposed surfaces of the fourth, central, and third bones. It transmits the perforating tarsal artery and vein and a branch of the deep peroneal nerve, which supplies the joints of the distal row of tarsal bones (see Fig. 16–1).

The large tuberosity of the plantar surface of the fourth tarsal is one of the points of attachment of the long plantar ligament, which extends from the plantar border of the calcaneus to the proximal end of the fourth metatarsal. Inflammation and swelling of the ligament are called curb. It pushes the overlying superficial digital flexor tendon, normally straight, into a curve, convex on the plantar surface (Fr. *courbe,* curve). The tendon should not be treated for a disease of the ligament. This desmitis associated with tearing of the plantar ligament is the result of abnormal stress that occurs at the moment of impact of the pelvic limb with the ground. Overflexion of the hock is resisted by the attachments of the common calcanean tendon to the tuber calcis and the distal attachments of the plantar ligament. Horses with abnormally overflexed hocks (sickle-hocked) are predisposed to this injury.[13]

Tarsal fractures are most common in the central and third tarsal bones of racing Standardbreds where they are subject to severe compressive and shearing forces.[25]

In the four standard views of the radiographs of the equine tarsus (lateromedial, dorsoplantar, dorsolateral-plantaromedial oblique, dorsomedial-plantarolateral oblique) identify all of the bones and the following features:[19]

Lateromedial View:
  Tarsocrural joint.
  Tibia: Articulation of cochlea with trochlea of talus.
        Intermediate ridge of cochlea in groove of trochlea of talus.

Talus: Trochlea with groove and medial and lateral ridges. Lateral ridge with prominent notch distally. Ridges usually superimposed.

Calcaneus: Tuber calcanei, sustentaculum tali.

Talocalcaneal joint (several articular surfaces).

Proximal and distal intertarsal joints.

Central and third tarsals exposed on dorsal surface.

Fourth and fused first and second tarsals usually overlap on plantar surfaces.

Tarsometatarsal joint, bases of metatarsals II, III, IV (II and IV overlap).

Dorsoplantar View:

Tarsocrural joint.

Tibia: Medial and lateral malleoli.

Cochlea: Medial and lateral grooves separated by oblique intermediate ridge with cranial blunt end lateral to caudal pointed end.

Talus: Trochlear ridges and oblique groove directed distolaterally.

Proximal and distal tubercles on medial side.

Calcaneus: Tuber calcanei, overlaps tibia.

Sustentaculum tali overlaps talus.

Proximal intertarsal joint.

Central tarsal: Exposed on medial surface. Overlaps fourth tarsal laterally. Concave proximal surface with plantar aspect more proximal and superimposed on talus.

Fourth tarsal: Exposed on lateral surface, overlaps central and third tarsals medially.

Distal intertarsal joint.

Third tarsal: Exposed on medial surface, overlaps fourth tarsal laterally. Plantar process superimposed in middle of distal row.

Fused first and second tarsals superimposed plantar to central and third tarsals.

Tarsometatarsal joint, base of metatarsals II, III, IV. Base of IV larger than II, both extend proximal to III, superimposed on distal tarsal bones.

Dorsolateral-Plantaromedial Oblique View:

Projects calcaneus and fourth tarsal on plantarolateral surface.

Projects medial ridge of trochlea on dorsomedial surface.

Tarsocrural joint.

Tibia: Medial and lateral malleoli.

Cochlea with cranial and caudal parts of intermediate ridge in groove of trochlea (view for lesions of osteochondrosis of the intermediate ridge). Because of the oblique view, the cranial end will appear closer to the medial malleolus.

Talus: Medial ridge of trochlea exposed on dorsomedial surface (view for soft tissue swelling of dorsomedial pouch of tarsocrural joint in "bog spavin"), lateral ridge superimposed on talus, distal tubercle medially.

Calcaneus: Tuber calcanei. Talocalcaneal joint. Radiolucent nonarticular area between distal talus and calcaneus.

Proximal and distal intertarsal joints.

Central and third tarsals exposed on dorsomedial surface (view for bone spavin—osteoarthrosis of distomedial tarsus). Ridge on dorsomedial surface of third tarsal.

Fourth tarsal: Plantar aspect exposed on plantarolateral surface.

Tarsal canal: Between central, third, and fourth tarsals.

Fused first and second tarsals overlapped by other bones.

Tarsometatarsal joint, bases of metatarsals II, III, IV. Base of II overlaps on III, base of IV exposed on plantarolateral surface.

Dorsomedial-Plantarolateral Oblique View:

Projects sustentaculum tali on plantaromedial surface.

Projects lateral trochlear ridge on dorsolateral surface.

Tarsocrural joint.

Tibia: Lateral malleolus, more blunt and craniolateral.

Articulation of cochlea with trochlea of talus.

Cranial aspect of intermediate ridge in trochlear groove.

Talus: Lateral trochlear ridge exposed on dorsolateral surface with prominent distal notch (view for lesions of osteochondrosis of ridge).

Medial trochlear ridge superimposed on lateral ridge.

Calcaneus: Tuber calcanei.

Sustentaculum tali exposed on plantaromedial surface.

Proximal and distal intertarsal joints.

Central and third tarsals exposed on dorsolateral surface. Overlap dorsal surface of fourth tarsal.

Fused first and second tarsals exposed on plantaromedial surface.

Fourth tarsal overlapped by other bones.

Tarsometatarsal joint, bases of metatarsals II, III, IV. Base of IV overlaps III, base of II exposed on plantaromedial surface.

16b. LIGAMENTOUS PREPARATION, HOCK, HORSE

Dorsal Surface. The tendon of the tibialis cranialis emerges between the branches of the peroneus tertius and bifurcates. The medial branch passes around the medial surface of the hock to the first tarsal. Note the dorsomedial pouch of the tarsocrural joint capsule on the medial side of the tendon of the peroneus tertius. This is the preferred site of puncture of the tarsocrural joint, which communicates with the proximal intertarsal joint. The other two joints, the distal intertarsal and the tarsometatarsal, are usually separate. The fan-shaped dorsal oblique ligament extends from the distal tubercle on the medial side of the talus to the front of the hock, where it spreads out to its attachments on the central and third tarsal and the second and third metatarsal bones.

Medial Surface. The medial branch of the tendon of the tibialis cranialis crosses the surface of the long medial collateral ligament. A synovial bursa (cunean bursa) lies between them. The tendon crosses the distal intertarsal joint and terminates on the first tarsal bone; therefore, the cunean bursa overlies the primary site of degenerative tarsal joint disease. Separate punctures should be made into the distal intertarsal and tarsometatarsal joints because of their inconstant communication. A 2.5 cm. 25 gauge needle is recommended.[16]

The distal intertarsal joint is entered through the T-shaped junction of the central, third, and fused first and second tarsal bones. This joint is palpable in some horses, but when it cannot be palpated, draw a line from the distal tubercle of the talus to the space between the proximal ends of the second and third metatarsal bones. On the extended hock, insert the needle at the intersection of this line with the distal border of the cunean tendon and direct it plantarolaterally.

The tarsometatarsal joint can be injected on the medial side, about 12 mm. (one finger's width) distal to the point of injection of the distal intertarsal joint. This is about level with the distal aspect of the chestnut. It is more easily punctured on the lateroplantar aspect of the hock between the fourth tarsal and fourth metatarsal bones by inserting a 19 gauge needle in a sagittal plane dorsodistally. If the needle is too far medial, it will enter the tarsal canal instead of the desired joint.

These puncture points are used for diagnostic purposes—withdrawal of fluid for examination and injection of anesthetic agents. They may also be used for injection of therapeutic or anti-inflammatory agents. Most of the operations formerly done on the hock for the treatment of tarsitis have been discarded as ineffective and have been replaced by more conservative measures, which may prolong the racing career of a horse for a short time but do not significantly alter the progressive course of the disease.

Behind the medial collateral ligament is the medioplantar pouch of the tarsocrural joint capsule. The narrow tendon of the medial digital flexor passes through a canal in the medial collateral ligament to join the tendon of the lateral digital flexor in the metatarsus (see Table 14–1). The latter tendon is surrounded by a long synovial sheath that extends about 7 cm. above and below the hock. Distention of the part above the hock is called thoroughpin (see Plate I).

Lateral Surface. In the long lateral collateral ligament is a groove containing the tendon of the lateral digital extensor. Distal to the hock, it inclines dorsally and joins the tendon of the long extensor. It is covered by a synovial sheath from the lateral malleolus through the metatarsal extensor retinaculum.

Plantar surface. Behind the origin of the lateral collateral ligament is the large lateroplantar pouch of the tarsocrural joint capsule. The long plantar ligament lies on the plantar border of the calcaneus. The tuber calcanei and the insertion of the gastrocnemius tendon are covered by a large bursa, which lies under the superficial digital flexor tendon from the distal fourth of the tibia to the middle of the hock. Capped hock, however, is usually limited to the subcutaneous calcanean bursa.[28]

Note the constant nutrient foramen at the junction of the proximal and middle thirds of the third metatarsal.[11] The interosseus arises from the plantar surface of the proximal end of the third metatarsal. The accessory (check) ligament of the deep digital flexor tendon is similar to that of the thoracic limb but is smaller and sometimes absent.

16c. DISSECTION, HOCK AND METATARSUS, HORSE

Anesthesia of the Hock. Nerve block anesthesia is not often used for the diagnosis of spavin. Tibial and peroneal nerve blocks in the distal part of the crus would anesthetize the joint, but superficial tissues are also innervated by the saphenous and caudal cutaneous sural nerves. Disease of the metatarsus and digit would have to be eliminated from consideration before the tibial and peroneal blocks were done. On the other hand, subcutaneous infiltration anesthesia of the tissues on the medial surface of the intertarsal and tarsometatarsal joints is a useful method. If the horse goes sound, the trouble is in the dorsal oblique or long medial collateral ligament.[17] It could also be in the cunean bursa. If medial infiltration does not eliminate the lameness, inject anesthetic into the tarsocrural joint. This is presumed to work by diffusion through the capsule into the nerves supplying the intertarsal and tarsometatarsal joints. If effective it indicates arthritis of the deep tissues.

Tibial and peroneal neurectomy are contraindicated because of the loss of proprioception, with the danger of tripping and falling, and because of atrophic degeneration of the hoof.

Anesthesia of the Metatarsus. There are three cutaneous nerves that extend as far distally as the fetlock and are not affected by blocking the tibial and deep peroneal nerves:

1. The saphenous nerve.
2. The superficial peroneal nerve.
3. The caudal cutaneous sural nerve.

The full distal extent of these nerves cannot be dissected grossly but has been demonstrated physiologically. All five nerves must be blocked to obtain surgical anesthesia of the metatarsus (see Figs. 16–1, 16–2; see also section 14d).

Anesthesia of the Digit. The plantar nerves (terminal branches of the tibial) course through the metatarsus in the medial and lateral grooves between the interosseus and the flexor tendons. The communicating branch between them crosses the plantar surface of the superficial flexor tendon. They are accompanied by small arteries. The plantar nerves supply a smaller part of the digit than the palmar nerves.

The dorsal metatarsal nerves, branches of the deep peroneal, supply the fetlock and the dorsal parts of the pastern joint and coffin joint and terminate in the dorsal laminar dermis.[10] The medial dorsal metatarsal nerve runs along the medial border of the long digital extensor tendon and then inclines backward to run closely dorsal and parallel to the splint bone. The lateral dorsal metatarsal nerve accompanies the dorsal metatarsal artery to the point where the latter perforates to the plantar surface of the bones. The nerve continues distally on the lateral side of the fetlock joint.

The plantar metatarsal nerves are from the deep branch of the lateral plantar that supplies the interosseus.They supply the plantar pouch of the fetlock joint. The medial plantar metatarsal nerve emerges at the distal end of the splint bone and joins in the innervation of the digit down to the laminar dermis. The lateral plantar metatarsal nerve often fails to reach the surface, but it may have a distribution like that of the medial nerve.

To obtain anesthesia of the digit, it is necessary to block all three nerves on each side.[8] The plantar nerve is blocked in the groove between the interosseus and the flexor tendons at the level of the end of the splint bone. Before blocking the lateral plantar nerve, the plantar communication should be palpated to make sure that the block is distal to the communication. The latter is smaller and more distal on the hind limb than on the forelimb and may be missing (see Figs. 16–1, 16–2).

To block the plantar metatarsal nerve, the needle is inserted in the hollow distal to the end of the splint bone for deep and superficial injections. The infiltration is then extended 2 to 3 cm. dorsal to the splint bone to block the dorsal metatarsal nerve on the side of the great metatarsal bone.[12]

Arteries and Veins. It will be recalled that the main artery to the digit in the forelimb is the medial palmar artery on the medial side of the flexor tendons. The main artery to the digit in the hind limb is the dorsal metatarsal artery, supplied by the cranial tibial through the dorsal pedal on the front of the hock. It passes obliquely distally under the lateral extensor tendon and reaches the dorsolateral groove between the third and fourth metatarsal bones. In the distal third of the interosseous space, the artery is continued by a segment called the perforating branch, which passes between the bones to the plantar surface of the third metatarsal bone and bifurcates. The medial and lateral digital arteries so formed pass back between the interosseus tendons to the space between the interosseus and deep flexor tendons. From this point, their distribution is the same as in the forelimb.

On the dorsomedial side of the hock is the large cranial branch of the medial saphenous vein. It is avoided in puncture of the tarsocrural joint capsule by inserting the needle on the plantar side of the vein.

Stringhalt. Note the relation of the lateral digital extensor tendon to the dorsal metatarsal artery. In the operation for stringhalt, the tendon is cut close to its junction with the long digital extensor tendon and pulled out through another incision proximal to the lateral malleolus. The mesotendon must be torn to do this. The extensor brevis lies in the triangle between the two tendons. A piece of the lateral digital extensor muscle about 7 to 10 cm. long is pulled out with the tendon and cut off.[1]

The overflexion of the limb that occurs in stringhalt may be related to abnormal activity of neuromuscular spindles or proprioceptive afferents in musculotendinous units. Removal of a portion of the long digital extensor muscle at its junction with the tendon may therefore be important in eliminating a source of excessive afferent impulses involved in this abnormal motor control. No lesions are observed at autopsy.

16d. LIVE HORSE

Palpate the following structures:

Medial and lateral malleoli (see Plate I).

Tuber calcanei. The attachments of the superficial digital flexor tendon to the tuber calcanei are sometimes ruptured, allowing the tendon to slip off.

Ridges of the trochlea of the talus. The lateral one is more prominent. The peroneus tertius tendon covers the medial ridge.

Long medial collateral ligament. It extends from the medial malleolus to the tubercle on the distal part of the talus, then to the medial surface of the central tarsal and the distal row of tarsal bones, then to the second and third metatarsals.

Long lateral collateral ligament. This extends from the lateral malleolus, to the prominent distal end of the lateral surface of the calcaneus, to the fourth tarsal and the third and fourth metatarsals.

Tendon of the lateral digital extensor. Palpate the tendon in the groove of the lateral malleolus. It cannot be palpated as it passes over the lateral surface of the hock because it is bound down in a groove of the long lateral collateral ligament by retinacula. Distal to the lateral ridge of the trochlea the tendon changes direction and can be palpated again in the metatarsus as it inclines dorsally to join the tendon of the long digital extensor. Palpate the two tendons in the proximal direction. They diverge, and the lateral extensor passes lateral to the trochlea while the long extensor passes between the ridges of the trochlea.

Tibialis cranialis. Trace the medial branch of the tendon as it crosses obliquely the medial surface of the hock to the first tarsal bone. The tendon must be relaxed to follow it to the termination. Palpate the limb that the horse is resting.

Long plantar ligament. This lies on the lateroplantar surface, from the plantar border of the calcaneus to the fourth tarsal and metatarsal bones. Differentiate the long plantar ligament from the superficial digital flexor tendon, which partly covers it.

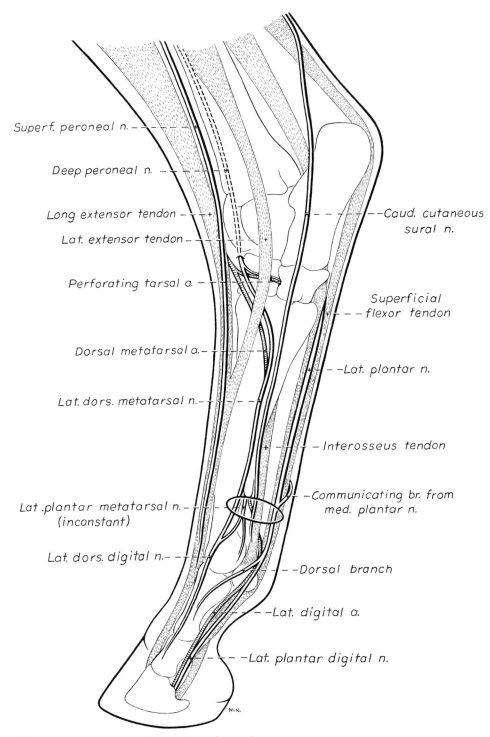

Superf. peroneal n. –

Deep peroneal n. –

Long extensor tendon –

Lat. extensor tendon –

Perforating tarsal a. –

–Caud. cutaneous
sural n.

Superficial
– flexor tendon

Dorsal metatarsal a. –

– Lat. plantar n.

Lat. dors. metatarsal n. –

– Interosseus tendon

– Communicating br. from
med. plantar n.

Lat. plantar metatarsal n. –
(inconstant)

Lat. dors. digital n. –

– Dorsal branch

– Lat. digital a.

– Lat. plantar digital n.

Figure 16–1. Left pelvic limb, horse, lateral aspect.

Tarsocrural joint capsule. The three pouches distended in hydrarthrosis (bog spavin) are (see Plate I):

1. Dorsomedial. This is bounded by the medial malleolus, the tendon of the peroneus tertius, the medial tendon of the tibialis cranialis, and the long medial collateral ligament. The cranial branch of the medial saphenous vein is superficial here. This is the preferred site for puncture of the tarsocrural joint. Insert the needle behind the vein and direct it from medial to lateral.

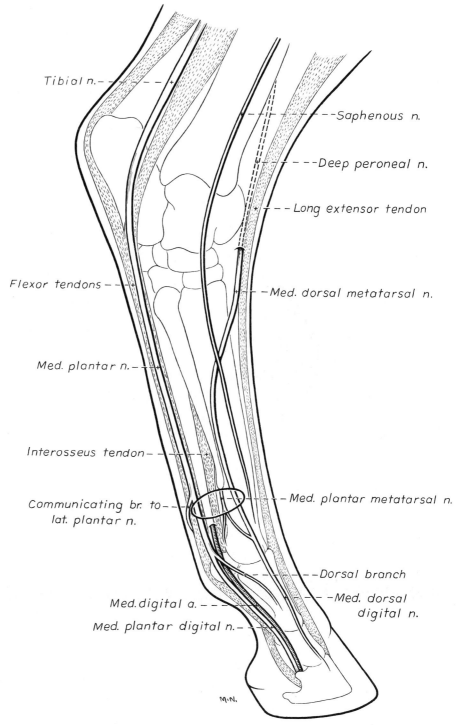

Figure 16–2. Left pelvic limb, horse, medial aspect.

2. Medioplantar. This pouch is between the long medial collateral ligament and the tendon of the lateral digital flexor, about at the level of the medial malleolus. The medioplantar pouch is punctured only if it is distended. The medial plantar vessels and nerve lie on the lateral flexor tendon here.

3. Lateroplantar. This pouch is between the calcaneus and the lateral malleolus. It is punctured only if it is distended.[27]

Distention of the tarsocrural capsule can be distinguished from a distended synovial sheath of the lateral digital flexor tendon by pushing on the swelling in the area of the medioplantar pouch. If the entire force is transmitted to the other hand in the region of the lateroplantar swelling, the synovial sheath is involved. It is called thoroughpin because the noncompressible fluid feels like a rigid pin when pressed from side to side. If pressure on both medioplantar and lateroplantar pouches causes distention of the dorsomedial pouch, and vice versa, the joint is involved. Swelling in the synovial sheath extends farther proximally than the distended plantar pouches of the tarsocrural joint.

Palpate the sites of the nerve blocks described in section 16c and shown in Figs. 16–1 and 16–2.

Cranial branch of the medial saphenous vein. This is subcutaneous on the medial side of the front of the hock. It is continued distally as the dorsal common digital vein, which crosses obliquely the medial surface of the proximal end of the large metatarsal bone and runs distally in the dorsal groove between the second and third metatarsal bones, then in the medial groove between the interosseus and the deep flexor tendon. It is the largest vein of the metatarsus, draining the digital veins through the distal plantar arch (see Plate I).

Dorsal metatarsal artery. This is the main artery to the hoof. It is supplied by the cranial tibial through the dorsal pedal on the front of the hock. Palpate the pulse where the artery crosses obliquely the proximal end of the lateral surface of the large metatarsal bone. It passes deep to the tendon of the lateral digital extensor and runs to the dorsal groove between the third and fourth metatarsal bones. In tenectomy for stringhalt, the tendon should be cut close to the long digital extensor tendon to avoid the artery (see Fig. 16–1).

16e. RADIOGRAPHS AND BONES OF HOCK, OX

There is a trochlea on each end of the talus. This permits flexion of the bovine hock in two joints, the tarsocrural and the proximal intertarsal. (Compare the horse.) The small bone lateral to the trochlea of the talus is the lateral malleolus, the distal end of the fibula, which articulates with the tibia, but never fuses with it, unlike its homologue in the horse. It also articulates with the talus and calcaneus.

Note the large bone composed of the fused central and fourth tarsals with a prominent proximal plantar process on the medial side. The first tarsal is small and separate, and the second and third bones are fused. Spavin also occurs in the ox, especially in draft animals and bulls.

The small round bone behind the proximal end of the metatarsal bone is not a rudimentary metatarsal but a sesamoid bone in the interosseus muscle.

In the four standard views of the bovine tarsus identify all of the bones and the following features:[21]

Lateromedial View:
  Tarsocrural joint.
  Tibia: Medial malleolus exposed on cranial surface. Intermediate ridge of cochlea. Articulation of cochlea with proximal trochlea of talus.
  Fibula: Lateral malleolus overlaps proximal trochlea, and articulates with calcaneus distal to level of trochlear groove.
  Talus: Proximal and distal trochleae with ridges. Radiolucent fossa on dorsal surface. Articulation with calcaneus on plantar surface (talocalcaneal joint).
  Calcaneus: Tuber calcanei, sustentaculum tali.
  Talocalcaneal joint. Radiolucent nonarticular area distal to joint.
  Proximal intertarsal joint.
  Fused central and fourth tarsals. Prominent plantaromedial process of central part projects proximally, superimposed on calcaneus, articulates with medial ridge of distal trochlea.
  Distal intertarsal joint.
  Fused second and third tarsals exposed on dorsal surface.
  First tarsal superimposed on fourth part of fused central and fourth tarsals and proximal plantar eminence of metatarsals III and IV.
  Tarsometatarsal joint, base of fused metatarsals III and IV.
  Sesamoid bone in third interosseus.

Dorsoplantar View:

    Tarsocrural joint.

    Tibia: Medial malleolus with distal projection.

        Cochlea with medial and lateral grooves and sagittal intermediate ridge.

    Fibula: Lateral malleolus, articulates with tibia and calcaneus.

    Talus: Proximal and distal trochleae with medial and lateral ridges.

    Calcaneus: Tuber calcanei superimposed on tibia.

        Sustentaculum tali superimposed on talus. Articulation with fibula and fourth tarsal laterally.

    Proximal intertarsal joint.

    Fused central and fourth tarsal. Central part exposed medially with proximal plantar process superimposed on talus, fourth part exposed laterally. (These are separate bones in the neonatal calf.)

    Distal intertarsal joint. Limited to medial half.

    Fused second and third tarsals exposed on medial surface.

    First tarsal superimposed on plantar side of tarsal bones medially.

    Tarsometatarsal joint, base of fused metatarsals III and IV.

Dorsolateral–Plantaromedial Oblique View:

    Projects calcaneus and fourth tarsal on plantarolateral surface.

    Projects medial malleolus and medial trochlear ridge of talus on dorsomedial surface.

    Tarsocrural joint.

    Tibia: Medial malleolus exposed on craniomedial surface. Cochlea with cranial part of intermediate ridge (view for lesions of osteochondrosis in young bulls).

    Fibula: Lateral malleolus superimposed on talus and calcaneus, articulation with latter.

    Talus: Proximal and distal trochleae with ridges, medial ridges exposed on dorsomedial surface.

    Calcaneus: Exposed on plantarolateral surface.

        Tuber calcanei, talocalcaneal and calcaneoquartal joints, articulation with lateral malleolus.

    Proximal intertarsal joint.

    Fused central and fourth tarsals. Central part exposed dorsomedially and fourth part plantarolaterally.

    Distal intertarsal joint.

    Fused second and third tarsals. Exposed on dorsomedial surface.

    First tarsal superimposed on fourth part of fused central and fourth tarsals.

    Tarsometatarsal joint, base of fused metatarsals III and IV, exposed plantarolateral aspect of IV.

Dorsomedial–Plantarolateral Oblique View:

    Projects sustentaculum tali and proximal plantar process of central tarsal on plantaromedial surface.

    Projects lateral ridges of trochleae of talus on dorsolateral surface.

    Tarsocrural joint.

    Tibia: Medial malleolus superimposed on talus.

        Cochlea, articulation of grooves with proximal trochlea of talus.

    Fibula: Lateral malleolus exposed on craniolateral surface, articulation with calcaneus.

    Talus: Proximal and distal trochleae with ridges. Lateral ridges exposed on dorsolateral surface.

    Calcaneus: Tuber calcanei. Sustentaculum tali exposed on plantaromedial surface.

    Talocalcaneal joint.

    Proximal intertarsal joint.

    Fused central and fourth tarsals. Proximal plantar process of central part exposed on plantaromedial surface, articulation with medial ridge of distal trochlea.

        Dorsolateral surface of fourth part exposed.

    Distal intertarsal joint.

    Fused second and third tarsals superimposed on first and fused central and fourth tarsals.

    First tarsal. Exposed on plantaromedial surface.

Tarsometatarsal joint, base of fused metatarsals III and IV, exposed plantaromedial aspect of III.

Sesamoid in third interosseus exposed on plantaromedial surface.[22]

16f. DISSECTION, METATARSUS, OX

Orient the specimen by means of the large cranial branch of the lateral saphenous vein, which lies on the dorsolateral surface. The saphenous veins differ markedly between species. The horse and cat are similar in having large medial saphenous veins with a prominent cranial branch on the dorsomedial surface of the hock. The ox and dog have large lateral saphenous veins with a large cranial branch on the dorsolateral side of the hock.

The disposition of the nerves on the digits is similar to that of the forelimb. The nerves in the

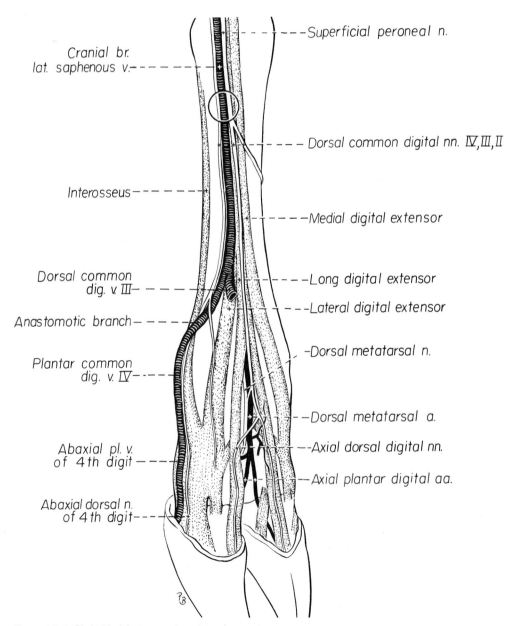

Figure 16–3. Right hind foot, cow dorsolateral aspect.

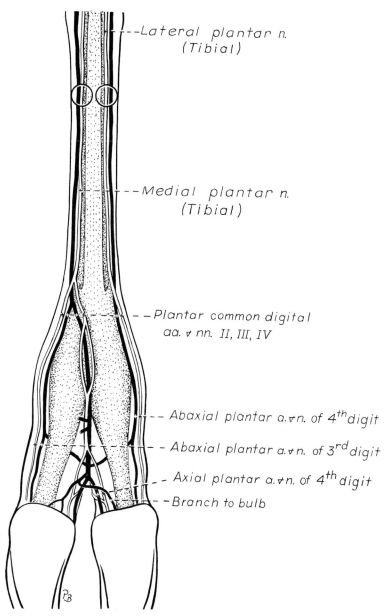

Figure 16–4. Right hind foot, cow, plantar aspect.

metatarsus, however, show some important differences, ignorance of which has led to failure in attempts to anesthetize the hind foot (Figs. 16–3 to 16–5).

The common digital nerves on the dorsal surface of the metatarsus are branches of the superficial peroneal. The two abaxial dorsal digital nerves cross the fetlock joints just dorsal to the digital veins as in the forelimb, but several cutaneous branches are given off high in the metatarsus. These branches run straight distally to the abaxial dorsal surface of P I and would not be blocked by injection of the abaxial dorsal digital nerves at the level of the fetlock joints as has been advocated. The dorsal common digital nerve III runs to the bifurcation of the long extensor tendon, gives off the two axial dorsal digital nerves and turns into the interdigital space, where it joins the dorsal metatarsal nerve.

The dorsal metatarsal nerve is the continuation of the deep peroneal. In the middle of the metatarsus it can be seen lying on the dorsal surface of the metatarsal bone, medial to the dorsal metatarsal artery. The long and lateral digital extensor tendons must be separated and the deep metatarsal

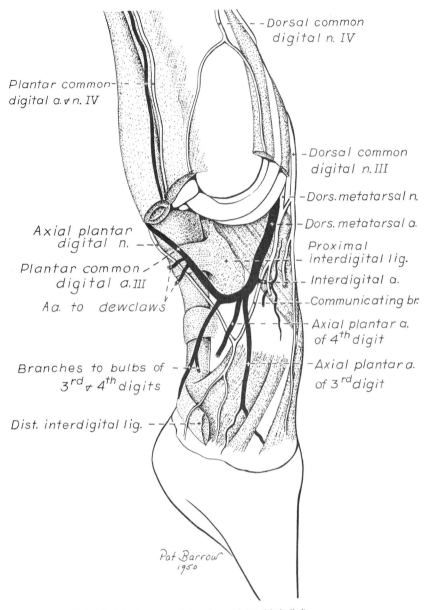

Plantar common-
digital a. ɑ n. IV

Dorsal common
digital n. IV

Dorsal common
digital n. III

Dors. metatarsal n.

Dors. metatarsal a.

Axial plantar
digital n.

Plantar common
digital a. III

Aa. to dewclaws

Proximal
interdigital lig.

Interdigital a.

Communicating br.

Axial plantar a.
of 4th digit

Branches to bulbs of
3rd ɑ 4th digits

Axial plantar a.
of 3rd digit

Dist. interdigital lig.

Pat Barrow
1950

Figure 16–5. Right hind foot, cow, axial surface of the third digit.

fascia incised to expose the artery and nerve. At the fetlock joints, the dorsal metatarsal nerve joins the dorsal common digital nerve III and communicates with the axial plantar digital nerves.

The plantar digital nerves are similar to the palmar digitals. The axial plantar digital nerves come from a branch of the medial plantar nerve.

To anesthetize the digits (but not the metatarsus and fetlock):

1. Block the superficial peroneal nerve a little above the middle of the metatarsus. The branches of the nerve lie subcutaneously on both sides of the cranial branch of the lateral saphenous vein, which is visible under the skin.

2. Block the dorsal metatarsal nerve in the groove on the dorsal surface of the metatarsal bone. This is done from the previous point of insertion by passing the needle between the extensor tendons. Test for puncture of the artery. This injection can also be made between the fetlock joints.

3. and 4. Block the medial and lateral plantar nerves just above the middle of the metatarsus. They lie on the borders of the flexor tendons, covered by deep fascia.

The blood supply of the metatarsus and digits differs from that of the forelimb in that the largest artery is the *dorsal metatarsal*. This anastomoses in the interdigital space with the plantar common digital, which gives off the large axial plantar digital arteries (see Fig. 16–5). The positions of the main arteries of each digit are similar to those in the forelimb:

1. The largest, the axial plantar digital, runs obliquely distodorsally on the axial surface to the foramen in the extensor process of P III.
2. A bulbar branch may be given off each axial plantar digital, or a common trunk from the plantar common digital may supply both bulbar branches.
3. The abaxial plantar digital artery is deep to the abaxial plantar digital nerve.

16g. LIVE COW

Work directly behind the cow or in front of the limb with one shoulder against the stifle. Palpate the following structures:

Medial and lateral malleoli.

Long medial and lateral collateral ligaments. Each passes from the malleolus to the tarsal attachment then forms an obtuse angle and descends vertically to the metatarsal attachment.

Proximal and distal trochleae of the talus.

Medial branch of the tendon of the tibialis cranialis.

Dorsomedial pouch of the tarsocrural joint. It has the same boundaries as in the horse, but is easier to puncture because there is no vein in the field. Palpate the pouch distal to the medial malleolus and medial to the tendon of the peroneus tertius. The needle is inserted in the mediolateral direction. The tarsocrural joint sac communicates only with the proximal intertarsal.

The three digital extensor tendons on the dorsal surface of the metatarsus. The one in the middle is the long digital extensor, the one that bifurcates at the fetlock.

The cranial branch of the lateral saphenous vein. This can be seen under the skin lateral to the extensor tendons. The lateral branch of the superficial peroneal nerve lies lateral to the vein. The rest of the nerve is on the extensor tendons medial to the vein (see Fig. 16–3).

Abaxial plantar digital veins. These lie, with the dorsal and plantar abaxial digital nerves, on the abaxial sesamoid bones at the level of the dewclaw. The artery here is too small and deep to palpate.

Intravenous local anesthesia of the distal metatarsus and digits can be performed after applying a tourniquet below the tarsus.[4, 5] Five superficial veins will distend in the metatarsus. The largest is (1) the cranial branch of the lateral saphenous vein where it courses on the lateral side of the extensor tendons (see Fig. 16–3). This vein divides at the distal third of the metatarsus into (2) the dorsal common digital vein III and (3) a short anastomotic branch to the lateral end of the distal deep plantar arch, where (4) the plantar common digital vein IV begins. On the medial side, (5) plantar common digital vein II arises from the other end of the distal deep plantar arch. Plantar common digital veins II and IV are continued as the abaxial plantar digital veins, which cross the sesamoid bones dorsal to the dewclaws. Anesthesia of the foot distal to the tourniquet is produced by injection of any one of these veins.

The angle formed between the dorsal border of the wall of the hoof and the ground is normally about 45° in the hind foot.

16h. BONES AND RADIOGRAPHS, HOCK, DOG AND CAT

Identify the bones in as many of the radiographs as possible. In the proximal row are the talus and calcaneus. Osteochondrosis occurs in the medial ridge of the trochlea in dogs. Osteotomy of the medial malleolus provides surgical access to this site.[20] The medial bone of the next row is the central, which is often fractured in the right tarsus of Greyhounds.[2] This is the outside limb on the counterclockwise track, where it is subject to compression forces. The fracture is in the dorsal plane, and a large fragment may be luxated dorsally. The third tarsal bone is also subject to luxation.[7]

The first tarsal bone is the medial one of the distal row and is about twice as long as the second. Attached to it is the first metatarsal, which may be only a rudiment, shorter than the first tarsal, if there is no dewclaw (first digit). The second and third tarsals articulate with the corresponding metatarsals. The fourth tarsal is the large bone on the lateral surface, which articulates with metatarsals IV and V. In the cat, the fifth metatarsal bone has a distinct proximal plantar process.

The epiphysis for the tuber calcanei unites with the calcaneus at 3 to 8 months in the dog, and 7 to 13 months in the cat. The epiphyses of the metatarsal bones are distal and unite at about the same time as in the metacarpus—5 to 7 months in the dog and 8 to 11 months in the cat.[23, 24]

In the skeleton, there is a groove on the dorsomedial surface of the proximal end of the third metatarsal bone for the proximal perforating branch, the continuation of the dorsal pedal artery, which is the principal blood supply to the paw. This artery runs obliquely across the dorsal surface of the central and third tarsal bones and should be considered in reduction of dorsal luxation of these bones. Pressure applied by a coaptation splint might compress the artery against the luxated bone (see Plate III).

Unlike the equine tarsocrural joint, that of the dog does not communicate with the joint between the first and second rows of tarsal bones. It does communicate with the proximal talocalcaneal joint and the tendon sheath of the lateral digital flexor. The recommended site for puncture of the tarsocrural joint in the dog is lateral.

Extend the hock and palpate the lateral malleolus and the lateral ridge of the trochlea. Insert the needle in a distoplantar direction just distal to the malleolus, lateral to the trochlea, and dorsal to the tendon of the peroneus longus. The latter runs dorsal to the lateral collateral ligament. Avoid the cranial branch of the lateral saphenous vein.[18]

Plantar ligaments extend from the calcaneus to the tarsal fibrocartilage, a thickening of the tarsometatarsal joint capsule. As in the horse, these act to prevent overflexion of the tarsus. Injury to these ligaments results in overflexion and a plantigrade gait.[9]

16i. ARTERIAL AND VENOUS DISSECTION, HOCK, DOG AND CAT

The lateral saphenous vein of the dog is a branch of the distal caudal femoral vein. It emerges from the deep surface of the popliteal lymph node between the biceps femoris and the semitendinosus. On the lateral surface of the distal part of the leg it divides into cranial and caudal branches. It is more firmly fixed for venipuncture at the proximal end where it is held on the gastrocnemius by the biceps and semitendinosus than it is at the usual site in the loose subcutaneous tissue of the leg (see Plate III).

In the cat, the medial saphenous vein is larger and more suitable for intravenous injection. It divides into cranial and caudal branches in the middle of the crus.

In the metatarsus, the largest arteries are the plantar metatarsals. These lie between the interossei deep to the deep digital flexor tendons. They originate from the proximal perforating branch, which passes through the space between the second and third metatarsal bones. The proximal perforating branch is the continuation of the dorsal pedal artery, which is the continuation of the cranial tibial artery. The largest artery of each digit is the axial plantar proper digital.

16j. LIVE DOG

Palpate the following structures:

> Trochlea of the talus. Palpate the lateral ridge and malleolus at the site of puncture of the tarsocrural joint (section 16h).
> Long medial and lateral collateral ligaments.
> Dorsal pedal artery. Take the pulse between the proximal ends of the second and third

metatarsal bones, where the dorsal pedal artery becomes the proximal perforating branch.

Lateral saphenous vein. Distend the vein and trace its branches.

References

1. Adams, O. R.: Lameness in Horses, 3rd ed. Lea & Febiger: Philadelphia, 1974.
2. Dee, J. F., J. Dee, and D. L. Piermattei: Classification, management, and repair of central tarsal fractures in the racing Greyhound. J. Am. Anim. Hosp. Assoc. *12* (1976):398–405.
3. De Moor, A., F. Verschooten, P. Desmet, et al.: Osteochondritis dissecans of the tibiotarsal joint in the horse. Eq. Vet. J. *4* (1972):139–143.
4. De Moor, A., F. Verschooten, P. Desmet, et al.: Intraveneuze lokale anesthesie van de distale delen van de ledematen bij het rund. Vlaams Dierg. Tijdsk. *42* (1973):1–7.
5. Estill, C. T.: Intravenous local anesthesia of the bovine lower leg. Vet. Med.—Small Anim. Clin. *72* (1977):1499–1502.
6. Habel, R. E.: Guide to the Dissection of Domestic Ruminants, 3rd ed. Ithaca, N.Y.: Habel, 1977.
7. Keene, R. B. and J. H. Yarborough: Lamenesses of the racing Greyhound. Vet. Scope *11* (1966):1–9.
8. Magda, I.: Lokalanästhesie. Anleitung für Tierärzte. Jena: Fischer, 1960.
9. Matthiesen, D. T.: Tarsal injuries in the dog and cat. Comp. Cont. Ed. *5* (1983):548–555.
10. Nilsson, S. A. Bidrag till kännedomen om fotens innervation hos häst. Skand. Vet. Tidskr. *38* (1948): 401–459.
11. Orsini, P. G., V. T. Rendano, and W. O. Sack: Ectopic nutrient foramina in the third metatarsal bone of the horse. Eq. Vet. J. *13* (1981):132–134.
12. Pohlmeyer, K. and R. Redecker: Die für die Klinik bedeutsamen Nerven an den Gliedmassen des Pferdes einschliesslich möglicher Varianten. Deutsche tierärztl. Wschr. *81* (1974):501–505, 537–541.
13. Rooney, J. R.: An hypothesis of the pathogenesis of curb in horses. Can. Vet. J. *22* (1981):300–301.
14. Sack, W. O.: The anatomy involved in the resection of the lateral extensor tendon in the horse. Film. JAVMA *160* (1972):1251.
15. Sack, W. O., and S. Ferraglio: Clinically important structures of the equine hock. JAVMA *172* (1978): 277–280.
16. Sack, W. O. and P. G. Orsini: Distal intertarsal and tarsometatarsal joints in the horse: injection sites and communication. JAVMA *179* (1981):355–359.
17. Schebitz, H.: Radiologic diagnosis and treatment of spavin. Proc. 11th Ann. Conv. Am. Ass. Eq. Pract. *11*(1965):207–222.
18. Schlüter, H., H. Wissdorf, and H. Wilkens: Beitrag zu den Gelenkkapselverhältnissen und zur Injektionsmöglichkeit am Tarsalgelenk des Hundes. Berl. Münch. tierärztl. Wochenschr. *83* (1970):360–363.
19. Shively, M. J. and J. E. Smallwood: Radiographic and xeroradiographic anatomy of the equine tarsus. Equine Pract. *2* (1980):19–36.
20. Sinibaldi, K. R.: Medial approach to the tarsus. J. Am. Anim. Hosp. Assoc. *15* (1979):77–83.
21. Smallwood, J. E. and M. J. Shively: Radiographic and xeroradiographic anatomy of the bovine tarsus. Bovine Pract. *2* (1981):28–46.
22. Smith, R. N.: The proximal metatarsal sesamoid of the domestic ruminants. Is it the vestige of a second metatarsal? Anat. Anz. *103* (1956):241.
23. Smith, R. N.: Fusion of ossification centres in the cat. J. Small Anim. Pract. *10* (1969):523–530.
24. Sumner-Smith, G.: Observations on epiphyseal fusion of the canine appendicular skeleton. J. Small Anim. Pract. *7* (1966):303–311.
25. Tulamo, R. M., L. R. Bramlage, and A. A. Gabel: Fractures of the central and third tarsal bones in horses. JAVMA *182* (1983):1234–1238.
26. Van Pelt, R. W.: Arthrocentesis and injection of the bovine tarsus. Vet. Med. *57* (1962):125–132.
27. Van Pelt, R. W.: Arthrocentesis and injection of the equine tarsus. JAVMA *148* (1966):367–377.
28. Van Pelt, R. W. and W. F. Riley: Traumatic subcutaneous calcaneal bursitis (capped hock) in the horse. JAVMA *153* (1968):1176–1180.
29. Wamberg, K.: Spat. Copenhagen: Mortensen, 1955. English summary pp. 116–128.

CHAPTER 17

LUNG: PERCUSSION AND AUSCULTATION

OBJECTIVES

1. To master the techniques of percussion.
   a. Hammer and pleximeter in large animals
   b. Finger-finger percussion in all species
2. To be able to recognize different degrees of resonance and to understand the reasons for different percussion sounds.
3. To be able to trace the boundaries of the normal area for percussion and auscultation of the lung in each species.
4. To learn the technique of determining the basal border of the lung by the method of maximum contrast. This will reveal:
   a. A reduced area of lung resonance caused by pneumonia in the ventral part of the lung, pleural transudate shown as a fluid level, an enlarged heart in the dog or horse, traumatic pericarditis in the cow, and abdominal organs of greater density than lung occupying the pleural cavity as a result of a ruptured diaphragm.
   b. Increased area of lung resonance caused by emphysema (heaves).
   c. Increased resonance resulting in a tympanitic sound over the lung area caused by pneumothorax. In small animals this is often caused by internal injury in a car accident. The thorax is compressed with the glottis closed, and the alveoli rupture through the pulmonary pleura.[1]
5. To be able to trace the diaphragmatic line of pleural reflection in each species and to be able to perform pleurocentesis at the proper point to reach the most ventral part of the pleural cavity without puncturing the heart or pericardium or injuring the intercostal vessels, or, in the horse, the superficial thoracic vein.
6. To be able to recognize the quality and extent of the normal breath sounds heard on auscultation in the dog, ox, and horse.
7. To be able to recognize the stenotic sound heard over the trachea and over the lung in pathological conditions.

Percussion of the lung, general considerations

The sound produced by percussion over the normal lung is derived from three sources.

1. *The noise of the impact* of the hammer or percussing finger. The word "noise" is used in the acoustic sense to denote a complex of irregular vibrations without musical quality. A tap is a noise. The noise of impact is of little diagnostic use because it is determined by the character of the striking and struck surfaces. It reveals nothing of the condition of the underlying organs. Therefore, the noise of impact is diminished as much as possible by using the cushion of the finger tip or a hammer with a rubber face.

2. *The sound of the vibration of the body wall.* Because the wall is elastic and because it overlies an air-filled cavity, it vibrates like a thick drumhead when struck. In areas where the body wall covers solid organs (liver, heart) or where the wall is too thickly muscled, it does not vibrate. To reduce the area of the body wall set in vibration and thus to increase the precision of the method, the blow must be light and confined to the intercostal spaces. Heavy percussion and percussion on the ribs evoke resonance from organs that are too far away from the point of impact for accuracy. The area of lung resonance is much enlarged by percussion on the ribs.[6]

3. *The resonance* of the underlying air-filled cavity. The sound waves of the complex noise of impact are transmitted through the body wall and radiate through the air in the thorax until they meet a solid organ or an opposed wall. From this they are reflected. Some of the waves, which happen to be of the right frequency, are returned in time to augment the sound of the vibration at the point of percussion. The irregularity of the thoracic cavity and the contained lung tissue interfere with resonance and muffle it.

The more prominent the noise of impact, the flatter the percussion sound (muscle, liver, heart). The more prominent the vibration of the wall and the resonance of the underlying organ, the more the percussion sound approaches a musical tone.

When the cavity percussed is regular in shape and smooth-walled, the resonance is improved, and the percussion sound becomes tympanitic. This is the nearest approach to a musical tone that we find. It occurs in percussion of gas-filled portions of the gut, the dorsal part of the rumen, and often the stomach of the dog. Pathologically, it is heard over small areas of normal lung walled off by hepatization, and over lung cavities. Generally, the pitch of the tympanitic sound is lower:

1. in large chambers (compare bass and snare drums)
2. in spherical chambers
3. in chambers with flaccid walls.

In summary, the normal percussion sound may be either flat or resonant. If it is resonant, it may vary from the rather dull sound heard over normal lungs to the tympanitic sound heard over the dorsal part of the rumen or equine cecum.

The finger percussion method is always used in small animal work and is considered the most accurate technique for large animals.[5] The middle finger of one hand is held firmly against the intercostal muscles and is struck between the distal interphalangeal joint and the nail with the tip of the middle finger of the other hand. In percussing large animals, the hammer and pleximeter have been preferred in the past. The pleximeter should be narrow enough to fit between the ribs and should be held firmly against the intercostal muscles. Whether hammer or finger is used, the blow is a light one from the wrist, and the hammer or finger is allowed to recoil immediately.

Work over the lung area only. The other organs will be percussed in later class periods. The object of this exercise is to learn the normal position of the lung by percussion (see Plates I to III). The cranial border of the lung area is the same in all animals, as is the dorsal border. The cranial limit is the tricipital line, from the caudal angle of the scapula to the olecranon. The dorsal border is on a line extending from the caudal angle of the scapula to the tuber coxae. The basal border, which intersects the other two, varies with the species. A general rule is that it ascends from the olecranon region to the next to the last intercostal space at the dorsal border. Percuss the area systematically, one intercostal space at a time. In determining the basal border of the lung, it is well for the beginner to start with two points in a single intercostal space—one point known to be over the lung and the other point known to be well outside the area of the lung. After establishing the difference in sound of these points of maximum contrast, the distance between them is gradually decreased by alternate percussion of the lung and non-lung areas until the border of the lung resonance is found. This line, as determined by light finger percussion during the greater part of the respiratory cycle, is 3 to 4 cm. above the actual border of the lung.[5] Rarely, a percussion blow coincides with maximum inspiration and yields a point of lung resonance caudoventral to the curve.

The diaphragmatic line of pleural reflection is the ventrocaudal limit of the costodiaphragmatic recess. It is clinically important as the caudal boundary of the pleural cavity for surgical purposes. Punctures or incisions caudoventral to this line will enter the peritoneal cavity. The course of the line varies in different species, but in general it passes along the eighth and ninth costal cartilages in the costal arch, then curves dorsally to the last rib. References to the middle of a rib in the descriptions of individual species mean midway between the back muscles and the costal arch. The part of the rib dorsal to the angle is not considered. The *angle of the rib* is formed at the lateral border of the back muscles, where the costal bone arches medially (see section 17c).

Pleurocentesis for the drainage of fluids from the pleural cavity is performed at the lowest safe point in the standing animal. This is in the costomediastinal recess caudal to the pericardium and cranial to the diaphragmatic line of pleural reflection. Thus, the optimum point for drainage of the pleural cavity varies slightly between the right and left sides and among species, according to the position of the heart and the pleural reflection. A general rule is to puncture the intercostal space somewhat dorsal to the costochondral junction and midway between the ribs to avoid the ventral intercostal vessels. Unlike the dorsal intercostal vessels, which hug the caudal border of the rib, the ventral ones are double and follow both cranial and caudal borders of the costal cartilage and the ventral end of the bony rib.

Auscultation of the Lung

Normal lung sounds are thought to result from the oscillations of respiratory tissue as air passes through them and from rapid fluctuations of gas pressure.[2, 4] They are produced by turbulent flow of air through larger airways. The minimum diameter of an airway capable of producing audible sounds is about 2 mm.[2] These sounds are attenuated as they are transmitted through the lung and thoracic wall to the listener and will vary with the position of the stethoscope on the thorax, the thickness of the thoracic wall, and the pattern of respiration. In a relaxed animal that is breathing slowly and that has a thick thoracic wall, normal breathing sounds may be inaudible or very quiet. An excited, panting, thin dog will have loud lung sounds on both inspiration and expiration. Normal lung sounds will be louder near the trachea and its bifurcation. They decrease in intensity toward the lung periphery. Normal breathing sounds resemble the nonmusical sound of wind blowing gently through the trees. A low volume, low pitch, clearly audible inspiratory phase is followed by a soft, short, lower pitched, poorly audible expiratory phase. These have been called vesicular sounds but do not come from terminal bronchioles and alveoli. They are normally generated in the larynx, trachea, and subdivisions of the bronchi down to the segmental bronchi in the adjacent lung. Loud breathing sounds, especially with a distinct expiratory component, are abnormal in a relaxed animal in good physical condition.

Abnormal sounds may be classified as discontinuous crackles or continuous wheezes. Discontinuous sounds or crackles are intermittent, discrete, non-musical, explosive sounds. They result from the sudden opening of obstructed airways, which creates an abrupt gas pressure change, or from a bursting of bubbles of secretions in airways. These are most commonly associated with bronchopneumonia, interstitial pneumonia, or pulmonary edema.

Continuous sounds or wheezes are musical, whistling sounds generated by air passing through an airway narrowed by spasm, mucosal edema, foreign bodies, neoplasia or tracheobronchial lymphadenopathy. They are usually associated with expiration. Inspiratory wheezing occurs with stenosis of the larynx, trachea, or principal bronchi.

17a. DISSECTION, THORAX, HORSE

The diaphragmatic line of pleural reflection is marked on the ribs. It follows the eighth and ninth costal cartilages, crosses the ninth rib above the costochondral junction, then curves dorsally, crossing the remaining ribs at successively greater distances from the costochondral junctions until it reaches the middle of the last rib, whence it curves mediocranially to join the mediastinum in the vertebral end of the last intercostal space. Pleurocentesis is done above the superficial thoracic vein in the seventh intercostal space. It is also possible to puncture the sixth space on the right side because of the more cranial position of the area of contact between the pericardium and thoracic wall.

The dorsal limit of the percussion and auscultation area is the lateral margin of the large spinal muscles, the most lateral of which terminates on the angles of the ribs. The muscles are not an obstacle to auscultation in emaciated animals. The cranial border is formed by the triceps muscle and varies with the position of the limb. In the usual standing position, the olecranon is in the transverse plane of the fifth costochondral junction. The *basal border* of the lung passes from the costochondral junction of the sixth rib, through the middle of the exposed part of the 11th or 12th rib, to the margin of the spinal muscles in the 16th intercostal space (see Plate I).

17b. DISSECTION, THORAX, CALF

The diaphragmatic line of pleural reflection, marked on the ribs, extends in a curve from the seventh or eighth costochondral junction, through the middle of the 11th rib, to the angle of the last rib. Pleurocentesis may be done in the sixth or seventh intercostal space on both sides, a short distance above the costochondral junction.

The dorsal limit of the percussion area is seen at the margin of the spinal muscles. In the standing adult animal, the olecranon is about at the sternal end of the fifth rib. The *basal border* of the lung runs from the costochondral junction of the sixth rib to the margin of the spinal muscles in the 11th intercostal space (see Plate II).

17c. DISSECTION, THORAX, DOG, AND CAT

Notice the difference between small and large animals in the knee of the rib (genu costae). A rib is composed of a costal bone and a costal cartilage. The knee of the rib in large animals is formed between the bone and the cartilage at the costochondral junction. In small animals it is a bend in the costal cartilage (see Plate III).

The diaphragmatic line of pleural reflection, marked on the ribs, runs from the knee of the eighth rib, across the 11th rib just above its costochondral junction, to the dorsal part of the 13th rib. Pleurocentesis is performed in the seventh or eighth intercostal space in the dog and in the eighth in the cat. Notice that the long axis of the heart forms a more acute angle with the sternum in the cat than in the dog.

The *basal border* of the lung curves from the costochondral junction of the sixth rib to the margin of the spinal muscles in the 11th intercostal space.

17d. LIVE HORSE

Percussion. The basal border of the lung percussion area, as determined by light, finger-to-finger percussion, begins at the sixth rib about two finger-breadths above the olecranon and runs dorsocaudally. At the tenth intercostal space the basal border intersects a dorsal plane through the shoulder joint. It can also be said to intersect the middle of the 11th rib. At the 14th space it intersects the dorsal plane of the tuber ischiadicum. Up to this point the line is straight, then it curves strongly to the point where the 16th intercostal space meets the back muscles.

The resonance of the normal lung decreases gradually as one approaches the basal border. Caudal to the dorsal third of the basal border of the right lung there is an abrupt change to the flat liver sound. This is a good place to learn the difference. Ventral to the middle of the basal border there may be a resonant area caused by gas in the dorsal colon, but this resonance has a lower pitch than that of the lung.

Auscultation. The normal lung sound is inspiratory. It is soft and hissing, and in the resting horse it is only audible in the region close to the triceps. If the horse is exercised, the sound becomes louder, and the lung may be outlined with the stethoscope. Listen to the trachea to hear the inspiratory and expiratory sound transmitted from the larynx.

Raise the superficial thoracic vein. It runs along the border of the deep pectoral muscle.

17e. LIVE COW

Percussion. The basal border of the percussion area is almost straight. It intersects the cranial border at the sixth costochondral junction. In the seventh intercostal space the basal border intersects the dorsal plane through the shoulder joint. In the 11th space the basal border meets the dorsal border at the muscles of the back. This is a small area, compared with that in other animals.

Caudal to the dorsal third of the basal border of the left lung, the resonance merges into the tympanitic sound of the upper part of the rumen, while in the dorsal third of the basal border of the right lung, the resonance ends abruptly at the liver. In the middle third of the basal border on both sides, the resonance ends abruptly because of the ingesta in the rumen and omasum.

Auscultation. The normal sound is much louder and harsher than in the horse. It is heard on inspiration and is loudest just caudal to the triceps. Outline the lung with the stethoscope. Listen to the trachea to hear the inspiratory and expiratory stenotic sound from the larynx.

17f. LIVE DOG AND CAT

Percussion. The basal border of the percussion area passes from the level of the olecranon at the sixth rib through the middle of the eighth rib, to intersect the dorsal border at the 11th intercostal space. The resonance is more clearly heard, in comparison with that in larger animals.

Auscultation. Outline the area of normal breathing sounds. They are more distinct in the axillary region and over the rest of the lateral thoracic wall in the sleeping or somnolent dog.

References

1. Kirk, R. W. (ed.) Current Veterinary Therapy IV, Small Animal Practice. Philadelphia: W. B. Saunders, 1971.
2. Kotilikoff, M. I. and J. R. Gillespie: Lung sounds in veterinary medicine. Part I. Terminology and mechanisms of sound production. Comp. Cont. Ed. *5* (1983):634–638.
3. Kotilikoff, M. I. and J. R. Gillespie: Lung sounds in veterinary medicine. Part II. Clinical information from lung sounds. Comp. Cont. Ed. *6* (1984):462–467.
4. Roudebush, P.: Lung Sounds. JAVMA *181* (1982):122–126.
5. Steck, W.: Technik und Ergebnisse der Finger-Finger Perkussion am Thorax bei Grosstieren. Schweiz. Arch. Tierheilkd. *102* (1960):641–649.
6. Steck, W.: Lungenschallperkussion und Brustwandschallperkussion bei Grosstieren. Schweiz. Arch. Tierheilkd. *104* (1962):59–66.
7. Walsh, F. E. and Murphy, H. S.: Figures illustrating the percussion and auscultation area over the lungs of the ox, together with adjacent structures. Iowa State Coll. Vet. Pract. Bull. *5* (1):1922.

CHAPTER 18

HEART: PERCUSSION AND AUSCULTATION

OBJECTIVES

1. To be able to visualize the position of the heart in the body with reference to external landmarks and to palpate the heart beat.
2. To be able to visualize the orientation of the heart chambers, valves, and great vessels with reference to right and left sides and the long axis of the body.
3. To be able to open the chambers of the heart systematically at necropsy without losing their continuity with the great vessels and without destroying valvular lesions.
4. To be able to determine by percussion whether the area of absolute cardiac dullness is normal in any individual dog, ox, or horse.
5. To be able to distinguish between the first and second heart sounds and to identify the time interval in which systolic and diastolic murmurs are heard.
6. To understand the point of maximum audibility for a murmur caused by a lesion of each heart valve.
7. To be able to state whether a murmur heard in a given time interval over a given point is caused by stenosis or insufficiency.
8. To be able to place a needle in the cardiac ventricles of small animals with minimum chance of error.

18a. DISSECTIONS, HEART

It is much easier to orient the heart at necropsy if it is not severed from the lungs and great vessels. If the trachea, esophagus, lungs, heart, and great vessels are removed as one mass, and the chambers of the heart are opened without destroying their connections with the vessels, much footless speculation can be avoided when it is necessary to describe the location of a lesion. Orient the heart so that the venae cavae are directed cranially and caudally in the same horizontal plane. The long axis of the heart is directed caudoventrally and slightly to the left. The right ventricle winds around the cranial surface of the heart from right to left. The relationship of the ventricles is as much cranial and caudal as it is right and left. To open the heart for examination of the chambers and valves, hold the pluck (thoracic viscera) up by the trachea and lay it down on its left side.[9] Recognize the right side of the heart by the smooth surface of the right atrium, the venae cavae and the base of the right auricle at the cranial end of the right atrium.

To open the pulmonary trunk, right ventricle, and atrium, place the left surface in your left hand. Turn the heart so the cranial surface faces you. Identify the pulmonary trunk on the left side of this surface (between the auricles) cranial to the paraconal interventricular groove. Cut into the pulmonary trunk and continue through the pulmonary valve and the right ventricle close to its attachment to the interventricular septum. This cut will begin along the cranial border of the paraconal interventricular groove. Turn the heart so the right surface faces you. Continue the cut through the right ventricle ventrally and then dorsally toward the base of the heart along the cranial border of the subsinuosal interventricular groove. At the dorsal end of this groove, continue the cut through the right atrioventricular valve, right atrium, and caudal vena cava. Cut any trabeculae septomarginales that attach the parietal wall of the right ventricle to the interventricular septum and reflect the parietal wall. Examine the following structures: the caudal and cranial venae cavae, coronary sinus, intervenous tubercle, fossa ovalis, interatrial septum, right auricle, right atrioventricular valve (septal, parietal, and angular cusps), right ventricle, conus arteriosus, interventricular septum, pulmonary valve, pulmonary trunk, site of ligamentum arteriosum, and pulmonary arteries.

To open the left atrium, ventricle, and aorta, lay the heart on its right surface. Recognize the left side of the heart by the left auricle caudal to the pulmonary trunk and the right auricle cranial to it. Make a straight vertical cut from the pulmonary veins that enter the left atrium dorsally, through the left atrium, left auricle, and the parietal wall of the left ventricle. This cuts the parietal cusp of the left atrioventricular valve. Examine the following structures: pulmonary veins, left atrium, interatrial septum, valve of foramen ovale, left auricle, left atrioventricular valve (septal and parietal cusps), and left ventricle (parietal wall and interventricular septum).

To open the aorta, pass your knife beneath the septal cusp of the left atrioventricular valve and out through the aortic valve into the aorta; cut through all of these tissues with a straight cut. This will also cut part of the wall of the left atrium and the pulmonary trunk. Examine the following structures: aortic valve, aortic sinuses, coronary arteries, brachiocephalic trunk (left subclavian artery in the dog and cat), and ligamentum arteriosum. The ligamentum arteriosum is the vestige of the ductus arteriosus found between the aorta and the pulmonary trunk, near the bifurcation of the latter. A patent ductus arteriosus is the most common clinically significant cardiac anomaly in the dog.[13] Examine the cusps of the atrioventricular valves. These are designated right AV and left AV rather than tricuspid and mitral to eliminate error.

The twist of the right ventricle around the cranial surface places the pulmonary valve on the left of the aortic valve and cranial to it.[4] For this reason, the pulmonary valve is auscultated on the left side. In the embryo, the originally unpaired distal part of the bulb of the heart and the arterial

Table 18–1. THE POSITION OF THE HEART

	Cranial Extent	Caudal Extent
Cat	4th space	7th rib
Dog	3rd rib	6th space
Pig	2nd rib	5th rib
Ruminant	2nd space	5th space
Horse	2nd space	6th space

trunk are divided by a spiral septum into the aorta and pulmonary trunk.[1] If this septum does not join the interventricular septum properly, the resulting four anomalies constitute the tetralogy of Fallot: pulmonary stenosis, aorta astride the interventricular septum and receiving blood from both ventricles, interventricular septal defect, and dilation and hypertrophy of the right ventricle, which results from the other three anomalies.[3]

18b,c,d. LIVE ANIMALS

It will save time if the fifth rib is located and marked. It is usually opposite the olecranon when the limb is vertical.

In *percussion* of the heart, two zones are described. (1) The area of absolute cardiac dullness corresponds to the area of contact of the pericardium with the thoracic wall. It gives a flat sound on light percussion. (2) The area of relative cardiac dullness is difficult to determine in animals. It is defined by somewhat stronger percussion and indicates the outline of the heart that is covered by the thin margin of the lung. For practical purposes, the absolute dullness may be used to test for hypertrophy, displacement, and pericardial effusion. It should be kept in mind, however, that it is not the outline of the heart as it would be seen in a lateral radiograph. The full craniocaudal extent in relation to the ribs is given for reference only in Table 18–1 (see Plates I to III).

The area of absolute dullness in the horse is a right triangle bounded by the triceps in front, the sternum below, and the lung along the hypotenuse. The object of percussion is to determine whether or not the heart is enlarged; i.e., whether or not the hypotenuse is displaced dorsocaudally. On the left side of the normal horse, dullness extends about 7 cm. above the olecranon in the fourth space and about 3 cm. above the olecranon in the fifth space. On the right, the dullness extends about 3 cm. above the olecranon in the fourth space only.

In the ox, the normal area of absolute dullness is too far cranial for percussion. The lower limits of lung resonance in the fourth and fifth spaces should be carefully explored. Traumatic pericarditis may produce absolute dullness in these spaces, extending above a dorsal plane through the shoulder joint (see Plate II).

Small dogs are most easily percussed by holding them in the sitting-up position and working on the ventral surface of the thorax. On the left side, the cardiac dullness extends out to the costochondral junctions in spaces four and five but not so far in six. On the right side, the dullness extends only 1 to 2 cm. from the sternum in spaces four and five.

In *auscultation,* the first heart sound heard in each cycle is caused by the closing of the right and left atrioventricular valves. The second sound is caused by the closing of the aortic and pulmonary valves. Systolic murmurs occur between the first and second heart sounds. Diastolic murmurs are much less common and occur after the second sound and before the first sound of the next cycle. Once it has been decided that a heart murmur is systolic or diastolic, it is necessary to determine which of four possible valvular conditions is the cause. The possibilities are listed in Table 18–2.

This determination is mainly an anatomical problem. By listening at the known point of maximum audibility for each valve, it may be possible to localize the murmur. The puncta maxima established for the valves do not necessarily correspond with the anatomical positions of the valves. The puncta maxima were determined by comparison of clinical and autopsy findings in valvular disease. In some cases the sound is conducted to a point on the thoracic wall that is not in the plane of the valve.

Table 18–2. HEART LESIONS AND MURMURS

Lesion	Time of Murmur	
	Systolic	*Diastolic*
Stenosis	aortic pulmonary	right AV left AV
Insufficiency	right AV left AV	aortic pulmonary

The locations of the puncta maxima may be summarized in general terms for all species as follows:

Left AV. Low in the left fifth intercostal space (fourth in the ox). This is dorsocaudal to the olecranon in the horse, medial to the medial epicondyle in the ox, and at the costochondral joint in the dog.

Aortic. High in the left fourth space, just below a dorsal plane passing through the shoulder joint.

Pulmonary. Low in the left third space.

Right AV. Low in the right third or fourth space.

An efficient procedure is to begin with the left AV valve, where the first sound is loudest, then gradually move the stethoscope cranially until the second sound reaches maximum intensity over the pulmonary valve. Return to the left AV valve and gradually move the stethoscope dorsally in the fourth space until the second sound reaches maximum intensity over the aortic valve.

Auscultation of the individual valves of the feline heart is difficult because the total length of the heart, about 4 cm., is the same as the diameter of the head of the stethoscope, and the heart rate is so fast that the first and second sounds can be distinguished only by their quality rather than their timing.[14]

The cardiac lesions that are not associated with valves also produce murmurs in certain locations. In the dog, the sound of an interventricular septal defect is heard regularly with maximum intensity on the right.[8] It is often accompanied by the murmur of a functional pulmonary stenosis on the left (see Chapter 19). A patent ductus arteriosus has a characteristic "machinery murmur" that increases in systole and decreases in diastole and is loudest in the third and fourth spaces on the left.[13]

Palpate the heartbeat. The maximum intensity is normally at the apex on the left. Valvular lesions and congenital defects may produce a palpable vibration instead of the beat, as in the left third and fourth spaces with patent ductus arteriosus. The intensity may be increased or the maximum intensity may be felt on the right side with enlargement or displacement of the heart.

Cardiac puncture for obtaining blood or the injection of drugs is usually done on the right side in the fourth or fifth intercostal space a few centimeters above the sternum, at about the level of the olecranon. The thin-walled right ventricle is accessible here in the notch between the right cranial and middle lobes of the lung. Left ventricular blood is accessible through the interventricular tum.[2] Puncture on the right side also avoids the large paraconal interventricular branch of the left coronary artery. If cardiac puncture is for resuscitation and is associated with cardiac massage, the left fifth intercostal space is preferred, where the puncture will be through the thicker left ventricle, which is less likely to bleed during the massage and produce cardiac tamponade.

References

1. Arey, L. B.: Developmental Anatomy, 7th ed. Philadelphia.: W. B. Saunders, 1965.
2. Buchanan, J. M. and R. P. Botts: Clinical effects of repeated cardiac punctures in dogs. JAVMA *161* (1972):814–818.
3. Clark, D. R., O. N. Ross, R. L. Hamlin, et. al.: Tetralogy of Fallot in the dog. JAVMA *150* (1968):463–471.
4. Habel, R. E.: Guide to the Dissection of Domestic Ruminants, 3rd ed. Ithaca, N.Y.: Habel, 1977.
5. Hahn, A. W.: Cardiac murmurs in the dog. Small Anim. Clin. *2* (1962):319–323.
6. Hamlin, R. L., R. J. Tashjian, and C. R. Smith: Diseases of the cardiovascular system. *In* Catcott, E. J. (ed.): Feline Medicine and Surgery. Wheaton, Ill.: Am. Vet. Publications, 1964.
7. Hamlin, R. L., D. L. Smetzer, and C. R. Smith: Congenital mitral insufficiency in the dog. JAVMA *146* (1965):1088–1100.
8. Hamlin, R.L.: Analysis of the cardiac silhouette in dorsoventral radiographs from dogs with heart disease. JAVMA *153* (1968):1446–1460.
9. King, J. M., D. C. Dodd, and M. E. Newson: Gross Necropsy Technique for Animals. Ithaca, N.Y.: Arnold Printing Corp., 1982.
10. Littlewort, M. C. G.: The clinical auscultation of the equine heart. Vet. Rec. *74* (1962):1247–1259.
11. Patterson, D. F. and D. H. Knight: Pathophysiology and clinical diagnosis of common cardiovascular diseases of the dog. Am. Anim. Hosp. Assoc. Proc. 38th Mtg. 1971:86–108.
12. Smetzer, D. L. and C. R. Smith: Diastolic heart sounds of horses. JAVMA *146* (1965):937–944.
13. Smetzer, D. L. and E. M. Breznock: Auscultatory diagnosis of patent ductus arteriosus in the dog. JAVMA *160* (1972):80–84.
14. Tilley, L. P. (ed.): Symposium on Feline Cardiology. Vet. Clin. North Am. 7, No. 2 (1977).

CHAPTER 19

THORACIC VISCERA

OBJECTIVES

1. To know the course and relations of the esophagus in the thorax and whether the surgical approach to each segment should be from the right or the left.
2. To understand the neuromuscular basis of the various kinds of megaesophagus in the dog and cat.
3. To understand what structures form the constricting ring around the esophagus in persistent right aortic arch and which of these may be cut to open the ring.
4. To be able to identify on radiographs the normal structures in and around the thorax and their variation with the stage of respiration, the cardiac cycle, the shape of the thorax, and the position of the animal.
5. To know the position of the normal openings in the diaphragm and its weak points.
6. To understand the fetal circulation, the changes that take place at birth, and the effect of various common anomalies on blood flow. To understand the functional closure of the valve of the foramen ovale and the significance of patency.
7. To be able to recognize enlargements of the four chambers of the heart and the great arteries in lateral and dorsoventral radiographs. To know the diagnostic significance of these enlargements.
8. To be able to find the lymph nodes examined routinely in post-mortem inspection of food animals and the nodes examined in final inspection of retained carcasses.

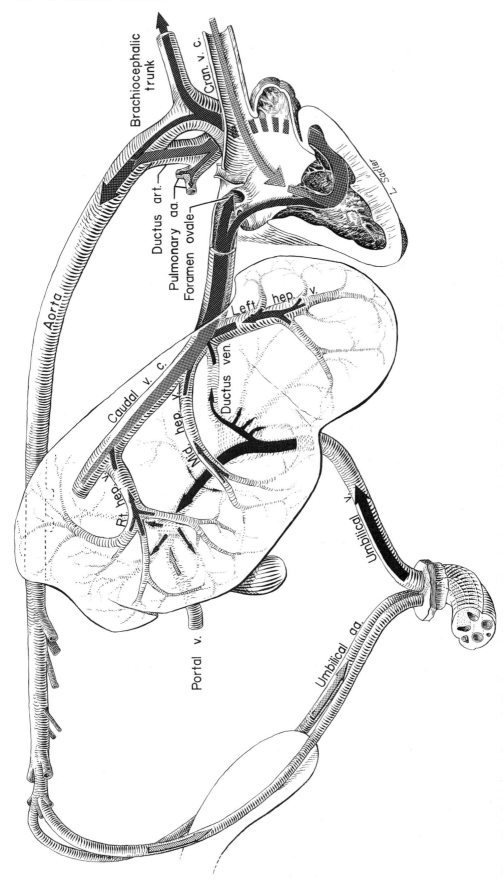

Figure 19–1. Fetal circulation, calf. Diaphragmatic surface of liver is shown, and right side of heart is opened. Flow from right ventricle into pulmonary trunk is indicated by interrupted tract. Maximum oxygen saturation is indicated by black arrows, with decreasing oxygen content in lighter shades of gray. Width of arrows is proportional to volume flow.

Notes on the Nomenclature: The large artery originating at the pulmonary valve is the pulmonary trunk. It bifurcates into right and left pulmonary arteries. All three are "main pulmonary arteries" in one sense or another, and therefore the last term should be dropped.

Various contrast media are used in radiology, but usually only one medium is used at a time.

19a. FETAL CIRCULATION, CALF

An understanding of the fetal circulation and the changes that occur after birth is useful in the diagnosis and surgical treatment of cardiac anomalies. The following normal data are based on experiments on fetal lambs.[10]

The blood from the placenta enters the fetus in the umbilical vein at 80 percent oxygen saturation. All species have one umbilical vein in the abdomen at term. Carnivora and ruminants have two umbilical veins in the cord, but these unite at the umbilicus. The pig and the horse have only one vein in the umbilical cord, the other having disappeared during gestation. The umbilical vein enters the liver between the quadrate and left lobes and joins the left end of the left intrahepatic branch of the portal vein. This junction is connected by a large shunt, the ductus venosus, to the caudal vena cava near the mouth of the left hepatic vein, so that about a ninth of the umbilical blood by-passes the liver. The ductus venosus is present at birth in the carnivores and ruminants but disappears during gestation in the horse. In the fetal pig, the ductus venosus is interrupted early, but a shunt is provided by anastomoses between afferent veins that sprout from the umbilical end of the ductus and efferent veins that sprout from the caval end.[2, 24, 25] After birth the ductus venosus is obliterated, and the intrahepatic part of the umbilical vein becomes the left extremity of the left branch of the portal vein (Fig. 19–1).

The blood in the vena cava caudal to the liver is about 26 percent saturated with oxygen, similar to that in the portal vein before it enters the liver. The admixture of umbilical blood raises the oxygen level to 67 percent in the caudal vena cava cranial to the liver. About three-fifths of the blood from the caudal vena cava is directed through the foramen ovale into the left atrium. The foramen is in the line of flow because its cranial border projects into the blood stream. The remainder of the blood from the caudal vena cava mixes with that of the cranial vena cava and passes into the right ventricle. Blood from the cranial vena cava is 31 percent saturated with oxygen. None of it passes through the foramen ovale because it is diverted into the ventricle by the intervenous tubercle and the stream from the caudal vena cava.

Closure of the foramen ovale at birth is caused by: (1) increased blood flow into the left atrium from the newly functional lungs, (2) decreased pressure in the right heart because of the expanded lung and closure of the umbilical vein, and (3) increased flow into the lungs resulting from reversed flow through the ductus arteriosus, which remains patent for a few hours or days. The pressure in the left atrium compresses the one-way valve of the foramen ovale against the wall of the left atrium (see Section 19c). Even though the valve may not be completely sealed for some days or weeks, it can leak only from right to left, and leakage occurs only if the pressure in the right atrium exceeds that in the left.

Clinical interatrial septal defect is not a persistent foramen ovale but a rare developmental failure of part of the septum. This permits flow from left to right, increasing the volume of blood pumped through the pulmonary valve. A relative or functional stenosis results and produces a murmur like that of a true stenosis. The right ventricle and pulmonary trunk are enlarged, but cardioangiography shows no constriction of the pulmonary valve, and the vessels in the lung are enlarged rather than diminished.[17] The signs of functional pulmonary stenosis are also produced by interventricular septal defect.[13]

The output of the right ventricle is about equal to that of the left in the fetus, and the thickness of the wall is about the same. Therefore the wall of the fetal right ventricle appears abnormally thick to one accustomed to necropsy of the adult. After birth the wall of the left ventricle grows in thickness faster than that of the right.

Blood leaving the fetal right ventricle in the pulmonary trunk is 52 percent saturated with oxygen. Only about one-fifth of it goes to the lungs; the rest passes through the ductus arteriosus into the aorta. The ductus is a muscular artery, unlike the elastic arteries it connects, and it constricts after birth. This constriction is caused by the direct stimulus of increased oxygen tension in the blood after breathing begins. Closure of the umbilical arteries causes increased pressure in the aorta, while expansion of the lungs causes lowered pressure in the pulmonary trunk; these factors result in a reversed flow of highly oxygenated blood in the ductus arteriosus. Closure is not complete for some hours or days, and the reversed flow continues. In the sheep, ox, and horse, it produces a loud continuous murmur in the left third intercostal space. In the pig, it is a systolic crescendo murmur. It is difficult to hear in puppies. After the transitional neonatal period, the ductus arteriosus is anatomically sealed. A persistently patent ductus, unlike a patent foramen ovale, causes heart disease.

Another, more rare, congenital anomaly of the aortic arches is a right aortic arch. In this condition, the embryonic right fourth aortic arch instead of the left forms the definitive aorta. It passes to the right of the trachea and esophagus. The pulmonary trunk and ductus arteriosus (left sixth aortic arch) take their normal course over the left side of the trachea and esophagus, and the ductus joins the aorta. The result is a vascular ring that constricts the esophagus and interferes with swallowing. The treatment is to cut the ductus arteriosus between ligatures. It may be patent. Less common vascular anomalies that produce partial or complete vascular rings over the esophagus in the dog are: a normal left fourth aortic arch as the aorta with an abnormal right sixth aortic arch as the ductus arteriosus; a normal left fourth aortic arch as the aorta with the right subclavian artery arising abnormally from the aorta at the site of the left subclavian artery and coursing cranioventrally to the right first rib (the right subclavian artery failed to migrate cranially to be a branch of the brachiocephalic trunk, and the right dorsal aortic root degenerated cranial to the right subclavian artery instead of caudal to it); a right fourth aortic arch as the aorta with the left subclavian artery arising abnormally from the right aorta at the abnormal site of the right subclavian artery instead of from the brachiocephalic trunk (with or without a left sixth arch ductus arteriosus); and a persistence of both aortic arches and dorsal aortic roots as aortas (double aortic arch).

To return to the flow of fetal blood through the foramen ovale into the left atrium, it is not much diluted by the blood from the pulmonary veins, which flows at about a fifth of the foramen ovale rate. Therefore the blood entering the aorta is 62 percent saturated with oxygen, and this is supplied to the coronary arteries, head, and thoracic limbs. Distal to the origin of the arteries to the head and thoracic limbs, the blood in the aorta is somewhat reduced in oxygenation by the large flow from the ductus arteriosus (52 percent O_2 sat.) so that the final oxygen saturation of blood flowing to the rest of the body and returning to the placenta is 58 percent. Two-thirds of the blood in the descending aorta enters the umbilical arteries.

All species have two umbilical arteries, which appear in the fetus to be the terminal branches of the aorta. Umbilical arteries and veins are both muscular vessels, difficult to distinguish grossly in the cord, and the spasm of their musculature is sufficient to close them when the cord is ruptured or bitten at birth. The ruminants and horse have an additional sphincter in the cord at the umbilicus. It is composed of longitudinal and circular smooth muscle fibers looped around the vessels, and it extends to the junction of the skin and amnion. The effect of the closure of the umbilical vessels on the pressures in the right and left chambers of the heart is an important cause of the changes that occur at birth. Two other causes are the decreased resistance in the pulmonary circulation and the increased oxygen tension. After birth the umbilical arteries of quadrupeds retract into the lateral ligaments of the bladder and become the round ligaments of the bladder.

19b. DISSECTION, THORAX, CALF

In the cranial mediastinum identify the cranial vena cava on the right and the brachiocephalic trunk on the left. The trachea and esophagus are dorsal to these vessels, with the esophagus on the left of the trachea. The cranial part of the cranial lobe of the right lung, although not in the mediastinum, occupies most of the space cranial to the heart by pushing the ventral part of the mediastinum against the left costal pleura. The only portion of the left lung cranial to the heart is the apex, located dorsally. The thoracic lobe of the thymus is in the cranial mediastinum on the left side of the esophagus and brachiocephalic trunk. It extends caudally to the aortic arch and pulmonary trunk. Cranially it is adjacent to the left costal pleura, but caudally it is covered on the left by the cranial parts of the cranial lobes of both lungs. Caudal to this, the heart is adjacent to the left wall at the third intercostal space, and its caudal left surface is covered by the caudal part of the left cranial lung lobe.

Pericardiocentesis is done at the left fifth interchondral space in the ox. Chronic suppurative pericarditis has been treated by resection of the fifth rib and cartilage for lavage and drainage. The left area of pericardial-thoracic wall contact is large in ruminants because of the larger cardiac notch in the left lung. Be aware of the curvature of the ribs and costal cartilages when considering the position of the heart relative to the rib cage. The interchondral space between costal cartilages extends cranially, so that it eventually is in line with the preceding intercostal space between the bony ribs. In directions for surgical approach be sure to distinguish between intercostal and interchondral levels.

The sternal attachment of the heart in ruminants and the horse is broad and firm—the sterno-pericardiac ligaments. In the dog, there is a loose diaphragmatic attachment—the phrenicopericardiac ligament, allowing mobility of the heart in the sagittal plane.

Note the position of the esophagus on the right side of the aortic arch as they cross.

19c. DISSECTION, CALF, HEART

Examine an opened fetal or newborn calf heart. In the right atrium, identify the foramen ovale. It is the opening in the embryonic septum secundum that leads to a channel between the septum secundum on the right and the septum primum on the left. The caudal border of the septum secundum forms the cranial border of this opening. It projects to the right into the blood stream entering from the caudal vena cava and diverts about three-fifths of it through the foramen ovale into the left atrium. When this foramen closes after birth and is obliterated, a small depression, the fossa ovalis, remains, and the remnant of the cranial border of the foramen is the intervenous tubercle.

Examine the interatrial septum in the left atrium. The valve of the foramen ovale extends across the cranial wall, forming the left wall of the tubular vascular channel from the right atrium. It ends in a fenestrated apex anchored by irregular cords. The valve of the foramen ovale is formed by the embryonic septum primum. The opening into the left atrium is the foramen secundum in that septum. This tubular valve is found in herbivores and differs from the simple flap of the primates, carnivores, and swine. After birth, this sleeve is collapsed against the wall of the left atrium by the higher pressure of blood from the pulmonary veins. This produces a functional closure, and sealing of the fenestrae begins. They are completely sealed in the foal at 15 days, and the tubular valve has disappeared at 30 to 40 days. The fenestrated end of the valve is usually sealed in the calf by 20 days.[27] A patent interatrial channel demonstrated by probing from the right atrium through the foramen ovale in the young animal at necropsy is of no clinical significance.

Identify the aorta, pulmonary trunk, and ductus arteriosus. Note that the segment of aorta between the origin of the brachiocephalic trunk and the entrance of the ductus arteriosus is smaller than the rest of the thoracic aorta and about the same size as the ductus. This segment is called the aortic isthmus. It is normal and results from the large volume of blood that enters the brachiocephalic trunk from the aorta and the large volume that passes through the ductus arteriosus from the pulmonary trunk to fill the descending thoracic aorta. After birth and closure of the ductus, the isthmus will expand to the size of the rest of the adjacent aorta. Do not open the pulmonary trunk, ductus arteriosus, and descending thoracic aorta and mistake them for an aorta arising from the right ventricle.

19d. DISSECTION, THORACIC LYMPH NODES, OX

The first two groups of lymph nodes are incised in the routine post-mortem inspection of the pluck (heart, lungs, and esophagus) of cattle. The other groups are incised in the final inspection of retained carcasses. Many small nodes have been omitted from this list.

1. *Tracheobronchial.* The left tracheobronchial node is located by drawing the left cranial lobe caudally and incising the tissues cranial to the left bronchus. The node lies between the arch of the aorta and the left pulmonary artery. On the right side, the cranial tracheobronchial node is the one commonly examined. It lies on the right side of the trachea cranial to the tracheal bronchus, the special bronchus of the right cranial lobe. There is a node in the ox that is related to the right principal bronchus, but it is small, inconstant, and seldom examined.

2. *Caudal mediastinal.* This is a group of very large elongated nodes lying in the mediastinum

between the aorta and esophagus. The most cranial node is at the aortic arch; the most caudal may be left in the carcass, attached to the diaphragm. Enlarged caudal mediastinal nodes in tuberculosis or lymphomatosis can cause choke or bloat by compression of the esophagus. They can also damage the vagal trunks on the esophagus and disturb gastric motility. They receive lymphatics from the abdominal surface of the diaphragm and the surface of the liver in addition to thoracic structures.

3. *Cranial mediastinal.* These nodes are distributed in the fat around the trachea, esophagus, and large vessels cranial to the heart. They are often left in the carcass.

4. *Thoracic aortic.* Small nodes on the dorsal surface of the aorta. They are relatively larger and more important in swine.

5. *Sternal.* The cranial sternal node is large and is not covered by the transverse thoracic muscle. It lies on the second costal cartilage. The caudal sternal nodes lie on the course of the internal thoracic vessels in the interchondral spaces, covered by the transverse thoracic muscle. The nodes in the fat around the sternal attachment of the pericardium are also included in the caudal sternal group. They are not covered by the muscle.

Perforations of the mediastinum have been reported in the adult horse, dog, cat, and in some old sheep. They do not occur in the ox, goat, or pig, or in very young animals of any species. Their dimensions range from 0.01 × 0.003 mm. to 0.77 × 0.56 mm. in the horse, and they are microscopic in the dog.[1] The significance of the openings lies in the possibility of a unilateral pneumothorax, pleural effusion, or infection becoming bilateral and fatal. There is some clinical evidence that this is a real danger in the horse, but even in that animal the openings are apparently closed by inflammatory processes. Dogs are usually not killed by acute experimental unilateral pneumothorax if the mediastinum is not disturbed. Cattle tolerate the unilateral pneumothorax associated with pericardial drainage.

19e. DISSECTION, THORAX, DOG, DORSAL VIEW

Identify in the cranial mediastinum: the cranial vena cava and azygous vein on the right; the brachiocephalic trunk with its left common carotid artery and its terminal branches—the right common carotid and right subclavian arteries; and the left subclavian artery arising from the aortic arch and coursing on the left side of the cranial mediastinum. The trachea and esophagus are dorsal to these vessels, with the esophagus dorsal or to the left of the trachea. The esophagus passes dorsal to the tracheal bifurcation and left principal bronchus and on the right side of the aortic arch. The latter relation is reversed when the aorta arises abnormally from the right fourth aortic arch. Fluoroscopic studies show some resistance to the passage of food at this point, and this is the usual site for cranial thoracic choke.

Identify the tracheal bifurcation and the principal bronchus to each lung. Because the bronchus to the right middle lobe branches ventrally from the principal bronchus, this is a source of pendant drainage and infection. Sternal recumbency is required for bronchography of this lobe. Find the pulmonary trunk at the left cranial part of the base of the heart on the left of the aorta. Trace the right pulmonary artery ventral to the tracheal bifurcation to the right lung and the left pulmonary artery beside or dorsal to the left principal bronchus. Identify the pulmonary veins from each lung entering the left atrium. Some dogs have a common venous drainage from the accessory and right caudal lung lobes. In lobectomy the branch to the healthy lung lobe must be avoided.

Trace the caudal vena cava, esophagus, and aorta to their respective hiatus at the diaphragm. Note the position of the accessory lobe of the right lung over the caudal vena cava, caudal to the heart, between the caudal mediastinum and the plica venae cavae.

Identify the aorta and azygous veins at and cranial to the aortic hiatus. The thoracic duct begins dorsally between the crura of the diaphragm as a cranial continuation of the cisterna chyli. It passes through the aortic hiatus, and in most dogs it courses cranially on the right of the thoracic vertebrae between the right side of the aorta and the ventral surface of the azygous vein. At about the sixth thoracic vertebra it passes between these vessels to the left side and into the cranial mediastinum. The level of crossing can vary from the fifth to the eleventh thoracic vertebra. It terminates by one or more branches in the left brachiocephalic vein or adjacent veins. Variations in the course, termination, and number of vessels that compose the duct are common. In most cats, the entire course to the cranial mediastinum is on the left side of the aorta.[15] One or more lymphatic collaterals may pass through the diaphragm and join the thoracic duct cranial to the hiatus.

Most of the lymph in the thoracic duct comes from the lymphatics in the liver and intestine. The volume is related to the diet and feeding habits of the animal. Chylothorax is most commonly associated with trauma or neoplastic invasion of the duct in the dog and cat.[3, 29] It can be diagnosed by analysis of the pleural fluid. In some cases lymphangiography will show the point of disruption of the duct. This is best performed by injecting an aqueous radiopaque medium into an intestinal lymphatic that is identified in the mesentery by feeding the animal a concentrated fat solution prior to surgery.[4, 23] Alternatively, subcutaneous injection of a dye between the digits of the hind paw will permit visualization of a lymphatic adjacent to the lateral saphenous vein, which can be cannulated and injected with an aqueous medium.[28]

If medical therapy is unsuccessful, the thoracic duct and all of its visible collaterals can be ligated as they emerge through the diaphragm. In the dog, the approach is through the right tenth intercostal space. The left tenth intercostal space is used in the cat.

19f. DIAPHRAGM (LIVER, KIDNEYS, AND STOMACH), DOG

Examine a specimen with the thoracic side of the diaphragm uppermost. Note the dome-like shape of the diaphragm as a whole. The tendinous center extends cranially to the plane of the sixth intercostal space. (This is the caudal extent of the heart.) The tendons of origin of the crura may be seen on both sides of the aorta at the level of the left kidney (third and fourth lumbar vertebrae). The crura (lumbar part) are separated from the costal part of the diaphragm by the V-shaped tendinous center. The caudal vena cava perforates the tendinous center on the right, and the esophagus passes through the right crus, which is much larger than the left. The liver is caudal to the right crus, and the fundus of the stomach is caudal to the left crus. Traumatic diaphragmatic hernias may occur anywhere in the diaphragm. The majority penetrate muscle rather than the normal openings, tendinous attachments, or points of embryonic closure—pleuroperitoneal membranes.[38, 40]

19g. RADIOGRAPHS, DOG AND CAT

Both dorsoventral and lateral views must be considered in radiographic examination of the thorax. Usually a left-right lateral view is used (patient in right recumbency) unless a lung lesion is suspected on the right side. The upper lung is usually better aerated, which may allow improved visualization of a parenchymal lesion.[36] Dorsoventral radiographs are usually made (patient in sternal recumbency), which permits more accurate and stable positioning of the thoracic viscera than dorsal recumbency.[8, 32] It is customary in human and veterinary radiology to read all dorsoventral or ventrodorsal radiographs in a ventrodorsal position.

Radiographs are usually made at the time of maximum inspiration.[34] The following features will be observed on a radiograph made on inspiration: increased pulmonary radiolucency, especially dorsally, with an increased radiolucent angle between the vertebrae and diaphragm on lateral view and between ribs and diaphragm on dorsoventral view; extension of left pleural cupula cranial to first rib; more extensive right pleural cupula dorsoventrally; wider area of accessory lung lobe caudal to the heart; enlarged dorsosternal lucency with less contact of right ventricle with the sternum; less overlap of diaphragm on the heart; dome of diaphragm more flat in lateral view and more dome-shaped in dorsoventral view and caudal to T 8; thinnner, more distinct caudal vena cava; and well defined aorta. In a radiograph made on expiration, the heart size will appear to be enlarged relative to the thorax. This is false cardiomegaly.

First examine the extrathoracic structures—vertebrae, diaphragm, ribs with costal cartilages, sternum. The shape of the diaphragm is the most variable, being influenced by the size, conformation, and position of the dog, the stage of respiration, distention of abdominal organs, and the line of projection of x-rays.[16] The right crus of the diaphragm is usually cranial to the left in right recumbency unless the stomach is enlarged; especially with gas. The crus on the recumbent side sags cranially from the pressure of the abdominal organs. The intercrural cleft is more prominent in large dogs. The dome-shaped ventral portion is called the cupula by radiologists. As dogs age, the costal cartilages calcify.

Examine in order the mediastinum, lungs, and pleural cavity. In examining the five parts of the mediastinum, consider the normal structures that occupy these spaces even though they may not be normally visible on radiographs.[26]

Cranial mediastinum. Lymph nodes (cranial mediastinal and sternal), vessels (cranial vena cava, brachiocephalic trunk, left subclavian artery), trachea, and esophagus. The great vessels cranial to the heart appear as one mass. The esophagus will be visible only if it contains air, which occasionally occurs during anesthesia. If a radiopaque substance such as barium sulfate is swallowed, the esophagus will be made visible.[39] It lies on the left of the trachea as far as the bifurcation, then passes dorsomedially over the left principal bronchus, crosses the right side of the aortic arch, and continues ventral to the aorta. The thymus is ventral and in dorsoventral view may extend into the left cranial thorax like the edge of a sail ("sail sign"). The cranioventral mediastinum deviates to the left because of the large portion of the right cranial lung lobe that extends across the cranial surface of the heart. In dorsoventral view, this may appear as a curved line passing caudally to the left from about the second thoracic vertebra to the silhouette of the pulmonary trunk. In dorsoventral view, fat in obese animals may expand the width of the mediastinum. Do not confuse this with a mass lesion. In dorsoventral view, the right border of the cranial mediastinum is the cranial vena cava. The left border is the esophagus or the left subclavian artery. Examine the caudal cervical and thoracic portions of the trachea. On strong inspiration the thoracic trachea widens and the cervical trachea narrows. The opposite effect occurs during expiration. Tracheal collapse most frequently occurs at the thoracic inlet and may require both inspiratory and expiratory radiographs to diagnose. Thoracic tracheal collapse may be evident only on radiographs made during expiration or during coughing. The acute angle, open caudally, between the trachea and vertebrae varies with breeds of dogs and is affected by space-occupying lesions. Cardiac enlargement elevates the trachea and closes this angle. Enlargement of the right atrium may put a hump in the trachea. If the neck is flexed in a normal dog, the trachea will be curved, with the convexity dorsal. The ventral edge of the longus colli may produce a shadow on the trachea. The trachea will be displaced ventrally by a dilated esophagus that is filled with food.

Dorsal Mediastinum. This lies dorsal to the heart and contains segments of the esophagus and thoracic duct, the tracheobronchial lymph nodes, the blood vessels passing to and from the heart, and the terminal part of the trachea.

The carina is the partition between the origins of the two principal bronchi. This is usually at or just caudal to the round radiolucent spot that is the origin of the lobar bronchus to the right cranial lung lobe.[7] Normally, the two principal bronchi are nearly superimposed and indistinguishable. The left may be slightly dorsal to the right. Atrial enlargement elevates the adjacent principal bronchus so that both principal bronchi become visible on lateral view (the V sign). In the early stages of a patent ductus arteriosus or left atrioventricular valvular insufficiency, the left atrium enlarges and may be seen in the fork formed by the displaced bronchi.

The large vessels are relatively opaque in contrast to the lungs on lateral view. The aorta arches dorsally and caudally from the base of the heart and runs just ventral to the vertebrae. The right and left pulmonary arteries arise from the bifurcation of the pulmonary trunk between the aorta and the bifurcation of the trachea. The left pulmonary artery may appear dorsal to the level of the bifurcation of the trachea, perhaps because it is held up by the ligamentum arteriosum. The right pulmonary artery passes ventral to the trachea to reach the right lung and may be seen end-on as a round dense spot. Pulmonary veins enter the caudodorsal contour of the heart. Ventral to the pulmonary veins, the caudal vena cava runs cranially and slightly ventrally from the liver to the right atrium.

Middle Mediastinum. The heart occupies the middle mediastinum.[30, 31] The heart usually extends over three intercostal spaces and is two-thirds the width of the thorax in dorsoventral view. It usually contacts the ventral thoracic wall in interchondral spaces four, five, and six and the three sternebrae ventrally. Excessive fat in the ventral mediastinum may elevate it off the sternum. In breeds of dogs with a deep thorax, the heart will be more vertical and narrow and have less sternal contact in lateral view and appear more round with a smaller width in a dorsoventral view. The heart will be larger relative to the thorax in young dogs and in radiographs made on expiration.

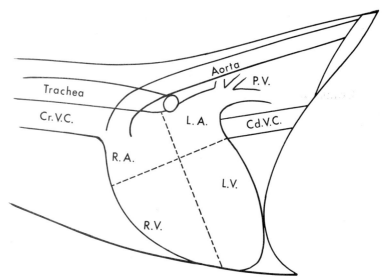

Figure 19–2. Diagram of a lateral radiograph of the canine thorax. *CdVC*, caudal vena cava; *CrVC*, cranial vena cava; *LA*, left atrium; *LV*, left ventricle; *PV*, pulmonary veins; *RA*, right atrium; *RV*, right ventricle.

Because of these variations, the relationship of the heart to the ribs is less significant for diagnosis than distortions of the outline of the heart. In cats, the heart has an oblique craniocaudal position, with extensive sternal contact.

The four chambers of the heart can be estimated in the lateral silhouette (Fig. 19–2) by drawing two lines. The first extends from the middle of the base of the heart to a point just cranial to the apex. The right side of the heart is cranial to this line and when enlarged will bulge the cranial cardiac border. A second line, perpendicular to the first and about one-quarter the distance from the base to the apex, defines the coronary groove between atria dorsally and ventricles ventrally. Normally there is a slight constriction where the cranial contour of the heart meets the cranial vena cava and where the caudal contour meets the pulmonary veins. These cranial and caudal profiles of the waist of the heart, become obliterated when the right and left sides of the heart enlarge respectively. In dorsoventral radiographs the apex is usually directed to the left. The right side is mildly curved, and the left is more straight. During systole the heart shadow is smaller, and the left ventricular border is more straight.

The parts of the heart that contribute to the normal silhouette have been identified by anatomical and cineangiographic studies. Enlargement of specific chambers and great vessels can be identified by examination of the silhouette in lateral and dorsoventral views.[12, 37] In lateral view the normal cardiac silhouette is made by the right auricle craniodorsally, the right ventricle cranioventrally, the left ventricle caudoventrally below the caudal vena cava, and the left atrium caudodorsally.[30] In dorsoventral view, the silhouette can be related to the face of a clock with 12 and 6 o'clock located where the median plane crosses the cranial and caudal borders respectively (see Fig. 19–3). The aortic arch is from 11 to 1, the pulmonary trunk from 1 to 2, the left ventricle from 2 to 7, the right ventricle from 7 to 9, and the right atrium from 9 to 11.[12] In the cat, the left auricle makes the silhouette from 2 to 3 and the left ventricle is at 3 to 7. The left side of the aorta is sometimes visible as it courses caudally above the base of the heart.

When the pulmonary trunk is enlarged from such conditions as post-stenotic dilation or heartworm infestation, it bulges at the prominent angle between the cranial and left borders. In the dog, the left auricle normally does not form part of the silhouette. Enlargement of the left auricle is seen in dorsoventral view as a bulge in the middle of the left side (2 to 3 o'clock). This occurs as an early change in a patent ductus arteriosus or left atrioventricular insufficiency (see Table 19–1). Left atrioventricular insufficiency is the most common acquired cardiac disease in the dog. The sequence of changes in the cardiac outline during the course of this disease are:[18] (1) enlargement of the left atrium, (2) enlargement of the left ventricle, (3) enlargement of the right ventricle, and (4) further

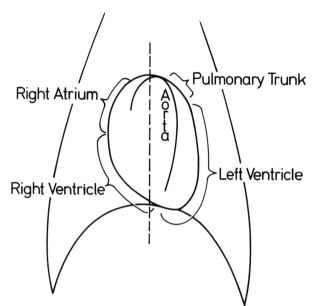

Figure 19–3. Diagram of a ventrodorsal radiograph of the canine thorax indicating the structures that form the normal cardiac silhouette.

enlargement of both ventricles, left atrium, and the pulmonary trunk. The silhouette is round, indicating heart failure.

In cardiac malformations, the enlargement of various chambers results from increased blood volume and muscle effort from septal defects and stenosis or insufficiency of valves. Aortic and pulmonary stenosis also result in a post-stenotic dilation of the affected vessel. The accepted explanation is that the constricted orifice greatly increases the velocity of systolic flow. This jet stream runs into a slower post-stenotic stream, and the energy of forward flow is converted to lateral pressure, resulting in eddies, turbulence, vibration of the wall, and an audible murmur. As the post-stenotic segment widens, the slowing effect increases and the dilation grows.[21]

Ventral Mediastinum. This short median septum connects the pericardium to the sternum. In obese dogs, fat in this part of the mediastinum lifts the heart off the sternum.

Caudal Mediastinum. Examine the descending thoracic aorta and the caudal vena cava. In dorsoventral view the caudal vena cava is on the right in its extension of the mediastinum, the plica

Table 19–1. RADIOGRAPHIC ANATOMY OF HEART LESIONS

Disease and Breed with High Incidence	Enlargement
Left AV insufficiency	Sequence: (1) LA, (2) LV, (3) RV, (4) pulmonary trunk
Aortic stenosis Newfoundland, Boxer, German Shepherd, Golden Retriever	LV and aorta
Patent ductus arteriosus Poodle (Miniature, Toy), Collie, Pomeranian, German Shepherd, Shetland Sheepdog, Cocker Spaniel	Preductal aorta, pulmonary trunk, LA, both ventricles
Tetralogy of Fallot Keeshond, Wire Fox Terrier	Right ventricle
Right AV insufficiency	RV, RA
Pulmonary stenosis Beagle, Chihuahua, English Bulldog, Fox Terrier, Old English Sheepdog, Schnauzer	RV, pulmonary trunk
Interatrial septal defect	RV, sometimes also pulmonary trunk
Interventricular septal defect Siberian Husky	If severe: RV, pulmonary trunk, LA, LV
Heartworms (in pulmonary arteries)	RV, pulmonary trunk, RA

venae cavae. The accessory lung lobe surrounds most of the caudal vena cava and extends into the V-shaped recess between the plica venae cavae on the right and the caudal mediastinum on the left. In dorsoventral view the caudal mediastinum between the accessory lobe of the right lung and the left caudal lobe is displaced to the left and may be seen as a line passing caudolaterally from the cardiac apex to the left side of the dome of the diaphragm. (This is not the phrenicopericardiac ligament.[6]) The esophagus and lymph nodes in the caudal mediastinum are not normally visible.

Lungs. Examine the pulmonary vessels and airway. Arteries diverge from the pulmonary trunk at the level of the carina in lateral view and at the left cranial border of the heart in dorsoventral view. In dorsoventral view the left pulmonary artery crosses the left ventricle at 4 o'clock; the right pulmonary artery crosses the right ventricle at 8 o'clock. In lateral view the left pulmonary artery (branch to left caudal lobe) is sometimes seen coursing dorsal and caudal to the carina, and the right pulmonary artery is seen on end ventral to the carina.

Pulmonary veins converge toward the left atrium at the caudodorsal heart shadow in lateral view and caudal to the level of the carina between principal bronchi over the center of the heart shadow in dorsoventral view. In dorsoventral view the left pulmonary vein crosses the left ventricle at 5 o'clock and the right pulmonary vein crosses the right ventricle at 7 o'clock.

Pulmonary arteries and veins follow bronchi toward the lung periphery. The artery is dorsal to the bronchus and vein in lateral view and lateral to the bronchus and vein in dorsoventral view. At the fourth intercostal space the artery and vein should be of equal size, and where the vessels cross the cardiac silhouette the diameter should be no larger than three-fourths of the width of the proximal end of the fourth rib.

In lateral view the radiolucent spot at the level of the carina is usually the bronchus to the right cranial lobe. This is slightly dorsal and cranial to the bronchus to the left cranial lobe (common opening to cranial and caudal parts of left cranial lobe). The right cranial lobar bronchus usually curves ventrally cranial to the heart, and the bronchus to the cranial part of the left cranial lobe courses straight toward the first rib. The right middle bronchus is caudal to the bronchus to the caudal part of the left cranial lobe. The left caudal bronchus is dorsal to the right caudal bronchus. The accessory bronchus is between the heart and diaphragm.

In lateral view, ventral to the level of the cranial vena cava, there is a cranial area that is partially radiolucent and a caudal area of greater radiolucency that borders on the heart. These are separated by a curved line passing caudoventrally. The cranial less radiolucent area contains mostly the thin cranial extension of the cranial part of the left cranial lobe and a small part of the right cranial lobe. The caudal, more radiolucent area contains the thin left cranial lobe and the thicker right cranial lobe that extends across the cranial surface of the heart.

The lobes of the lungs that contact the borders of the heart shadow are:

> Cranial heart border. Right cranial lobe.
> Middle heart border
> > Left: Caudal part of left cranial lobe, cranial surface of left caudal lobe.
> > Right: Middle lobe.
> Caudal heart border. Right accessory lobe (between heart and diaphragm).

Radiodense lesions of lobes that border on the heart will obliterate the normal cardiac silhouette.

The caudal lobes extend into the costodiaphragmatic recess. Between the heart and the diaphragm on lateral view are the two caudal lobes and the accessory lobe.

The interstitial connective tissue of the lung becomes more visible as linear and nodular densities as the animal ages.

Pleural Cavity. Normally there is no pleural space visible on radiographs. The pulmonary pleura lies adjacent to the parietal pleura of the thoracic wall and mediastinum. If fluid accumulates in the pleural cavity, it separates the lung from the parietal pleura and penetrates between the lobes, delineating them and creating a "leafing effect" in lateral views.

Do not be confused by linear opacities produced by folds of skin. These can be seen in either view and can usually be followed beyond the limits of the thorax.

In thoracic surgery the following approaches are used to obtain access to specific viscera in the thorax: patent ductus arteriosus—left fourth intercostal space, hilus of lung for lobectomy—left or right sixth intercostal space, caudal esophagus—left eighth to tenth intercostal space, cranial esophagus—right fifth to sixth intercostal space. The right side is selected for the cranial esophagus despite the position of the cranial vena cava because, if more caudal exposure of the esophagus is necessary, only the azygous vein crosses the esophagus on the right, and it can be ligated. The aorta crosses the esophagus on the left.

Megaesophagus and regurgitation have many causes in the dog. Congenital causes include esophageal obstructions from segmental hypoplasia with stenosis and vascular ring malformations over the base of the heart. The megaesophagus occurs cranial to the obstruction. A congenital idiopathic functional disorder results in megaesophagus from the caudal cervical region through the thorax.[9, 11, 20] This neuromuscular esophageal defect has been called achalasia due to the failure of the gastroesophageal sphincter to relax. This is not the primary defect but part of the entire esophageal disorder that prevents normal primary peristalsis that is responsible for initiating this gastroesophageal sphincter relaxation.

In the dog, the esophageal tunica muscularis is entirely striated except for the terminal 1 to 2 cm. of the inner layer, which is smooth muscle. In the cat, the transition from striated to smooth muscle begins in the inner layer between the middle and caudal thirds and in the outer layer between the fourth and last fifth of the esophagus. The striated muscle is innervated directly by neurons with cell bodies in the nucleus ambiguus in the medulla and axons in the vagus nerve and its esophageal branches.[22] Smooth muscle is innervated by parasympathetic preganglionic neurons with cell bodies in the parasympathetic nucleus of the vagus nerve in the medulla and axons in the vagus nerve and its esophageal branches and second neurons with cell bodies in ganglia in the wall of the esophagus. Sympathetic neurons that innervate the esophagus are located in the cranial and middle cervical ganglia and cervicothoracic, thoracic sympathetic trunk, and cranial mesenteric ganglia. Visceral afferent neurons of the esophagus course through branches of the vagus and glossopharyngeal nerves and segmental spinal nerves. Their cell bodies are in the distal ganglia of the vagus and glossopharyngeal nerves and spinal ganglia of the cervical and cranial thoracic spinal nerves. The neural component in the wall of the esophagus is complex, and its function is poorly understood. Although bilateral experimental lesions in the nucleus ambiguus or cervical portion of the vagus nerves will produce a megaesophagus similar to this idiopathic disorder, no consistent lesions have been found in this clinical disease. If the disorder is recognized early and the affected puppy is trained to eat in an erect posture standing on its pelvic limbs, the clinical disorder may be alleviated and functional recovery sometimes follows.[19, 35]

Acquired megaesophagus can result from obstructions by foreign bodies and from inflammatory or neoplastic lesions. Neuromuscular disorders include myasthenia gravis, botulism, polymyositis, and an idiopathic disorder of adult dogs of large breeds.[20]

References

1. Agduhr, E.: Morphologische Beweise für das Vorhandensein intra-vitaler Kommunicationen zwischen den Kavitäten der Pleurasäcke bei einer Reihe von Säugetieren. Anat. Anz. *64* (1927):276–298.

2. Barnes, R. J. et al.: On the presence of a ductus venosus in the fetal pig in late gestation. J. Dev. Physiol. *1* (1979):105–110.

3. Berg, J.: Chylothorax in the dog and cat. Comp. Cont. Ed. *4* (1982):986–991.

4. Birchard, S. J., H. D. Cantwell, and R. M. Bright: Lymphangiography and ligation of the canine thoracic duct: a study in normal dogs and three dogs with chylothorax. J. Am. Anim. Hosp. Assoc. *18* (1982):769–777.

5. Buchanan, J. W.: Radiographic aspects of patent ductus arteriosus in dogs before and after surgery. Acta Radiol. (suppl.) *319* (1972):271–278.

6. Burk, R. L.: Radiographic definition of the phrenicopericardiac ligament. J. Am. Vet. Radiol. Soc. *17* (1976):216–218.

7. Burk, R. L., L. A. Corwin, R. J. Bahr, et al.: The right cranial lung lobe bronchus of the dog: its identification in a lateral chest radiograph. J. Am. Vet. Radiol. Soc. *19* (1978):210–212.

8. Carlisle, C. H. and D. E. Thrall: A comparison of normal feline thoracic radiographs made in dorsal versus ventral recumbency. Vet. Radiol. *23* (1982):3–9.

9. Clifford, D. H., J. G. Pirsch, and M. L. Mauldin: Comparison of motor nuclei of the vagus nerve in dogs with and without esophageal achalasia. Soc. Exp. Biol. Med. Proc. *142* (1973):878–882.

10. Dawes, G. S.: Foetal and Neonatal Physiology, a Comparative Study of the Changes at Birth. Chicago: Yearbook, 1968.

11. Diamant, N., M. Szczepanski, and H. Mui: Manometric characteristics of idiopathic megaesophagus in the dog: an unsuitable model for achalasia in man. Gastroenterology *65* (1973):216–223.

12. Ettinger, S. J. and P. F. Suter: Canine Cardiology. Philadelphia: W. B. Saunders, 1970.

13. Eyster, G. E., et al.: Pulmonary artery banding for ventricular septal defect in dogs and cats. JAVMA *170* (1977):434–438.

14. Farrow, C. S.: Equine thoracic radiology. JAVMA *179* (1981):776–781.

15. Forsythe, W. B.: Surgical anatomy of the thoracic duct in the cat. Feline Pract. *10* (1980):38–40.

16. Grandage, J.: The radiology of the dog's diaphragm. J. Small Anim. Pract. *15* (1974):1–17.

17. Hamlin, R. L., C. R. Smith, and D. L. Smetzer: Ostium secundum type interatrial septal defects in the dog. JAVMA *143* (1963):149–157.

18. Hamlin, R. L.: Prognostic value of changes in the cardiac silhouette in dogs with mitral insufficiency. JAVMA *153* (1968):1436–1445.

19. Harvey, C. E., J. A. O'Brien, V. R. Durie, et al.: Megaesophagus in the dog: a clinical survey of 79 cases. JAVMA *165* (1974):443–446.

20. Hoffer, R. E.: Diseases of the esophagus. *In*: Kirk, R. W. (ed.): Current Veterinary Therapy VI: Small Animal Practice. Philadelphia: W. B. Saunders, 1977.

21. Holman, E. and W. Peniston: Hydrodynamic factors in the production of aneurysms. Am. J. Surg. *90* (1955):200–209.

22. Hudson, L. C.: The origins of innervation of the esophagus and the caudal pharyngeal muscles with histochemical and ultrastructural observations on the esophagus of the dog. Ph.D. Thesis, Cornell University, 1983.

23. Kagan, K. G. and E. M. Breznock: Variations in the canine thoracic duct system and the effects of surgical occlusion demonstrated by rapid aqueous lymphography, using an intestinal lymphatic trunk. Am. J. Vet. Res. *40* (1979):948–958.

24. Kaman, J.: Der Umbau des Ductus venosus des Schweines I. Pränatales Stadium. Anat. Anz. *122* (1968):252–266.

25. Kaman, J.: Der Umbau des Ductus venosus des Sch-Schweines II. Postnatales Stadium. Anat. Anz. *122* (1968):476–486.

26. Myer, W.: Radiography review: the mediastinum. J. Am. Vet. Rad. Soc. *19* (1978):197–202.

27. Ottaway, C. W.: The anatomical closure of the foramen ovale in the equine and bovine heart. Vet. Jour. *100* (1944):111–118, 130–134.

28. Quick, C. B. and H. P. Jander: Aqueous lymphangiography of the canine thoracic duct. J. Am. Vet. Radiol. Soc. *19* (1978):178–180.

29. Quick, C. B.: Chylothorax: a review. J. Am. Anim. Hosp. Assoc. *16* (1980):23–29.

30. Rhodes, W. H., D. F. Patterson, and D. K. Detweiler: Radiographic anatomy of the canine heart. Part I. JAVMA *137* (1960):283–289.

31. Rhodes, W. H., D. F. Patterson, and D. K. Detweiler: Radiographic anatomy of the canine heart. Part II. JAVMA *143* (1963):137–148.

32. Ruehl, W. W., Jr. and D. E. Thrall: The effect of dorsal versus ventral recumbency on the radiographic appearance of the canine thorax. Vet. Radiol. *22* (1981):10–16.

33. Schaller, O.: Anatomische Grundlagen der Roentgen Darstellung des Hundeherzens. Acta Anat. *17* (1953):273–347.

34. Silverman, S. and P. F. Suter: Influence of inspiration and expiration on canine thoracic radiographs. JAVMA *166* (1975):502–510.

35. Sokolovsky, V.: Achalasia and paralysis of the canine esophagus. JAVMA *160* (1972):943–955.

36. Spencer, C. P., N. Ackerman, and J. K. Burt: The canine lateral thoracic radiograph. Vet. Radiol. *22* (1981):262–266.

37. Suter, P. F.: The radiographic diagnosis of canine and feline heart disease. Comp. Cont. Ed. *3* (1981):441–453.

38. Toomey, A. and M. J. Bojrab: Traumatic diaphragmatic hernias. Comp. Cont. Ed. *2* (1980):866–871.

39. Watrous, B. F. and P. F. Suter: Normal swallowing in the dog: a cineradiographic study. Vet. Radiol. *20* (1970):99–109.

40. Wilson, G. P., C. D. Newton, and J. K. Burt: A review of 116 diaphragmatic hernias in dogs and cats. JAVMA *159* (1971):1142–1146.

CHAPTER 20

VERTEBRAL COLUMN
AND SPINAL CORD

OBJECTIVES

1. To be able to use the vertebral formulae of the various species of domestic animals to identify the vertebrae by serial palpation in either the cranial or caudal direction and to identify the intervertebral discs and spinal nerves.
2. To be able to diagnose the location of an injury of the spinal cord by means of the diagnostic reflexes and reactions.
3. To understand the relation of the lumbar, sacral, and caudal segments of the spinal cord to the vertebrae and to correlate signs of injured cord segments and spinal nerves with skeletal lesions.
4. To be able to use the radiological anatomy of the vertebrae in the diagnosis of fractures, dislocations, and disc lesions of the dog and cat.
5. To understand the age and sequence of union of the vertebral epiphyses in the dog.
6. To know where the spinal cord and the dura mater end in each species. The dural tube containing the arachnoid and the cerebrospinal fluid is longer than the cord. It is important in epidural injections to know in which species it is possible to injure the cord or inject the anesthetic into the cerebrospinal fluid at the usual site of epidural injection.
7. To be able to palpate the landmarks for epidural injection in each species.
8. To understand the mechanism whereby epidural anesthesia used in obstetrics stops straining.
9. To be able to palpate the middle caudal artery to take the pulse in the horse and cow.
10. To be able to palpate the sites of injection for abdominal wall anesthesia in ruminants and to understand what nerves are injected for various surgical purposes.
11. To know the landmarks to obtain cerebrospinal fluid by lumbosacral puncture and the precautions or limitations of its use in each species.

Note on the Nomenclature. Because the term coccyx, from a resemblance to the beak of a cuckoo, is applicable only to the fused rudimentary tail bones of man, we use the term caudal in the restricted sense to refer to the vertebrae, arteries, veins, nerves, and muscles of the tail, with the exception of m. coccygeus and m. rectococcygeus.

Introduction. Certain fundamental facts about the vertebral column and the spinal nerves should be memorized to provide the framework for the clinical anatomy of this region. The vertebral formulae of domestic animals can be remembered more easily if the species are arranged in order of evolutionary specialization, as in Table 20–1. It also aids memory to set aside the constants and concentrate on the variables. All mammals, with few exceptions, have seven cervical vertebrae. The number of caudal vertebrae, about 20, is individually variable and irrelevant and may be ignored. The remaining series of significant numbers of thoracic, lumbar, and sacral vertebrae are listed in Table 20–1. Most Arabian horses and donkeys and a few Morgan horses have only five lumbar vertebrae.

Table 20–1. SPECIES VARIATIONS OF THE VERTEBRAL FORMULA

Species	Thoracic	Lumbar	Sacral
Dog and cat	13	7	3
Swine	14–15	6–7	4
Sheep	13	6–7	4
Ox	13	6	5
Horse	18	6	5

Another basic principle is the relation of the ribs to the vertebrae of the same number. The head of a rib articulates with the cranial end of the body of the vertebra of the same number. It may help to remember that the tubercle of a rib projects caudally and articulates with the transverse process of the vertebra of the same number (see Fig. 20–1).

All of the spinal nerves, except the cervical nerves, emerge from the intervertebral foramen caudal to the vertebra of the same number or from a lateral vertebral foramen in the caudal part of the arch of that vertebra. In the cervical region, where there are eight pairs of nerves for seven cervical vertebrae, all the nerves emerge cranial to the vertebrae of the same number, except the eighth, which passes between C 7 and T 1, and the first, which passes through the lateral vertebral foramen in the arch of the atlas.

A concept necessary for the correlation of nervous signs with lesions of the vertebral column is the relative cranial displacement of the segments of the spinal cord with respect to the vertebrae. The central nervous system develops faster than the skeleton, and the spinal cord reaches its definitive length while the vertebral column is still growing. The vertebral epiphyses are not fused until about 1 year of age. In the adult dog, as a result of this unequal growth rate, most of the segments of the thoracic cord lie about one vertebra cranial to the vertebra of the same number. In the caudal thoracic and cranial lumbar regions the segments of the cord lie in the vertebrae of the same number, but the remaining lumbar, sacral, and caudal segments are increasingly cranial to the corresponding vertebrae as shown in Tables 20–3 to 20–6. Consequently their nerve roots, which in the early embryo passed transversely outward through the intervertebral foramina, must course caudally in the vertebral canal for increasing distances to reach their foramina. The order of the degree of displacement in different species is shown in Table 20–2. Different investigators have reported terminations

Table 20–2. RELATION OF THE END OF THE SPINAL CORD TO THE VERTEBRAE

Species	Vertebrae
Man	L1–2
Dog	L 6–7
Ruminants	S 1
Swine	S 1—2
Horse	S 2
Cat	L 7–S 3

of the cord in the cat ranging from L 5 to Cd 3, mostly between L 7 and S 3. This may be due to a lack of data on age.

A useful rule to use for adult domestic animals is that the sacral segments are located in the vertebral foramen of L 5 in the dog, L 6 in the cat and ox, and L 6 and S 1 in the horse. This site is farther caudal in young animals and varies between some breeds of dogs. In small breeds, these segments are usually in one more vertebra caudal.

In the horse, the thoracolumbar vertebrae are held fairly rigid by the contraction of the axial muscles during locomotion.[23] Flexion and extension are minimal, and most occurs at the lumbosacral articulation.[46] Movement at this joint helps contribute to the length of the stride. There is little sacroiliac movement, and a diarthrodial joint commonly develops between the transverse processes of L 6 and the wings of the sacrum and between the fifth and sixth lumbar transverse processes.[42] The rarity of disc protrusion and spondylosis in this species may be a reflection of this relative inflexibility of the vertebral column. A problem does occur when the spinous processes of the vertebrae are too close and override and impinge on each other.[22, 24] The dorsal tip of each process often has a separate ossification center that fuses with the rest of the spinous process between 7 and 15 years, or it may never fuse. The highest process is usually at T 4 or T 5. Back pain may also be associated with injury to the epaxial muscles or supraspinous ligament or excessive stress at the sacroiliac articulation. Evidence of back pain includes a stiff gait in the hind limbs or restricted hind limb activity, poor performance, change in temperament, reluctance to jump or back, and resentment of saddling, grooming, or palpation.[24, 25]

20a. SECTION, FIRST CAUDAL INTERSPACE, HORSE

The vertebral canal is triangular, with the caudal nerves lying on the floor. The injection is made into the fat-filled space dorsal to the nerves. Each is covered with a sheath, the epineurium, which is continous with the dura. If the needle is inserted perpendicular to the joint and passses through the canal, it will enter the anulus fibrosus, which surrounds the nucleus pulposus. The nucleus is not so well defined in the horse as in the young dog. Although intervertebral disc degeneration occurs in older horses, protrusion into the vertebral canal is rare.

There are five arteries in the tail; the small, paired dorsolateral and ventrolateral arteries are deep to the sacrocaudalis dorsalis lateralis and sacrocaudalis ventralis lateralis. The largest artery is the middle caudal, between the small sacrocaudales ventrales mediales.

20b. DISSECTION OF LUMBOSACRAL SPACE, HORSE

The supraspinous ligament continues from the spinous process of L 6 to the sacral spinous processes. The interspinous ligament separates the epaxial muscles on the median plane. The yellow ligament covers the epidural space between the arch of L6 and S 1. Usually the last few sacral spinal cord segments are in the canal between the sixth lumbar vertebra and the sacrum in addition to the

Table 20–3. RELATION OF THE LAST SEGMENTS OF THE SPINAL CORD TO THE VERTEBRAE IN THE ADULT HORSE[39]

Segments	Vertebrae				
	L 5	L 6	S 1	S 2	S 3
L 6	X				
S 1		X			
S 2		X			
S 3		X			
S 4			X		
S 5			X		
Caudal segments			X	X	
End of dura mater					X

spinal nerves of the cauda equina (Table 20–3). It is usually necessary to penetrate the spinal cord to reach the subarachnoid space ventral to it to obtain an adequate amount of CSF for analysis. The internal ventral vertebral venous plexus passes over the lateral aspect of the intervertebral disc adjacent to the intervertebral foramen.

20c. LIVE HORSE

Epidural anesthesia is administered between the sacrum and first caudal vertebra or between the first and second caudal vertebrae. The point of injection is in the palpable depression formed on the dorsal surface when the tail is raised. Usually no motion of the sacrocaudal joint can be palpated and therefore it is easier to make the injection in the joint between Cd 1 and Cd 2. Insert the needle at a 45° angle to inject over the body of the first caudal vertebra. Only skin, muscle, and fascia cover the vertebral canal between vertebrae; there is no yellow ligament here (see Plate I).

Middle caudal artery. Palpate lightly about 15 cm. from the root of the tail. The pulse is more easily felt if the artery can be pressed laterally against one of the medial ventral sacrocaudal muscles.

The lumbosacral space cannot be felt but is located by adjacent landmarks, which should be palpated. A transverse line across the caudal aspect of each tuber coxae crosses the median plane approximately at the site of needle insertion. If each tuber sacrale can be palpated, a transverse line across their cranial edges is at the same level. The spine of S 1 is too short to feel. The spine of L 6 is shorter than that of L 5, and this depression should not be mistaken for the lumbosacral space. Note the long interspinous space between L 6 and S 1.

20d. VERTEBRAL COLUMN, OX

T 13 to L 3, Paravertebral anesthesia. Locate the last thoracic vertebra. It is the last one that bears a costal fovea on the craniolateral aspect of the body. The last rib extends obliquely caudolaterally from this fovea, forming an acute angle with the first lumbar transverse process. Note that the lumbar transverse processes do not extend straight laterally but curve cranially. Just caudoventral to the transverse process of each vertebrae, the spinal nerve emerges from the caudal vertebral notch or lateral foramen of the vertebra of the same number (see Section 7i). The nerve runs obliquely caudo-laterally (see Fig. 20–1).

These spinal nerves can be anesthetized where they leave the intervertebral foramen by an injection 5 cm from the midline on a line connecting the caudal border of each pair of transverse processes or·the caudal border of the last rib for T 13. Other sites for anesthetizing these nerves will be described (see Section 20f).

L 1 and L 2, lumbar epidural anesthesia. Draw a transverse line connecting the cranial edges of the tips of the transverse processes of the second lumbar vertebra. The space between the spinous processes is 1.5 to 2 cm. caudal to this line. The transverse processes are used as landmarks because the thick supraspinous ligament often prevents direct palpation of the summits of the spinous processes. Note the size of the interarcuate space through which the needle is inserted. The interarcuate space is closed by the yellow ligament which can be felt as the needle punctures it to enter the epidural space.

Sacrocaudal epidural anesthesia. Observe that the vertebral canal in the last three vertebrae of the sacrum is narrow, only 2 to 3 cm. wide; whereas the canal in L 4 to S 2 is larger. A much smaller volume of anesthetic is required to block the last three sacral nerves for obstetrical purposes than is needed to anesthetize the lumbar nerves for operations on the limb, inguinal region, scrotum, penis, or udder. If the volume of anesthetic solution is increased above the obstetrical dose, it also blocks the motor nerves of the hind limb as it infiltrates cranially, and the cow goes down when the roots of the femoral nerve, L 4 to L 6, are reached. Occasionally enough volume is used to reach the 13th thoracic spinal nerves. This will put the cow down and anesthetize the abdominal wall for surgical purposes.

The purpose of epidural anesthesia in obstetrics is to anesthetize the birth canal by blocking the sacral nerves. This eliminates the stimulus for the reflex abdominal press caused by the entry of the

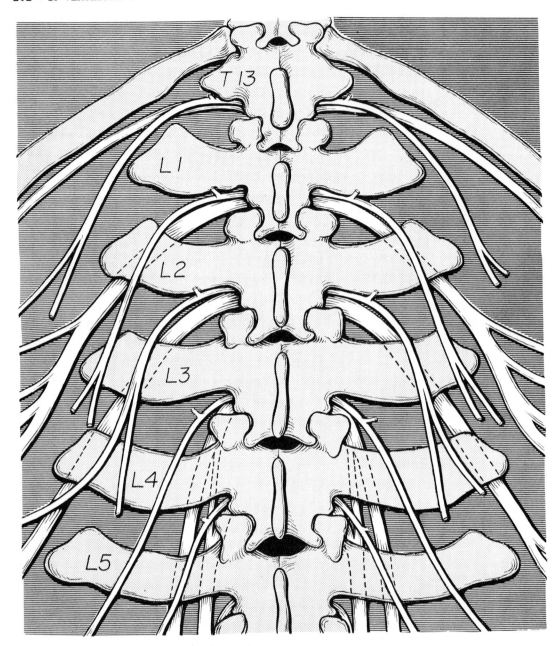

Figure 20–1. Lumbar nerves, cow, dorsal aspect.

fetal head or feet into the vagina. Straining is stopped by blocking the sensory limb of the reflex arc—not by blocking the motor nerves of the abdominal muscles or uterus. The motor nerves to the rectum and perineal muscles are blocked, and this prevents defecation and relieves tension around the obstetrician's upper arm.

The anesthetic solution flows along connective tissue planes and vascular channels and often does not penetrate the epidural fat uniformly. It may not reach all the spinal nerves bilaterally, especially if the cow is down.[36]

20e. SKELETON, OX

The caudal vertebrae in the ox are well developed. The spinous processes are large; articular processes (non-functional) are present; and there are hemal processes on the ventral surface. The right and left hemal processes of Cd 2–5 may fuse to form hemal arches. Therefore the pulse in the middle caudal artery must be palpated between the hemal processes of succeeding vertebrae, or about 18 cm. from the root of the tail.

Tail bleeding is done from the middle caudal vein between hemal processes. The middle caudal artery and vein usually run side-by-side as far caudally as the fourth caudal vertebra, but it is impossible to determine which one is on the left or right.[16] Caudal to Cd 4 they assume a dorsoventral relationship, with the artery usually ventral. Because of this variability, the artery is often punctured and hematomata are frequent. It is recommended that the tail be raised and the needle be inserted on the ventral midline at the level of Cd 2 and Cd 3.

Observe the prominence of the spinous process of Cd 1, separated by a depression from the crest of the sacrum. The epidural injection is made between Cd 1 and Cd 2. The opening between the vertebrae is 2 cm. wide, 2.5 cm. in the craniocaudal direction, and 2 to 4 cm. under the surface of the skin. Note the relation of this interspinous space to the tuber ischiadicum. It is 10 to 11 cm. cranial to the caudal prominence of the tuber ischiadicum. Occasionally the needle strikes the intervertebral disc, which plugs the lumen and prevents injection until the needle is withdrawn slightly (see Plate II).

A transverse plane through the tubera coxarum intersects the caudal part of the spinous process of the sixth lumbar vertebra. The depression between the spinous process and the sacral crest is usually palpable. It serves as a landmark in counting lumbar spines and as the site of lumbosacral puncture. Note the distance from the summit of the spinous process to the floor of the vertebral canal through the lumbosacral space (6 to 9 cm., depending on breed).

The lumbosacral space is the preferred location for epidural anesthesia in the sheep. A line connecting the tubera coxarum intersects the last lumbar spinous process, and the injection is made caudal to that.

Note on the Nomenclature. The iliac crest includes the tuber coxae and tuber sacrale. The tuber coxae is composed of the cranial ventral iliac spine and, in large animals, a thickened additional portion of the iliac crest. The tuber sacrale is broadened to form cranial and caudal dorsal iliac spines in carnivores, swine, and sheep.

20f. DISSECTION, LUMBAR NERVES, OX

On the dorsal surface of the intertransverse muscles, the dorsal branches of the costoabdominal (13th thoracic) and first three lumbar nerves may be seen running obliquely caudolaterally. They supply the muscles and skin of the loin, and the skin of the paralumbar fossa. The large ventral branches are ventral to the intertransverse muscles. The ventral branches of T 13, L 1, and L 2 course obliquely caudolaterally to the skin, muscles, and peritoneum of the abdominal wall. Each nerve is directed more caudally than the preceding one. The costoabdominal nerve does not follow its rib as closely as the other thoracic nerves do, but runs near the tip of the first lumbar transverse process. The first lumbar nerve crosses the tip of the second transverse process. The second lumbar nerve crosses the tip of the *fourth* transverse process. The dorsal branch of the third lumbar nerve crosses the fifth transverse process near its tip. The ventral branches of L 3 and L 4 run straight caudally along the bodies of the vertebrae (see Fig. 20–1).

In anesthetizing the flank, one is primarily concerned with the dorsal and ventral branches of T 13 to L 2. If the incision is to be made in the caudal part of the paralumbar fossa, the dorsal branch of L 3 should be blocked also. If the incision is to be close to the last rib, T 12 should be blocked.

An epidural procedure for anesthetizing the flank is described in Section 20g. Paravertebral anesthesia at the level of the intervertebral foramina[12] (see Section 20d) also paralyzes the muscles of the back on the side of the operation causing a lateral curvature of the vertebral column in the standing cow that makes the viscera bulge out of the flank incision. It also blocks the rami communicantes to the sympathetic ganglia with unknown consequences for visceral circulation. These side effects can be avoided by a paravertebral procedure that blocks nerves T 13, L 1, and L 2 where they cross the tips of transverse processes 1, 2, and 4.[8] This does not affect the visceral rami communicantes or the branches to the muscles of the back. The infiltration is made ventral to the tip of the transverse process to block the ventral branch and subcutaneously over the tip to block the dorsal branch. Because of variation in the course of the nerves, it is recommended that the same technique of injection be applied to the tip of the third transverse process.

These nerves can also be blocked by superficial and deep injections of anesthetic along a line caudal and parallel to the last rib and along a horizontal line just distal to the tips of the transverse processes. The two lines connect dorsally in the angle made by the last rib and transverse process of L 1.

In anesthesia of the udder (see Section 27b) the ventral branches of L 1–4 are involved. Because L 3 and L 4 run caudally close to the bodies of the vertebrae, they are blocked by a vertical injection 3 cm. from the midline, on a transverse plane through the cranial edges of the transverse processes of L 5, to a depth just ventral to the transverse processes.

20g. SECTION BETWEEN LUMBAR VERTEBRAE 1 AND 2, OX

Site of lumbar epidural anesthesia.[31, 40, 41] To block the left T 13, L 1, and L 2 spinal nerves, the needle is inserted 1 to 2 cm. to the right side of the summit of the spine of L 2 and the supraspinous ligament. The needle is inclined about 12° from the median plane to pass through the yellow ligament on the left of the median plane. The tip of the needle will be in the epidural fat in position to infiltrate the roots of the left spinal nerves T 13, L 1, and L 2. This will be helped by directing the bevel cranially and laterally. The depth of the insertion is about 6 to 9 cm. A disadvantage of this technique is the lateral flexion of the vertebral column that often results with the convexity directed toward the anesthetized side.

20h. DISSECTION, CAUDAL NERVES, CALF

At the lumbosacral space, the spinal cord is present, enclosed in the dura. At the first caudal interspace, the caudal nerves, vertebral venous plexus, and fat are exposed in the canal.

20i. SAGITTAL SECTION, SACRUM, OX

The dural sheath extends to the fourth or fifth sacral vertebra. At that point, the caudal nerves emerge from the common sheath and continue separately, each in its epineurium and surrounded by fat of the epidural space, in which the anesthetic is placed. The spinal cord ends as the conus medullaris, which extends through the first sacral vertebra in the adult ox and through the third in the calf (Table 20–4).

Note that the subarachnoid space, containing spinal fluid, extends into the sacrum. In diagnostic lumbosacral puncture, the needle is inserted through the supraspinous ligament and directed toward the center of the lumbosacral space. The needle must be advanced carefully through the yellow ligament, epidural fat, and dura mater until cerebrospinal fluid can be withdrawn. The pressure of

Table 20–4. RELATION OF THE LAST SEGMENTS OF THE SPINAL CORD TO THE VERTEBRAE IN THE ADULT COW[39]

Segments	Vertebrae					
	L 5	L 6	S 1	S 2	S 3	S 4
L 6	X					
S 1	X	X				
S 2		X				
S 3		X				
S 4		X				
S 5		X				
Caudal segments			X			
End of dura mater						X

the spinal fluid may not be great enough to force it out of the needle in the normal ox. Flow can be increased by occlusion of the external jugular veins or by elevation of the forequarters. The total depth varies from 6 to 9 cm., depending on the breed. In the adult animal, the danger to the spinal cord is not great, but it is always possible to injure sacral nerves or the caudal segments of the conus medullaris. In yearlings and calves, the sacral segments of the cord could be damaged.

20j. LIVE COW.

Paravertebral Anesthesia. Palpate the first to fifth lumbar transverse processes. The sixth is not palpable. If the first cannot be palpated, the intersection of the last rib and the lateral border of the iliocostalis may be taken to indicate the plane of injection. Visualize the course and point of injection of the nerves described in section 20f.

Lumbar Epidural Anesthesia. Locate the space between the spinous processes of L 1 and L 2 by drawing a line across the cranial edges of the tips of the transverse processes of L 2. The space is 1.5 cm. caudal to the line. Visualize the insertion of the needle as described in section 20g.

Sacrocaudal Epidural Anesthesia. The injection is usually made into the first caudal interspace. This is located by the following methods:

1. Grasp the tail and move it up and down. The first movable joint is usually between the first and second caudal vertebrae.
2. Observe the dorsal contour of the tail head. The first prominence caudal to the sacral crest is the first caudal spinous process.
3. A transverse plane 10 to 11 cm. cranial to the caudal prominence of the tuber ischiadicum should intersect the space between Cd 1 and Cd 2.

Middle caudal artery. About 18 cm. from the root of the tail, palpate the two medial ventral sacrocaudal muscles. The artery lies between them, accompanied by a vein. In palpating the pulse, the artery may easily be occluded by too much pressure.

20k. SKELETON, SWINE

Epidural anesthesia in swine, as in the sheep and the dog and cat, is administered through the lumbosacral space. This space is 2.5 to 5 cm. caudal to a transverse plane through the tubera coxarum (cranial ventral iliac spines). In fat animals, it may be difficult to palpate the tuber coxae; it is in the transverse plane of the fold of the flank.[15] The depth of injection varies with the size of the animal, from 5 to 9 cm. The needle is inserted carefully until it is felt to puncture the yellow ligament. The dimensions of the lumbosacral space are about 2 cm. craniocaudally and 3 cm. transversely. The canal is 1 cm. in diameter dorsoventrally.

20l. DISSECTION, SACRUM, SWINE

Spinal cord is present in the canal at the lumbosacral space. The conus ends at S 1 or S 2, and the dura mater and subarachnoid space extend to S 3. Fat is usually present in the epidural space, which is much larger than the dural sac. It is possible, however, to insert the needle too far and inject the anesthetic into the cerebrospinal fluid.

20m. SKELETON AND RADIOGRAPHS, DOG AND CAT

The field of a lateral vertebral radiograph should be limited to a few vertebrae close to the central beam to avoid distortion.[10]

In addition to the spinous, transverse, and articular processes seen in the cervical vertebrae, the mammillary processes are present from the third thoracic to the caudal vertebrae and the accessory processes project caudally from the pedicles in the caudal thoracic and lumbar regions. Mammillary and accessory processes are important in exposure of the vertebrae for laminectomy. Muscle attachments must be severed from them and they serve as landmarks.[34]

The mammillary processes project from the transverse processes as far back as the anticlinal vertebra, T 11, where they become projections of the cranial articular processes. There is also a marked change in the articular processes at this point. Cranial to T 11 the articular surfaces are flat and meet in an oblique dorsal plane, readily visible in the lateral view, but not in the dorsoventral. Beginning with T 11, the plane of articulation is sagittal; that is, the cranial processes clasp the lateral surfaces of the caudal processes of the preceding vertebra, and the joint line is clear in the dorsoventral view.

In a lateral radiograph of the thoracolumbar region, T 11 may be recognized by its vertical spinous process and large rounded articular processes on both ends. Identify T 13 by the attachment of the last rib and note that the ribs overlap. The lumbar vertebral transverse processes project cranially beside the intervertebral discs. These should not be confused with a mineralized nucleus pulposus. The seventh lumbar vertebra is smaller than the other lumbar vertebrae and is between the wings of the ilia.

Examine the ends of the vertebral bodies for exostoses. Ventral spurs are probably harmless, but if the exostosis extends dorsolaterally to the intervertebral foramen and compresses the spinal nerve, it may produce clinical signs.

Examine the intervertebral discs in the lateral view. They are normally radiolucent. Calcification of the disc is not evidence of protrusion, but a calcified protrusion seen in the vertebral canal is clinically significant. Failing that, the plain radiograph can only indicate protrusion of a disc by a narrowing of the radiolucent zone. To evaluate the width of a disc, the dog must be anesthetized and the direction of the x-rays must be parallel to the plane of the disc in question. A narrow disc is significant only if it is clear that the discs on either side are of normal width.[10]

The union of the vertebral epiphyses begins in the seventh to ninth month with the axis and the distal caudal vertebrae.[18] Union progresses from both ends of the vertebral column toward T 4, T 5, or T 6, which are the last to unite at 11 to 14 months. Note the relation of the lumbosacral space to the cranial dorsal iliac spines. These are easily palpated in the dog and cat. The spinous process of L 7 is shorter than that of L 6. Lumbosacral epidural anesthesia is useful for surgery on the hind limb, and the sacrocaudal method is especially useful for docking.

20n. DISSECTION, LUMBAR AND SACRAL VERTEBRAL CANAL, DOG

The conus medullaris ends between the sixth and seventh lumbar vertebrae (Table 20–5). The spinal nerves course progressively more caudally from L 2 to the caudal nerves as they run successively longer distances in the vertebral canal to their respective foramina. The last two lumbar and the sacral and caudal nerves run parallel on the sides of the conus medullaris and form the cauda equina. The dura mater, containing the arachnoid and the cerebrospinal fluid, extends into S 1. Injection of

Table 20–5. RELATION OF THE LAST SEGMENTS OF THE SPINAL CORD TO THE VERTEBRAE IN THE ADULT DOG[14]

Segments	Vertebrae					
	L 3	L 4	L 5	L 6	L 7	S 1
L 4	X	X				
L 5		X				
L 6		X				
L 7		X	X			
S 1			X			
S 2			X			
S 3			X			
Caudal segments				X		
End of dura mater						X

Table 20–6. RELATION OF THE LAST SEGMENTS OF THE SPINAL CORD TO THE VERTEBRAE
IN THE CAT

Segments	Vertebrae						
	L 5	L 6	L 7	S 1	S 2	S 3	Cd 1
L 6	X	X					
L 7	X	X	X				
S 1	X	X	X				
S 2		X	X	X			
S 3		X	X	X			
Caudal segments		X	X	X	X	X	
End of dura mater							X

radiopaque medium into the subarachnoid space for a myelogram may be done at L 5–6.[9] The great variability in the relation of the segments of the spinal cord to the vertebrae in the cat is shown in Table 20–6. Some of the variation may be due to differences in age.

At the lumbosacral junction the vertebral canal contains all the caudal and sacral nerves and the seventh lumbar spinal nerves pass through the intervertebral foramina. Fractures of the seventh lumbar vertebra may cause paralysis of the tail, anus, and bladder with atonia, areflexia, and analgesia. If the seventh lumbar spinal nerves are also injured, sciatic nerve paresis will be observed in the limbs. Trauma to the pelvis that injures the sacral plexus and the sciatic nerve or the spinal nerves that contribute to it produces similar signs but spares the function of the tail. Tail paralysis implicates a lesion in the vertebral canal.

Lumbosacral stenosis is a slowly progressive narrowing of the vertebral canal at this site by encroachment of the adjacent structures: intervertebral disc, ligaments, articular processes, and vertebral bodies.[33, 44] It is more common in older dogs of large breeds. Clinical signs result from compression of the spinal nerves at this site and include: pain; hyperesthesia; self-mutilation; incontinence; tail paresis; anal paresis; lameness; and pelvic limb atrophy, paresis, and ataxia. Myelography may not be helpful because the dural sac and its subarachnoid space are so small at this site. Epidurography normally may show filling defects due to the epidural fat.[13] Intraosseous vertebral venography is performed by injecting radiopaque dye into the body of a caudal vertebra (usually Cd 4) or L 7 while the abdomen is compressed.[4, 30] Normally this will show the internal ventral vertebral venous plexus on the floor of the vertebral canal. Compression of this plexus may be observed at the lumbosacral articulation in dogs with stenosis.

20o. INTERVERTEBRAL DISCS T 13 TO L 1, DOG

The internal pressure of the disc causes the nucleus pulposus to bulge on the cut surface. When the disc degenerates, the thin dorsal part of the anulus fibrosus may stretch because of partial rupture of the inner layers, permitting the disc to bulge on the floor of the vertebral canal and injure the cord or nerve roots by compression. In another type of disc lesion the anulus ruptures completely, and the degenerate, often calcified nuclear material is extruded into the vertebral canal, resulting in a severe extradural inflammatory reaction as well as compression of the spinal cord and compromise of its blood supply. The incidence of disc protrusion in the cervical region is about 15 percent and in the thoracolumbar region (T 9 to S 1) about 85 percent.[17] They occur most often in the disc between T 13 and L 1. They almost never occur in the region between T 1 and T 9, possibly because of the intercapital ligament, which is found there. It connects the heads of each pair of ribs, passing over the dorsal surface of the disc, between the disc and the dorsal longitudinal ligament.

20p. LIVE DOG AND CAT

Palpate the spinous processes of the thoracic and lumbar vertebrae and the transverse processes of the lumbar vertebrae. Find the spine of T 13 from the attachment of the last rib.

Palpate the lumbosacral space for epidural injection. The thumb and third finger are placed on the cranial dorsal iliac spines, while the index finger palpates the space caudal to the last lumbar spinous process. Do not mistake the shorter spine of L 7 for the space. The needle is inserted perpendicular to the skin until it is felt to pop through the yellow ligament (see Plate III).

Diagnostic Reflexes and Reactions

These tests are used to locate a lesion in the spinal cord or in the peripheral nerves. A reflex is a test of all three parts of the reflex arc: the afferent nerve, the nucleus in the central nervous system, and the efferent nerve. It is obvious that failure of the reflex may be caused by a lesion in any part of the arc. Reflexes elicited by stimulation of the skin have the afferent and efferent limbs of the arc in different nerves. Tendon reflexes are simpler; the afferent and efferent impulses are carried in the same nerve.

A general rule is that the more complete and localized the nervous dysfunction, the more peripheral is the lesion.[32] For example, if the only nervous signs present are anesthesia and flaccid paralysis of one limb, the lesion is probably outside the central nervous system. Conversely, widespread nervous disorder—as opposed to complete lack of function—suggests a brain lesion.

A complete neurological examination should begin with a study of the history and behavior of the animal when presented. The animal should be observed from a distance both at rest and in motion.

The functions of the cranial nerves should be examined systematically from I through XII by the tests and observations discussed in the chapters on the head. The results must be recorded in writing. All reflexes and reactions must be tested on both sides of the animal.

Spinal Reflexes

The following reflexes are arranged for a segmental study of the spinal cord and the peripheral nerves indicated. Because of the normal spinal cord displacement, the terminal segments of the spinal cord do not lie in the vertebrae of the same number (see Tables 20–2 to 20–6). For example, in the dog neurological signs of damage to the second sacral segment of the spinal cord or its nerve could be caused by a vertebral lesion anywhere between L 5 and S 3. Protrusion of the disc between L 6 and L 7 might compress the caudal segments of the cord and any spinal nerve that emerges caudal to the sixth lumbar vertebra.

A few practical generalizations may be made about the neurological diagnosis of the location of a disc protrusion or other focal spinal cord lesion. Upper motor neuron disease is characterized by spasticity and hyperreflexia; lower motor neuron disease, by flaccid (pronounced flack-sid) paralysis, areflexia, and neurogenic atrophy. Lesions between C 1 and C 5 cause signs of upper motor neuron disease in the limbs. Lesions between C 6 and T 1 cause signs of lower motor neuron disease of the forelimbs and signs of upper motor neuron disease of the hind limbs. Disc protrusions in the dog are rare between T 1 and T 9. They are most common between T 11 and L 2, where the effect on the hind limbs is the spasticity of upper motor neuron disease. Protrusions of discs between vertebrae L 3 and S 1 may injure the cord segments L 4 to Cd 5 or the spinal nerves L 3 to Cd 5 in the vertebral canal, causing signs of lower motor neuron disease in the muscles of the hind limb, perineum, and tail.

The flexor reflexes of the limbs and the patellar and perineal reflexes are seen in all normal animals, although they may be inhibited temporarily by excitement or fear. Their absence is diagnostically significant.[3] The other reflexes are either inconstant or pathological, but they reveal two important facts when elicited: (1) the peripheral nerves and segments of the cord involved in the reflex are functioning and (2) the reflex activity of the cord at this level is increased, a release phenomenon indicating a lesion of the upper motor neurons.

Tendon reflexes are elicited by a sharp stretch of the muscle. To do this, the joint concerned must be held in such a position that moderate tension is exerted on the muscle before the stimulus is given.[43]

1. Flexor Reflex of Forelimb. Cord segments C 6 to T 1 and musculocutaneous, axillary, part of radial, median, and ulnar nerves. Pinch a toe or press on the coronet in the large animal. The limb is flexed. In the recumbent animal, if the flexor reflex is accompanied by an involuntary crossed extensor reflex of the opposite limb, there is an upper motor neuron lesion above C 6.[29]

2. Extensor Reflex of Forelimb. Cord segments C 7 to T 1. Afferent nerves: median and ulnar. Efferent nerve: radial. In the recumbent small animal, an extensor reflex elicited by sudden pressure on the foot pads is a pathological response indicating an upper motor neuron lesion of the cord above C 6.[3,47] The normal postural extensor thrust in the upright animal is discussed under reactions.

3. Triceps Reflex. Cord segments C 7 to T 1 and the radial nerve. Hold the paw with the carpus extended and the elbow in 90° flexion. Strike the triceps tendon just above the olecranon. The elbow is extended in a short jerk by contraction of the triceps. This reflex is often not elicited in normal animals.

4. Extensor Carpi Radialis Reflex. Cord segments C 7 to T 1 and the radial nerve. Hold the forelimb relaxed in partial extension. Strike the extensor carpi radialis muscle lightly in the proximal forearm. This will elicit an extension of the carpus in many normal animals.[43]

5. Biceps Reflex. Cord segments C 6–7 and the musculocutaneous nerve. (Contributions from C 8 also occur.[5]) With the elbow extended, place a finger on the distal ends of the biceps and brachialis. Tapping this finger will elicit a slight flexion of the elbow, which is more easily palpated than seen.[9] This reflex is often not present in normal animals.

6. Patellar Reflex. Cord segments L 4 to L 6 and the femoral nerve. With the animal lying on its side, the limb supported from the medial side of the stifle, and the stifle in moderate flexion, lightly strike the patellar ligament with a blunt instrument. The side of your hand can be used in large animals. The stifle is extended. This is the most constant tendon reflex.

7. Flexor Reflex of Hind Limb. Cord segments L 1 to S 1 in small animals, to S 2 in large animals; hip flexion involves the lumbar nerves to the iliopsoas muscle and the femoral and obturator nerves; flexion of the other joints involves only L 6 to S 1–2 and the sciatic nerve.

8. Extensor Reflex of Hind Limb. Cord segments L 4 to S 1–2 and the femoral and sciatic nerves. Same as in forelimb, reflex number 2, a pathological reflex.

9. Cranial Tibial and Digital Extensor Reflex. Cord segments L 6 to S 1 and the peroneal nerve. With the small animal in lateral recumbency, extend the hock and strike the plantar surface of the tuber calcanei. This stretches the cranial tibial and digital extensor muscles, which respond by slight flexion of the hock and extension of the digits. It is often not elicited in normal animals.[3]

10. Common Calcanean Tendon Reflex. Cord segments L 6 to S 1–2 and the tibial nerve. Hold the hock in 90° flexion and strike the tendon just above the tuber calcanei. The response is a slight extension of the hock. This is often not elicited in normal animals.[3] In the standing large animal, the gastrocnemius can be seen to contract, although the foot remains stationary.

11. Scratch Reflex. Afferent: cord segments and nerves T 2 to L 2. Efferent: cord segments L 1 to S 1 and the nerves of the hind limb. In the small animal, scratch the saddle region. The hind limb is flexed and extended. This reflex is often inhibited in the normal animal but is frequently present in the dog with a transverse thoracolumbar spinal cord lesion. It is useful because it tests so many segments of the spinal cord.

12. Cutaneous Trunci Reflex. Afferent: thoracic and lumbar segments of the cord and their nerves. Efferent: cord segments C 8 to T 1 and the lateral thoracic nerve. Touch the hair along the costal arch of the large animal. Stimulate the skin along the back of a small animal with a pin or forceps. The cutaneous muscle contracts. This reflex is constant in the normal horse. In small animals, it is often not elicited by stimuli caudal to the mid-lumbar region. It may require vigorous stimulation to elicit this reflex in the normal dog, and occasionally it is completely absent. Because this reflex requires an ascending spinal cord pathway from the peripheral sensory neuron to the lower motor neuron of the lateral thoracic nerve, it may be useful in localizing a transverse spinal cord lesion. This is especially helpful in stoic dogs in which a line of analgesia cannot be assessed. This reflex will be absent caudal to a line two to three vertebrae caudal to the transverse lesion.[52] Stimulation of the skin on one side elicits a bilateral cutaneous trunci response in small animals.

13. Perineal Reflex. Large animal: cord segments S 3 to S 5 and caudal segments. Small animal: S 1 to S 3 and caudal segments. The nerves are the pudendal, caudal rectal, and caudal. Touch the skin of the perineum, underside of the tail, or the anus. The sphincter ani contracts, the vulva is raised, and the tail is clamped down (except in the female during estrus). The anus is the most sensitive reflexogenic zone. It remains effective when stimulation of other parts of the perineum do not elicit a reflex. This reflex will be absent in animals with bladder paralysis due to lesions in the lower motor neurons.

Postural Reactions

The following reactions are more complex than the spinal reflexes. When normal they indicate the integrity of the peripheral nerves, local segments of the spinal cord, ascending and descending tracts, brain stem, cerebellum, and cerebral cortex. They occur in all normal animals.[9, 29]

1. Righting Reaction. This should be observed when the animal is released from a position of lateral recumbency.

2. Proprioceptive Positioning—Correction of Posture. In the standing animal, cross one forefoot in front of the other or abduct one foot to an abnormal posture or place the paw on its dorsal surface. The normal animal will return the foot to the usual position.

3. Tonic Neck Reactions. If the nose is elevated, the extensor tonus is increased in the fore-limbs and decreased in the hind limbs. If the head is turned to one side, extensor tonus is increased in the forelimb on that side.

4. Postural Extensor Thrust. If a small animal is held in the upright position blindfolded and lowered until the front or hind foot pads touch a supporting surface, the limbs extend and support the weight. If the animal can see the supporting surface, the test becomes an optical placing reaction. In the standing large animal, if the flexor reflex is elicited from one limb, a postural extensor reaction takes the weight on the opposite limb.

5. Placing Reactions. If a small animal is held as in reaction number 4 and brought to the edge of a table so that the dorsal surfaces of the feet touch it, the feet will be placed on the table and will support the weight. This is the tactile placing reaction. If the animal is not blindfolded, it will place the feet on the table without prior contact. This is the optical placing reaction.

6. Hopping Reaction. The animal is held with three limbs flexed and the fourth standing on the ground. The center of gravity is shifted, and the animal hops with the supporting limb to keep it under the body. This is the most reliable of the postural reactions for small animals. To test the forelimb hopping, stand over the animal, facing in the same direction, and lift the abdomen with the left hand until the pelvic limbs are just off the ground. Pick up the right forelimb with your right hand and hop the dog to the left on the left forelimb. It will start to hop laterally as soon as the trunk starts to move over it. Reverse the position of your hands and hop the dog back to the right on the right forelimb. Keep repeating this to compare the responses in the forelimbs with each other. For the hind limbs, stand on the left side of the dog and place your left hand between the forelimbs under the sternum. Elevate the sternum until the forelimbs are just off the ground. With your right hand, raise the left pelvic limb and hop the dog to the right on its right pelvic limb. Reverse your position and hop the animal to its left on the left pelvic limb and compare the pelvic limb responses with each other. In a less cooperative or a heavy animal, the same responses can be observed by standing beside the animal and lifting both limbs on one side and hopping the dog in the direction of the supporting limbs.

7. Circling. In large animals, similar observations can be made by watching the animal walk slowly in a small circle. Abnormal reactions include delay in protraction of a limb, excessive abduction of a limb, crossing over of a limb or stepping on the opposite foot, and stiffness in the limb motion. If the delay in protraction is severe, the animal will pivot on that limb and sway to the side.

8. Sway. This tests the large animal's strength and coordination. As the animal is walking, it is pulled by the tail to either side. The normal animal resists this and maintains its coordination.

References

1. Allam, M. W., D. G. Lee, F. E. Nulsen, et al.: The anatomy of the brachial plexus of the dog. Anat. Rec. *114*(1952):173–179.
2. Arnold, J. P. and R. L. Kitchell: Experimental studies of the innervation of the abdominal wall of cattle. Am. J. Vet. Res. *18*(1957):229–240.
3. Bässler, H. P.: Die Reflexuntersuchung beim Hund. Arch. exp. Veterinärmedizin. *15*(1961):100–140.

4. Blevins, W. E.: Transosseous vertebral venography: a diagnostic aid in lumbosacral disease. Vet. Radiol. 21(1980):50–54.

5. Bowne, J. G.: Neuroanatomy of the Brachial Plexus of the Dog. Ph.D. Thesis, Iowa State University, 1959.

6. Bradley, R. L., S. J. Withrow, R. B. Heath, et al.: Epidural analgesia in the dog. Vet. Surg. 9(1980):153–156.

7. Brook, G. B.: Spinal (epidural) anesthesia in the domestic animals. Vet. Rec. 15(1935):553, 581, 597, 631, 659.

8. Cakala, S.: A technic for the paravertebral lumbar block in cattle. Cornell Vet. 51(1961):64–67.

9. de Lahunta, A.: Veterinary Neuroanatomy and Clinical Neurology. 2nd ed. Philadelphia: W. B. Saunders, 1983.

10. Douglas, S. W. and H. D. Williamson: Veterinary Radiological Interpretation. Philadelphia: Lea & Febiger, 1970.

11. Dukes, H. H.: The Physiology of Domestic Animals. Ithaca, N. Y.: Comstock, 1955.

12. Farquharson, J.: Paravertebral lumbar anesthesia in the bovine species. JAVMA 97 (1940):54–57.

13. Feeney, D. A. and M. Wise: Epidurography in the normal dog: technic and radiographic findings. Vet. Rad. 22(1981):35–39.

14. Fletcher, T.: Anatomical studies of the spinal cord segments in the dog. Ph.D. Thesis, University of Minnesota, 1964.

15. Getty, R.: Epidural anesthesia in the hog—its technique and applications. Proc. AVMA 1963:88–98.

16. Ghoshal, N. G. and R. Getty: Applied anatomy of the sacrococcygeal region of the ox as related to tail bleeding. Vet. Med.—Small Anim. Clin. 62(1967): 255–264.

17. Hansen, H. J.: Pathogenesis of disc degeneration and rupture. In Pettit, G. D. (ed.): Intervertebral Disc Protrusion in the Dog. New York: Appleton-Century-Crofts, 1966, pp. 21–50.

18. Hare, W. C. D.: Zur Ossifikation und Vereinigung der Wirbelepiphysen beim Hund. Wiener tierärztl. Msch. 48(1961):210–215.

19. Heath, E. H. and V. S. Myers.: Topographic anatomy for caudal anesthesia in the horse. Vet. Med.—Small Anim. Clin. 67(1972):1237–1239.

20. Hopkins, G. S.: The correlation of anatomy and epidural anesthesia in the domestic animals. Cornell Vet. 25(1935):263–270.

21. Huddleston, O. L. and White, C. S.: Segmental motor innervation of the tibialis anterior and gastrocnemius-plantaris muscles in the dog. Am. J. Physiol. 138(1943):772–775.

22. Jeffcott, L. B.: Disorders of the thoracolumbar spine of the horse—a survey of 443 cases. Eq. Vet. J. 12(1980):197–210.

23. Jeffcott, L. B. and G. Dalin: Natural rigidity of the horse's backbone. Eq. Vet. J. 12(1980):101–108.

24. Jeffcott, L. B.: Diagnosis of back problems in the horse. Comp. Cont. Ed. 3(1981):S134–S143.

25. Jeffcott, L. B. and G. Dalin: Bibliography of thoracolumbar conditions in the horse. Eq. Vet. J. 15(1983):155–157.

26. Jefferson, A.: Aspects of the segmental innervation of the cat's hind limb. J. Comp. Neurol. 100(1954):569–596.

27. Klide, A. M. and L. R. Soma.: Epidural analgesia in the dog and cat. JAVMA 153(1968):165–173.

28. McClure, R. C., M. J. Dallman, and P. D. Garrett: Cat Anatomy, an Atlas, Text, and Dissection Guide. Philadelphia: Lea & Febiger, 1973.

29. McGrath, J. T.: Neurologic Examination of the Dog with Clinicopathologic Observations, 2nd ed. Philadelphia: Lea & Febiger, 1960.

30. McNeel, S. V. and J. P. Morgan: Intraosseous vertebral venography: a technic for examination of the canine lumbosacral junction. J. Am. Vet. Radiol. Soc. 19(1978):168–175.

31. Magda, I. I., N. E. Shalduga, and V. M. Voskoboinikov: Some remarks in connection with rumenotomy. Veterinariya, 29(1952):47–51. (Abstr.) JAVMA 122 (1953):326.

32. Mettler, F. A.: Some neurologic derangements of animals. Cornell Vet. 36(1946):195–200.

33. Oliver, J. E., Jr., R. R. Selcer, and S. Simpson: Cauda equina compression from lumbosacral malarticulation and malformation in the dog. JAVMA 173(1978):207–212.

34. Piermattei, D. L. and R. G. Greeley: An Atlas of Surgical Approaches to the Bones of the Dog and Cat. Philadelphia: W. B. Saunders, 1966.

35. Rooney, J. R.: Autopsy of the Horse. Baltimore: Williams and Wilkins, 1970, p. 56.

36. Schreiber, J. and O. Schaller: Anatomische Studien über die extradurale Anästhesie bei Rind und Hund. Wiener tierärztl. Msch. 41(1954):386–436.

37. Schreiber, J.: Die Leitungsanästhesie der Rumpfnerven beim Rind, Wiener tierärztl. Msch. 42(1955):471–491.

38. Schürmann, H. T.: Die Topographie des Rückenmarkes bei der Katze. Diss. Hanover, 1951.

39. Seiferle, E.: Zur Rückenmarkstopographie von Pferd und Rind. Zschr. Anat. 110(1939):371–384. (Abstr.) JAVMA 118(1951):379–383.

40. Skarda, R. T. and W. W. Muir: Segmental lumbar epidural analgesia in cattle. Aust. J. Vet. Res. 40(1979):52–57.

41. St. Clair, L. E. and H. J. Hardenbrook: Lumbar epidural anesthesia in cattle. JAVMA 129(1956):405–409.

42. Stecher, R. M.: Lateral facets and lateral joints in the lumbar spine of the horse—a descriptive and statistical study. Am. J. Vet. Res. 23(1962):939–947.

43. Steinberg, H. S.: Myotatic reflexes. Comp. Cont. Ed. 4 (1982):895–901.

44. Tarvin, G. and R. G. Prata: Lumbosacral stenosis in dogs. JAVMA 177(1980):154–159.

45. Thompson, R. G.: Vertebral body osteophytes in bulls. Pathol. Vet. (Suppl) 6(1969):1–47.

46. Townsend, H. G. G., D. H. Leach, and P. B. Fretz: Kinematics of the equine thoracolumbar spine, Eq. Vet. J. 15(1983):117–122.

47. Verwer, M. A. J.: Het neurologisch onderzoek van de hond. Tijdschr. Diergen. 82(1957):445–482.

48. Weber, W.: Anatomie für die Praxis 3. Anatomisch—Klinische Untersuchungen über die Punktions—und Anästhesiestellen des Rückenmarkes und über die Lage des Gehirnes beim Rind. Schweiz. Arch. Tierheilkd. 84(1942):161–173.

49. Weber, W.: Die Rückenmarkspunktionsstellen beim Schwein. Schweiz. Arch. Tierheilkd. 85(1943):101–105.

50. Westhues, M.: Verhalten des Liquordruckes bei der hohen Sakralanästhesie. (Abstr.) Schweiz. Arch. Tierheilkd. 90(1948):46.

51. Ziegler, H.: Zur Anatomie der Liquorpunktionsstellen bei Haustieren. Schweiz. Arch. Tierheilkd. 87-(1945):247.

52. Bailey, C. S., R. L. Kitchell, S. S. Haghighi, and R. D. Johnson: Cutaneous innervation of the thorax and abdomen of the dog. Am. J. Vet. Res. 45(1984):1689–1698.

CHAPTER 21

ABDOMINAL MUSCLES, INGUINAL REGION

OBJECTIVES

1. To be able to identify the muscle layers of the lateral abdominal wall by the direction of the fibers as a surgical incision is made through them. To do this, one must know the difference in the caudal extent of the transverse abdominal muscle in large and small animals and the line of junction of the fleshy muscle with its aponeurosis in the transverse and oblique muscles.
2. To understand the sheath of the rectus abdominis and to be able to use it in closure of paramedian abdominal incisions.
3. To know the blood supply of the abdominal wall.
4. To understand the structures in the umbilical cord and their intra-abdominal course in order to trace infectious processes.
5. To understand the structure of the inguinal canal and rings in each species.
6. To be able to palpate the superficial inguinal ring in each species and the external pudendal artery in the horse and dog.
7. To be able to palpate the spermatic cord from the scrotum to the superficial inguinal ring.
8. To understand the stages in the descent of the testis and the normal time of descent in each species.
9. To be able to palpate the vaginal ring and deep inguinal ring per rectum in large animals, to know the difference between them, and to be able to diagnose the position of a cryptorchid testis by the structures present at the vaginal ring.
10. To understand the inguinal approach for cryptorchid surgery and to be able to find an abdominal cryptorchid testis by tracing its attachments. To understand what the vaginal tunic surrounds in the normal and cryptorchid male.
11. To be able to avoid damage during surgery to the nerves and vessels passing through the inguinal canal as well as the external iliac vessels passing just caudal to the aponeurosis of the external oblique.
12. To understand the diagnostic significance of inflammation of the superficial inguinal lymph nodes and to be able to palpate these in the dog.

Note on the Nomenclature. The inguinal ligament was defined in the English literature of human and large animal anatomy as the caudal border of the aponeurosis of the external oblique muscle, extending from the tuber coxae to the pubic tubercle or prepubic tendon. In the dog and cat, the caudal border of the aponeurosis is not attached to the tuber coxae but courses cranioventral to the ilium until it reaches its pelvic attachment. In the dog, it is attached with the tendon of the pectineus on the iliopubic eminence. In the cat, its only attachment to the pelvis is on the medial half of the pecten of the pubis. Therefore, the homology with the human inguinal ligament is dubious, and the term caudal border of the aponeurosis of the external oblique will be used here.

The prepubic tendon is essentially the common tendon of termination of the two rectus abdominis muscles.[13] It incorporates the caudal end of the linea alba and gives attachment to the oblique abdominal muscles and the pectineus. It is attached to the cranial branches of the pubic bones. In addition to the longitudinal fibers, it contains transverse fibers extending from one iliopubic eminence to the other. In the horse and ox, the longitudinal fibers predominate because the caudal part of the rectus is tendinous. In the dog, the transverse fibers predominate because the rectus continues as a fleshy muscle to its termination on them and on the pubis.

The mesorchium is the homologue of the mesovarium. It is a fold of serous membrane containing the testicular vessels and nerves. It extends from the origin of the testicular vessels to the testis. In the spermatic cord proximal to the epididymis, the thin part of the mesorchium connecting the vascular part and the mesoductus deferens to the parietal lamina of the vaginal tunic may be called the mesofuniculus.

The vaginal process is the embryonic evagination of the peritoneum, which becomes the vaginal tunic after the descent of the testis. In the bitch it remains a vaginal process.

21a. INGUINAL REGION, HORSE

The main interest in the inguinal canal in the horse is connected with the castration of cryptorchid colts. Examine the inguinal canal and vaginal ring from the inside of the peritoneal cavity. The vaginal ring is formed by the peritoneum where it evaginates through the inguinal canal to form the vaginal tunic. This occurs at the lateral end of the deep inguinal ring. On rectal examination of an adult stallion the vaginal ring can be located about 10 cm. cranioventral and slightly lateral to the palpable external iliac artery. The ductus deferens is more readily palpated at the ring than the testicular vessels. The testicular vessels are joined here by the ductus deferens, and their serous coverings are continuous with the visceral lamina of the vaginal tunic on the spermatic cord. Identify the abdominal muscles and note their relationship to the vaginal tunic and inguinal canal. Note that the transversus abdominis in the large animals does not extend back to the inguinal region.

The deep inguinal ring is a long slit (palpable per rectum through the peritoneum) running dorsolaterally between the caudal border of the fleshy internal oblique and the inner surface of the aponeurosis of the external oblique. The latter curves dorsally to the pelvis around the caudolateral abdominal wall. The medial angle of the deep ring is at the thick, palpable lateral border of the prepubic tendon. This tendon is concealed by the caudal part of the aponeurosis of the external oblique, which decussates with the contralateral aponeurosis at its termination on the internal surface of the prepubic tendon. The pectineus, originating from the transverse fibers of the prepubic tendon, bulges under the aponeurosis. The external pudendal artery enters the deep ring at the medial angle. (The external pudendal vein of the horse passes through a separate foramen in the origin of the gracilis.) The lateral angle of the deep ring is limited by the origin of the internal oblique from the iliac fascia and from the aponeurosis of the external oblique. The vaginal tunic and the cremaster muscle pass through the lateral angle of the deep ring. Examine the superficial inguinal ring, which is a slit in the aponeurosis of the external oblique. The medial angle coincides with that of the deep ring so that the medial wall of the inguinal canal is very short. The superficial ring is directed craniolaterally, making the lateral angles of the two rings widely separated so that the lateral part of the inguinal canal is about 15 cm. long. Only the medial crus of the superficial ring presents a free border. The lateral crus is directly continuous through the femoral lamina of the aponeurosis with the medial femoral fascia. When the limb is abducted, the ring is opened. In palpating the ring in the live horse the palm of the hand should be turned toward the abdomen to palpate the medial crus. If the palm is turned toward the thigh, the ring will not be felt as the fingers pass into the inguinal canal. The canal is a narrow slit between the oblique muscles. The caudolateral wall is the aponeurosis of the external oblique; the craniomedial wall is the fleshy internal oblique, which attaches to the prepubic tendon medially. The vaginal tunic runs obliquely through the canal from the lateral angle of the deep ring to the medial angle of the superficial ring.

21b. INGUINAL REGION, EQUINE FETUS

A review of the descent of the testis is necessary for an understanding of cryptorchidism. The gonad first appears as a swelling on the ventromedial surface of the long mesonephros. The mesonephric duct runs caudally, lateral to the gonad, then turns medially to enter the urogenital sinus. This bend is an important landmark, the future tail of the epididymis. Cranial to this point the mesonephric duct becomes greatly elongated and convoluted to form the duct of the epididymis. The caudal part of the mesonephric duct becomes the ductus deferens. All of these structures are covered by peritoneum, and as the mesonephros regresses the testis comes to be suspended by a peritoneal fold, the mesorchium. The testicular artery comes directly from the aorta to the testis in the mesorchium.

A mesenchymal tract develops between the caudal pole of the testis and the bend in the mesonephric duct. This tract, covered by a fold of peritoneum that is continuous with the mesorchium, is the proper ligament of the testis, the first segment of the gubernaculum testis. From the bend in the mesonephric duct to the inguinal region and out into the body wall, other segments of the gubernaculum develop *in situ* and link up to form a continuous cylindrical mesenchymal mass into the genital swelling. In the fetus it is not a fibrous cord as it is often described but jelly-like. The intra-abdominal part projects into the peritoneal cavity, covered by a peritoneal fold. The extra-abdominal part develops in the body wall before the muscles appear, and the muscles form the inguinal canal around it. The distal end grows to form a large gubernacular bulb.

The mechanical action of the gubernaculum in the descent of the testis has been greatly clarified.[5, 8, 21] The vaginal process of the peritoneum begins to form at a very early stage (45 days of gestation in the horse), long before the testis reaches the vaginal ring (270 days in the horse). The vaginal process invades the gubernacular mesenchyme as an incompletely circular slit lined with mesothelium. It separates a peripheral layer from the cranial, medial, and lateral sides of the central gubernaculum proper, which remains attached by a mesentery-like caudal strip to the peripheral layer. The relation of the vaginal process to the gubernaculum proper is the same as the relation of the vaginal tunic to the spermatic cord. The gubernacular mesenchyme around the outside of the vaginal process contains the cremaster muscle.

The vaginal process continues to invade the gubernacular mesenchyme, and the latter continues to grow toward the scrotum but is not attached there. It cannot exert traction from the bottom of the scrotum, but its bulbous enlargement outside the inguinal canal may provide anchorage. Measurements in pig and calf fetuses show that during the descent of the testis to the inguinal canal the intra-abdominal gubernaculum undergoes an absolute shortening while the extra-abdominal part is growing longer.[21]

The main function of the gubernaculum is to swell, dilate the vaginal ring and inguinal canal, and guide the testis in its descent. Most of the swelling takes place in the extra-abdominal part, but in the final stage the cranial part of the gubernaculum swells to a diameter as great as that of the testis. The gubernacular swelling is caused partly by active cell division but mostly by an increase in intercellular fluid.[21] The latter becomes strongly metachromatic, indicating an increase in mucopolysaccharides.

The passage through the canal occurs rapidly in the calf and pig, slowly in the horse. When the gubernaculum swells, enlarging the vaginal ring and the inguinal canal and decreasing their resistance to passage of the testis, the loop formed by the tail of the epididymis and the ductus deferens enters the canal first, followed by the testis and the rest of the epididymis. These structures always remain covered by the visceral peritoneum, continuous with that on the gubernaculum below and on the mesorchium and mesoductus deferens above. The ductus deferens and testicular vessels are elongated. The testis descends into the scrotum as the gubernaculum is converted from a large mass of mucous connective tissue to the short fibrous ligaments of the testis and of the tail of the epididymis. This is an absolute decrease in length, which in the pig is from 24 mm. to 4 mm.[21] Studies have shown that an unidentified testicular factor is necessary for the gubernacular outgrowth and swelling. Testosterone is only partly involved in this development. However, the gubernacular regression that follows descent of the testis through the canal is testosterone-dependent.[7]

In pigs, high abdominal cryptorchidism can be caused by abnormal intra-abdominal swelling of the gubernaculum, low abdominal cryptorchidism by insufficient or excessive swelling, and inguinal herniation by excessive swelling followed by regression of the gubernaculum and descent of the testis.[22, 23]

There is an added complication in the horse that may contribute to the high incidence of cryptorchidism in that species. The gonads are greatly enlarged by an increase in interstitial cells in the fetus. The testis must become smaller in diameter by reduction of these cells before it can pass the inguinal canal. At 150 days of gestation the horse testis is 6 cm. × 3 cm. and weighs 20 g. At 250 days it has enlarged to 5 cm. in diameter and weighs 50 g. By the time it begins its passage through the vaginal ring it has elongated to 10 cm.; the diameter is 2.5 cm.; and the weight is 30 g.[8]

The normal time of descent is about 80 days of gestation in the pig and 106 days of gestation in the calf. It is much later in the dog and horse, occurring near term. Descent through the canal occurs at 3 to 4 days after birth in the dog, but it takes up to 35 days to reach the scrotum.[6] About half of newborn foals examined post-mortem have the testes descended. Palpation of the scrotum is not a reliable method to determine descent in the foal because the gubernacular bulb feels like a testis for the first three weeks after birth. Later, a gubernaculum can be recognized by regression, a testis by growth.

Figure 21–1 is a dissection of an equine fetus with one testis not descended. The vaginal ring on that side contains three elongated structures: the large white proper ligament of the testis (first segment of gubernaculum), the epididymis covered by mesorchium, and the ductus deferens. The latter emerges from the vaginal ring attached to the free border of the mesoductus. It passes around the cranial side of the umbilical artery to the urethra. In the inguinal canal the proper ligament of the testis joins the middle of the loop where the tail of the epididymis is continuous with the ductus deferens. Across this junction the ligament is continuous with the rest of the gubernaculum, which draws the loop into the canal. The gubernaculum and the loop can be used to locate the testis in the abdominal cavity in cryptorchid castration. In the normal adult, the proper ligament of the testis is very short and thick, holding the tail of the epididymis in close contact with the testis. The rest of the gubernaculum becomes the ligament of the tail of the epididymis in the distal free border of the mesofuniculus.

Diagnosis of cryptorchidism in the horse involves palpation of the scrotum and inguinal region, rectal palpation, and exploratory surgery. If the testis is not palpable in the scrotum or subcutaneously in the inguinal region, it is either in the inguinal canal or intra-abdominal. It is often impossible to locate an intra-abdominal testis per rectum, but palpation of the vaginal ring may be diagnostic.[19] If there is nothing passing through the vaginal ring but the gubernaculum (and that may be regressed so that it cannot be felt), the testis and epididymis are entirely intra-abdominal. If the vaginal ring cannot be palpated, the testis and epididymis are intra-abdominal, and the vaginal process is probably inverted. If there are three structures passing through the vaginal ring, as in Figure 21–1 (the tail of the epididymis, the ductus deferens, and the proper ligament of the testis), the testis and the rest of the epididymis are intra-abdominal. If only two structures are passing through the vaginal ring (the ductus deferens and the mesorchium), the testis and epididymis are in the inguinal canal or external to it.

To explore the inguinal canal an incision is made over the superficial inguinal ring. This exposes a large plexus of external pudendal vessels. Careful visual exploration of the exposed superficial inguinal ring reveals the infravaginal part of the gubernaculum on the craniomedial border of the ring. The gubernaculum will be regressed to a fibrous band 0.5 to 2 cm. wide. Traction on this will deliver the vaginal process through the ring.[10, 20] Incision of the parietal layer of the process will expose either the gubernaculum or the loop formed by the tail of the epididymis and the ductus deferens, covered by the visceral layer of the vaginal process. Gentle traction on either of these will

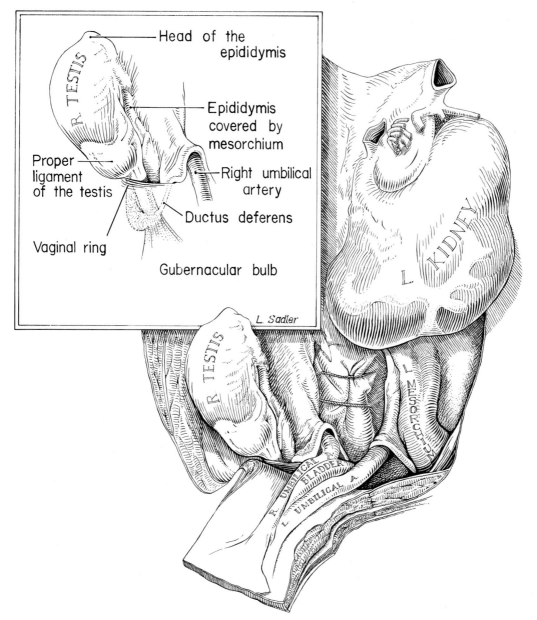

Figure 21–1. Dissection of equine fetus. The left testis has descended; the right testis is retained and is rotated laterally, so that the epididymis is concealed by the testis and mesorchium. The right kidney was removed and the rectum is retracted by sutures.

deliver the testis and the rest of the epididymis through the incision in the parietal layer of the vaginal process.[20]

If the gubernaculum cannot be found visually, the canal is explored caudally and laterally toward the deep inguinal ring. The vaginal ring is dorsolateral to the site of the incision. If the vaginal process is not found, sponge forceps are passed through the canal and vaginal ring to grasp and draw out the peritoneum of the process, which may be inverted into the abdominal cavity. The vaginal process is then opened as previously described.[1]

A careful anatomical identification of the hypoplastic testis is necessary to avoid the mistake of removing the tail of the epididymis with a part of the gubernaculum and leaving the testis in the abdomen. The tail of the epididymis is often widely separated from the testis by an elongated proper ligament. The vaginal ring may have to be widened to remove the testis. If it is necessary to invade the abdomen to find the testis, this is best done through a grid laparotomy in the flank, rather than through the inguinal canal.[10] The genital fold of peritoneum dorsal to the bladder contains the ductus deferens of each side. The ductus should be found here and traced cranially to the retained testis.

Inguinal hernias in stallions are usually indirect, with the herniated viscus within the vaginal tunic.[17] Most involve small intestine that has passed through a normal-sized vaginal ring, causing strangulation and colic. These can be diagnosed by palpation in the inguinal canal or through the rectum. Careful examination of the inguinal canal is necessary in all cases of colic. Congenital hernias may not cause clinical signs; therefore, it is important to palpate the inguinal canal and vaginal tunic in the standing horse before castration.[14]

21c. LIVE HORSE

Palpate the superficial inguinal ring by placing the palm of your hand on the ventrolateral abdominal wall and reaching caudally toward the prepubic tendon. Feel the depression at the medial crus of the superficial inguinal ring. The external pudendal artery can be palpated crossing the caudal aspect of this crus and, in the intact male, the spermatic cord.

Palpate the abdominal wall and appreciate the structure of the muscles that compose it at the various surgical sites.

21d. INGUINAL REGION, BULL

Identify the peritoneum, vaginal ring and vaginal tunic, mesoductus deferens, and mesorchium. Identify the external oblique, internal oblique, and transversus muscles. Observe that the transversus does not extend back to the inguinal region. Locate the lateral border of the rectus and the prepubic tendon. Note the linea alba. The caudal border of the aponeurosis of the external oblique extends from the tuber coxae to the prepubic tendon. The internal oblique originates mainly from the tuber coxae but also from the iliac fascia. With the exception of the direct attachment to the tuber coxae, the abdominal muscles are attached to the pelvis by the prepubic tendon, the linea alba, the caudal border of the external oblique, and the iliac fascia.

The aponeurosis of the external oblique forms the caudal wall of the inguinal canal. Caudal to the aponeurosis, between it and the pelvis, are the lacunae through which the external iliac vessels and the iliopsoas muscle pass to reach the thigh. The external iliac becomes the femoral artery at the origin of the deep femoral artery. The latter passes medially, gives off the pudendoepigastric trunk, and runs caudally. The pudendoepigastric gives off the caudal epigastric, which crosses the inguinal ring and enters the rectus, and the external pudendal artery, which crosses the caudal border of the aponeurosis of the external oblique and passes through the medial angle of the inguinal ring with the external pudendal vein and genitofemoral nerve.

There are two kinds of inguinal hernias. The most common type in domestic animals passes through the vaginal ring and follows the vaginal canal to the scrotum. This is called an indirect hernia in human surgery, because it takes the long route through the inguinal canal. It is uncommon in man because the vaginal canal is normally obliterated. A direct inguinal hernia is more common in man. It passes through the short medial part of the inguinal canal, medial to the caudal epigastric artery, and outside the vaginal tunic.

21e. INGUINAL REGION, CALF

The caudal border of the internal oblique and the lateral border of the rectus may be seen through the peritoneum. The mesoductus deferens crosses the round ligament of the bladder (umbilical artery) and enters the vaginal ring with the mesorchium. From the ventral surface, the vaginal tunic can be seen in its course through the inguinal canal. The superficial inguinal lymph nodes lie caudal to the vaginal tunic. It should be emphasized that in none of the domestic animals does the lymphatic drainage of the testis pass through the superficial inguinal nodes. The lymphatics of the testis are in the spermatic cord and go directly to the medial iliac and lumbar nodes. Swelling of the superficial inguinal nodes does not necessarily indicate orchitis.

21f. UMBILICAL REGION, BOVINE FETUS

In the bovine fetus four structures pass through the abdominal wall at the umbilicus: the urachus, two arteries, and a vein. The urachus comes from the apex of the bladder, with which it communicates, and courses to the umbilicus in the middle ligament of the bladder. The two umbilical arteries come from the internal iliacs, pass by the bladder in its lateral ligaments, and accompany the urachus to the umbilicus. The two umbilical veins in the umbilical cord join to form a single vein that passes into the abdomen and courses cranially in the falciform ligament to the liver. Umbilical hernias in calves are often complicated by abscesses. These infections may involve the vessels or urachus in the umbilical cord, which provides a route of extension into the abdomen. Infection in the umbilical vein may be a source of a liver abscess. Infection in the urachus may extend to the bladder.

21g. DISSECTION, LATERAL ABDOMINAL WALL, OX

Note the dorsal borders of the external and internal abdominal oblique muscles and the caudal border of the transversus abdominis. In the ox, the origin of the transversus abdominis from the lumbar transverse processes is aponeurotic as well as the ventral part of the muscle. The paralumbar fossa is a surgical area in the dorsal part of the flank. It is bounded by the tips of the lumbar transverse processes, the last rib, and a prominent muscular ridge formed by the part of the internal oblique that extends from the tuber coxae to the ventral end of the last rib. Palpate these structures in the live cow. The blood supply of this region comes from the costoabdominal and lumbar arteries and from the circumflex iliac artery at the tuber coxae.

The transverse and oblique muscles form a purely aponeurotic zone of the abdominal wall that begins medial to the stifle and extends forward for a variable distance along the lateral border of the rectus. Hernias sometimes result from injury in this region.

21h. DISSECTION, UMBILICAL REGION, PIG

Beginning from the inside of the abdomen, identify the following layers:

1. Peritoneum.

2. Retroperitoneal fat and the transversus muscle. The aponeurosis of the transversus is the internal lamina of the sheath of the rectus.

3. The rectus abdominis is easily recognized by the longitudinal direction of the fibers. The epigastric vessels lie on the dorsal surface.

4. The aponeurosis of the internal oblique. This is separable only at the lateral border of the rectus because its dorsal surface is fused with the tendinous intersections of the rectus. The ventral surface is fused with the aponeurosis of the external oblique.

5. Aponeurosis of the external oblique. The fused aponeuroses of the oblique muscles form the external lamina of the sheath of the rectus and furnish the site for the main row of sutures in herniorrhaphy.

6. Abdominal cutaneous muscle.

7. Mammary gland.

8. Subcutaneous fat.

9. Skin.

Inguinal hernias are common in female pigs. This has been related to abnormalities of the reproductive organs that are comparable to freemartinism in cattle.[9]

21i. DISSECTION, ABDOMINAL WALL, MALE DOG

The superficial inguinal ring in the dog is almost sagittal in direction. As in other species it is a slit in the aponeurosis of the external oblique. The medial and lateral crura meet behind the ring in a complex junction with the tendon of origin of the pectineus and the prepubic tendon at the iliopubic eminence. This point is easily palpated in the live dog.[15] The prepubic tendon continues the line of tension of the caudal border of the aponeurosis of the external oblique from the pectineus tendon to the ventral pubic tubercle and gives attachment to the lateral part of the rectus. The vaginal tunic emerges from the cranial end of the ring. It can be palpated from the scrotum to the ring in the live dog.

The external pudendal vessels are at the caudal end of the ring. The external pudendal artery supplies the external genitalia and gives rise to the caudal superficial epigastric artery. This supplies the caudal abdominal region. Note the superficial inguinal lymph node on the external pudendal vessels. Inguinal hernias should be repaired carefully to avoid constriction by sutures of the external pudendal vein and the lymphatics in the caudal angle of the ring. Occlusion causes edema of the ventral abdominal wall and hind limb. Care should also be taken to avoid injury to the large external iliac vessels, separated only by the narrow caudal border of the aponeurosis of the external oblique from the inguinal ring.

Study the sheath of the rectus. In the usual operative field, the external lamina is formed by the fused aponeuroses of both oblique muscles. The deep lamina is formed by the aponeurosis of the transversus. (In the cranial part of the sheath, a lamina from the internal oblique passes deep to the rectus, and in the caudal part, the transversus becomes superficial to the rectus.)

Cryptorchidism has been recognized sporadically in numerous breeds in which inheritance is not thought to be a predominant factor except for the Miniature Schnauzer.[11, 16] Testicular neoplasms are common in cryptorchid testes.

21j. DISSECTION, ABDOMINAL WALL, FEMALE DOG

On the deep surface of the rectus abdominis are the caudal and cranial epigastric vessels. In the superficial fascia at the cranial end of the rectus are the cranial superficial epigastric vessels. The ventral abdominal wall is supplied by four sets of arteries and veins: the cranial epigastric and cranial superficial epigastric from the internal thoracic, and the caudal epigastric and caudal superficial epigastric from the pudendoepigastric and external pudendal.

The deep inguinal ring is formed as in the other species with slight modifications. The transversus abdominis extends back to the inguinal ring and joins the internal oblique at the craniomedial border. The medial angle is formed by the fleshy rectus abdominis. The caudolateral border is the aponeurosis of the external oblique. The bitch has a vaginal process accompanied by the round ligament of the uterus in the inguinal canal. Inguinal hernias are more common in female dogs.

On the cranial part of the abdominal floor is a median fold of peritoneum, the falciform ligament of the liver. It contains in its concave dorsal free border a thin cord, the ligamentum teres hepatis, the vestige of the umbilical vein. This is visible only in puppies. The falciform ligament represents the cranial part of the ventral mesentery of the embryo. Its only surgical importance is that it is often filled with fat and bulges out of laparotomy incisions on the midline cranial to the umbilicus. Caudal to the umbilicus is another peritoneal fold, the middle ligament of the bladder. Either of these vestigial structures may be removed without harm.

21k. LIVE DOG

Palpate the femoral artery in the femoral triangle cranial to the pectineus. Follow it proximally to the abdominal wall, where it emerges caudal to the aponeurosis of termination of the external oblique abdominal muscle. It is the continuation of the external iliac artery.

Palpate the superficial inguinal ring by abducting the pelvic limb of the recumbent dog.[15] Locate the iliopubic eminence at the origin of the pectineus. Feel the taut band that extends cranially from this eminence on the abdominal wall. This is the medial crus of the superficial inguinal ring. The external pudendal artery can be palpated crossing this crus. In the intact male the spermatic cord and cremaster can also be palpated. Follow the spermatic cord and cremaster to the testis in the scrotum.

Palpate the superficial inguinal lymph nodes in the subcutaneous tissue a few centimeters cranioventral to the superficial inguinal ring. In the male they can be felt in the skin fold that suspends the penis. They are caudal to the bulb of the glans. In the female they are deep to the inguinal mammary gland and may be difficult to locate. In the young puppy after the testis emerges from the inguinal canal, the testis and superficial inguinal lymph nodes are similar in size and can be confused on palpation. The testis is usually more movable.

References

1. Adams, O. R.: An improved method of diagnosis and castration of cryptorchid horses. JAVMA *145* (1964):439–446.
2. Adams, B.: Surgical approaches to and exploration of the equine abdomen. Vet. Clin. North Am. *4* (1982):89–104.
3. Arey, L. B.: Developmental Anatomy, 7th ed. Philadelphia W. B. Saunders, 1965.
4. Ashdown R. R.: The anatomy of the inguinal canal in the domesticated mammals. Vet. Rec. *75* (1963):1345–1351.
5. Backhouse, K. M. and H. Butler: The gubernaculum testis of the pig. J. Anat. *94* (1960):107–120.
6. Baumans, V., G. Dijkstra, and C. J. G. Wensing: Testicular descent in the dog. Zbl. Vet. Med. C. *10* (1981):97–110.
7. Baumans, V.: Regulation of Testicular Descent in the Dog. University of Utrecht, 1982.
8. Bergin, W. C., H. T. Gier, G. B. Marion, et al.: A developmental concept of equine cryptorchism. Biol. Reprod. *3* (1970):82–92.
9. Colenbrander, B. and C. J. G. Wensing: Studies on phenotypically female pigs with hernia inguinalis and ovarian aplasia. Koninkl. Ned. Akad. Wetensch. Proc. Ser. C. *78* (1975):33–46.
10. Collier, M. A.: Equine cryptorchidectomy: surgical considerations and approaches. Mod. Vet. Pract. *61* (1980):511–515.
11. Cox, V. S., L. J. Wallace, and O. R. Jessen: An anatomic and genetic study of canine cryptorchidism. Teratology *18* (1978):233–240.
12. Evans, H. E. and G. C. Christensen: Miller's Anatomy of the Dog, 2nd ed. Philadelphia: W. B. Saunders, 1979.
13. Getty, R.: Sisson and Grossman's The Anatomy of the Domestic Animals, 5th ed. Philadelphia: W. B. Saunders, 1975.
14. Goetz, T. E., C. H. Boulton, and J. R. Coffman: Inguinal and scrotal hernias in colts and stallions. Comp. Cont. Ed. *3* (1981):S272–S276.
15. McCarthy, P. H.: The anatomy of the superficial inguinal ring and its contained and adjacent structures in the live Greyhound—a study by palpation. J. Small Anim. Pract. *17* (1976):507–518.
16. Pendergrass, T. W. and H. M. Hayes, Jr.: Cryptorchidism and related defects in dogs: epidemiologic comparisons with man. Teratology *12* (1975):51–55.
17. Schneider, R. K., D. W. Milne, and C. W. Kohn: Acquired inguinal hernia in the horse: a review of 27 cases. JAVMA *108* (1982):317–320.
18. Seiferle, E.: Über die Leistengegend der Haussäugetiere. Schweizer Arch. Tierheilkd. *75* (1933):281–301.
19. Stickle, P. L. and J. F. Fessler: Retrospective study of 350 cases of equine cryptorchidism. JAVMA *172* (1978):343–346.
20. Valdez, H., T. S. Taylor, S. A. McLaughlin, et al.: Abdominal cryptorchidectomy in the horse, using inguinal extension. JAVMA *174* (1979):1110–1112.
21. Wensing, C. J. G.: Testicular descent in some domestic mammals. I. Anatomical aspect of testicular descent. Koninkl. Ned. Akad. Wetensch. Proc. Ser. C *71* (1968):423–434.
22. Wensing C. J. G.: Abnormalities of testicular descent. Koninkl. Ned. Akad. Wetensch. Proc. Ser. C *76* (1973):373–381.
23. Wensing, C. J. G. and B. Colenbrander. Cryptorchidism and inguinal hernia. Koninkl. Ned. Akad. Wetensch. Proc. Ser. C *76* (1973):489–494.
24. Wensing, C. J. G.: Testicular descent in some domestic mammals. II. The nature of the gubernacular change during the process of testicular descent in the pig. Koninkl. Ned. Akad. Wetensch. Proc. Ser. C *76* (1973):190–202.

CHAPTER 22

STOMACH

OBJECTIVES

1. To be able to relate the bovine stomach to the abdominal wall and to recognize a possible distention of the stomach from distortion of the outline of the body as viewed from the rear of the cow.
2. To be able to trocarize the distended stomach of the horse or cow.
3. To be able to recognize by palpation at laparotomy the external features of the ruminant stomach with the animal in the standing position or in dorsal recumbency for abomasopexy. To be able to recognize the internal features of the rumen and reticulum at rumenotomy and to palpate the omasum and abomasum through the rumen wall.
4. To understand the attachments of the lesser and greater omenta in all the domestic animals and how to reflect the greater omentum to find the organs it covers. To understand the hepatoduodenal ligament.
5. To understand the normal attachments and relations of the abomasum and its possible displacements. To know how to diagnose abomasal displacements and volvulus by auscultation and exploratory laparotomy.
6. To be able to use the greater omentum in the reduction of abomasal displacement.
7. To be able to interpret the functional significance of the movements of the rumen palpated in the left paralumbar fossa.
8. To be able to distinguish the normal rumen percussion sound from the sound of a displaced abomasum.
9. To be able to apply pressure in the right place to elicit pain from traumatic inflammation of the reticulum. To be able to auscultate the contractions of the reticulum.
10. To be able to apply pressure to the omasum to elicit pain and to be able to auscultate the omasum.
11. To understand the functions of the ruminant stomach that are regulated by the vagus nerve, and the probable causes of vagal disorders. To understand the reason for bradycardia in some cattle with indigestion.
12. To be able to position a dog for a radiograph of the stomach, and to be able to interpret the radiograph.
13. To be able to perform a gastrotomy on the dog with proper precautions regarding the blood and nerve supplies.
14. To be able to diagnose the direction of gastric volvulus in the dog and to understand its effect on the spleen.
15. To be able to find the epiploic foramen through a laparotomy and to know where the major vessels that supply the liver are located.

Note on the Nomenclature. Volvulus and torsion are often used synonymously, but the rotation of a loop formed by the stomach or intestine is usually called a volvulus in human medicine.[38] It often causes a torsion (twist on the long axis) of the mesenteric vessels, and in canine gastric volvulus, a torsion of the esophagus.

22a. STOMACH, HORSE

Note on the Nomenclature. The fundus is often confused with the body of the stomach. The fundus is only the blind sac that projects dorsal to the level of the cardiac orifice on the left. The body is the main part of the stomach. The pig has a dorsal diverticulum of the fundus directed caudally and to the right. In the horse, the fundus and adjacent part of the body are lined by nonglandular stratified squamous epithelium.

The stomach of the horse is not accessible for examination from the exterior in the normal state (see Plate I). When the stomach is distended and the stomach tube fails, a trocar may be inserted high in the left 17th intercostal space and directed toward the right elbow.

Note the small lumen and thick musculature of the terminal part of the esophagus. The cardiac sphincter is much thicker and better defined than in the other animals. The horse rarely vomits. Gastric ulcers occur in young foals and may cause pain that can be localized to the stomach in the right and left paracostal regions. These foals often lie on their back with their limbs flexed, presumably to relieve pain.[29]

22b. RUMINANT STOMACH PREPARATIONS

Note on the Nomenclature. No domestic animal has more than one stomach. The ruminants have one stomach with four compartments. No part of the stomach develops from the esophagus. The terms monogastric and polygastric, frequently encountered in the literature, are nonsense. We may contrast the simple stomach with the ruminant stomach, or complex stomach.

Study the compartments and their relations to each other. Inflated stomachs do not give a true picture of the relative size of the parts or their position when confined by the abdominal wall.

The most cranial part of the rumen, between the reticulum and the cranial pillar, is the atrium (cranial sac). The rest of the rumen is divided by the longitudinal pillars into dorsal and ventral sacs. The dorsal sac lies farther toward the left than the ventral sac. At the caudal end of the dorsal sac is the caudodorsal blind sac. The cranial end of the ventral sac is the recess of the rumen, and the caudal end, the caudoventral blind sac.

Review the attachments of the lesser and greater omenta on the stomach. Distinguish the omenta from the omental bursa. The bursa is a potential cavity enclosed by the greater and lesser omenta, the stomach, and the liver. It includes the vestibule and the caudal recess.

The lesser omentum passes from the visceral surface of the liver to the lesser curvature of the reticulum, base of the omasum, and lesser curvature of the abomasum, covering the parietal surface of the omasum. It forms the right wall of the vestibule of the omental bursa and ends caudodorsally in a free border, the hepatoduodenal ligament, which is the ventral boundary of the epiploic foramen (omental foramen).

The greater omentum has complex attachments and is best understood by considering first the condition in the dog, then the development in the ruminant embryo. The greater omentum in all species originates from the dorsal body wall at the root of the celiac artery, where it is continuous with the mesentery. The left lobe of the pancreas is enclosed in the dorsal attachment. In the dog, the greater omentum passes ventrally between the stomach and intestines, then caudally on the ventral surface of the intestinal mass as the deep wall of the caudal recess of the omental bursa. Near the pelvis it reflects cranially on itself as the superficial wall and extends to the greater curvature of the stomach. The caudal recess of the omental bursa is closed on the sides by continuity of the deep and superficial walls. The spleen is attached on the left side, and on the right the greater omentum is continuous with the mesoduodenum at the caudal border of the epiploic foramen. Cranially, the caudal recess of the omental bursa is continuous with the vestibule, and the latter with the peritoneal cavity through the epiploic foramen. The foramen is a slit between the liver and the peritoneal fold where the greater omentum is reflected to become the mesoduodenum. The foramen is bounded dorsally by the caudal vena cava and ventrally by the hepatoduodenal ligament containing the bile duct, hepatic artery, and portal vein. Compression of the vessels in the hepatoduodenal ligament will stop the flow of blood to the liver for surgical purposes.

In the dog and cat, the caudal fold of the greater omentum can be picked up and drawn forward to expose the intestines. The difference in the ruminant is only that the greater omentum has firm attachments on both sides in the caudal part of the abdomen. On the left the greater omentum is attached to the caudal groove of the rumen, and on the right it is adhered to the medial surface of the descending duodenum and its mesoduodenum. Thus the greater omentum forms a sling ventral to the intestines. The space in which they lie is the supraomental recess. When the peritoneal cavity is opened from the right flank, all of the intestines except the descending duodenum are usually concealed by the greater omentum. To reach them it is necessary to draw the omentum cranially, as in the dog, but the omentum is not so easily displaced.

The reason for the caudal attachment of the greater omentum in ruminants is shown in the schematic diagrams of its development (see Fig. 22–1). The dorsal mesogastrium is attached along the greater curvature of the stomach primordium everywhere except at the fundus. Here the line of attachment leaves the future dorsal sac of the rumen free and follows the future caudal groove so that only the ventral sac is covered by omentum. Over the primordium of the abomasum the greater omentum elongates and reflects on itself to form a sac. When the rumen primordium is forced to turn caudally by space limitations in the craniodorsal abdominal cavity, it carries the attachment of the greater omentum with it. On the right the omentum adheres to the descending duodenum. In the diagrams the dorsal attachment of the omentum is greatly elongated; actually it is very short. The attachment to the stomach in the adult follows the line established in the embryo: along the right longitudinal groove, around the caudal groove, cranially in the left longitudinal groove, across the cranial sac to the greater curvature of the reticulum, to the greater curvature of the abomasum, which it follows back to the right side and up to the epiploic foramen along the duodenum. The attachment to the duodenum is on the opposite side from the attachment of the lesser omentum.

The pylorus may be recognized during surgery by the adjacent cushion of fat in the attached greater omentum, which forms a prominence, the so-called pig's ear. On the parietal surface the pylorus appears to be a blind pouch separated from the duodenum by a band of subserous fat.

The reticulo-omasal orifice, at the ventral end of the reticular groove, opens into the omasal groove. This in turn conducts to the omasoabomasal orifice. The transfer of ingesta from the ruminoreticular cavity to the abomasum is an active cyclic process, requiring coordinated contraction and relaxation of the reticulum, reticulo-omasal orifice, and omasum.[35] Paralysis of the omasum results in a fatal stasis of ingesta in the ruminoreticulum and omasum.

The abomasum is a long, thin-walled sac that is capable of distention to enormous size when atonic. It is attached to the omasum around the omasoabomasal orifice. The fundus of the abomasum is attached on the left side to the reticulum and to the atrium and ventral sac of the rumen by bands of smooth muscle. These bands are covered by the attachment of the greater omentum to form palpable ligaments. One of these, called the reticuloabomasal ligament, is a landmark for abdominal exploration.[33] Because of these attachments, severe displacements of the abomasum to the left or right often involve the reticulum and omasum.

When the abomasum is distended, it bends in the middle and forms a loop between the omasum and the cranial duodenum. The greater curvature, with the line of attachment of the greater omentum, is on the outside of the loop. The lesser omentum is on the inside and serves as the axis for rotation if volvulus occurs. The crest of the loop may slip under the rumen and creep up the left side toward the left flank (left displacement of the abomasum, LDA, see Fig. 22–2). It is buoyed up by the gas trapped at the top of the loop and may be pushed along by alternate contraction and relaxation of the atrium of the rumen.[32]

The loop of abomasum may simply dilate caudally in a sagittal plane on the right side with the pyloric part dorsal (right displacement, RDA), or it may undergo volvulus through 180 to 450° usually counterclockwise as viewed from the rear or the right side of the cow (see Figs. 22–3 and 22–4).[14] The site of volvulus, where the duodenum is wrapped around the axis of the stomach, is often at the reticulo-omasal junction. Torsion may occur here, either through the reticulum or be-

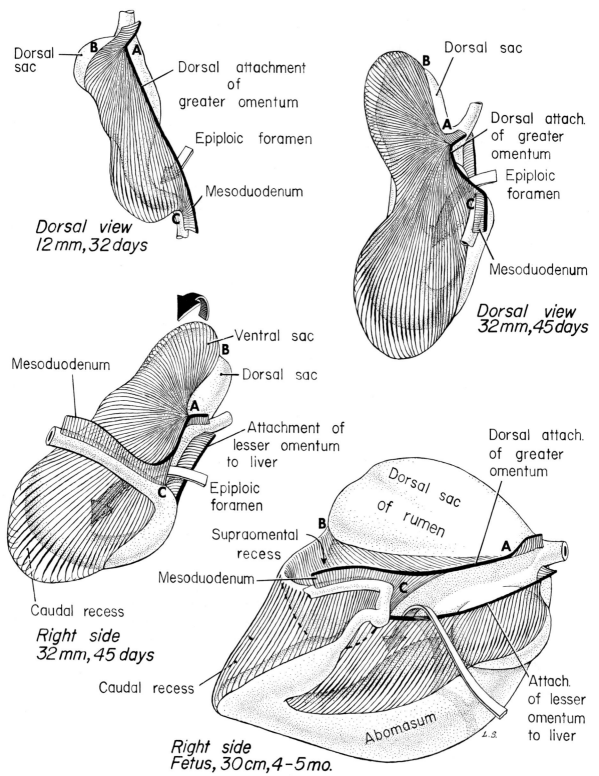

Dorsal sac

B **A**

Dorsal attachment of greater omentum

Epiploic foramen

Mesoduodenum

C

Dorsal view
12 mm, 32 days

Dorsal sac

B

A

Dorsal attach. of greater omentum

Epiploic foramen

C

Mesoduodenum

Dorsal view
32 mm, 45 days

Mesoduodenum

Ventral sac

B

Dorsal sac

A

Attachment of lesser omentum to liver

C

Epiploic foramen

Supraomental recess

Mesoduodenum

Caudal recess

Right side
32 mm, 45 days

Caudal recess

Dorsal attach. of greater omentum

Dorsal sac of rumen

B

A

C

Abomasum

Attach. of lesser omentum to liver

L.S.

Right side
Fetus, 30 cm, 4–5 mo.

Figure 22–1. Diagrams of the development of the bovine stomach and omental bursa. *A,* cardiac region; *B,* caudal groove of rumen; *C,* caudal border of the epiploic foramen where the greater omentum is continuous with the mesoduodenum. The supra-omental recess contains the intestines.

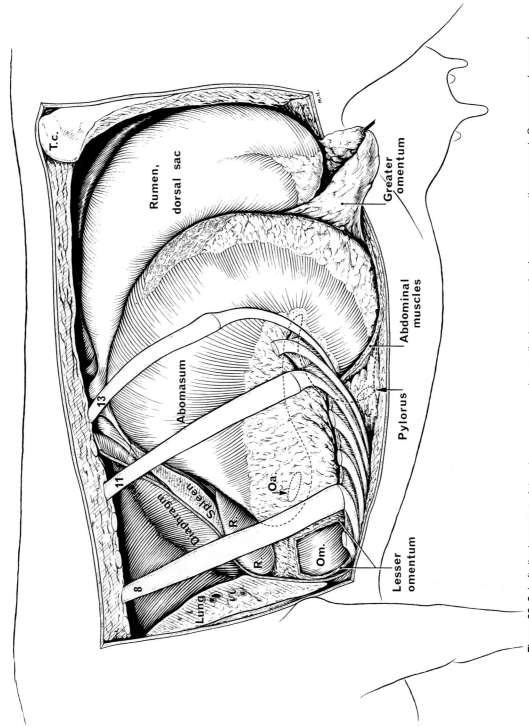

Figure 22–2. Left displacement of the abomasum, cow. Lung, diaphragm, and spleen were partly removed. *Oa,* omasoabomasal orifice; *Om,* omasum; *R,* reticulum; *Tc,* tuber coxae; *8, 11, 13,* ribs of like number.[32]

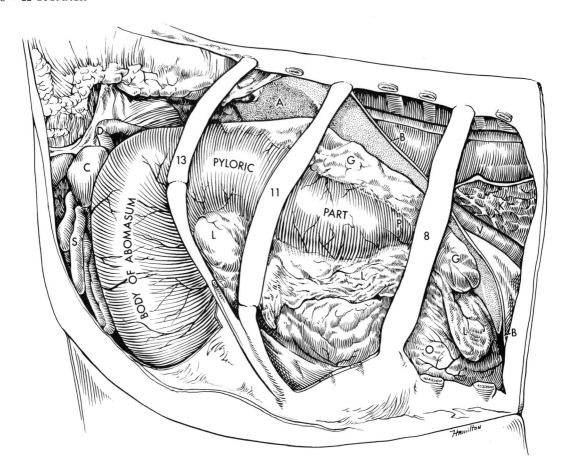

Figure 22–3. Right displacement of the abomasum with counterclockwise valvules, cow. Lung and diaphragm were partly removed. The abomasum probably extended farther dorsally before death. *A,* depression formed by the abomasum on the diaphragmatic surface of the medially displaced liver; *B,* cut edge of the diaphragm; *C,* cecum; *D,* caudal flexure of the duodenum; *G,* greater omentum; *K,* lung, cut surface; *L,* lesser omentum; *O,* omasum covered by lesser omentum; *P,* pylorus; *S,* jejunum; *V, caudal vena cava; 8, 11, 13,* ribs of like number.[14] (See Fig. 22–4,4.)

tween the reticulum and omasum, with serious damage to the vagal trunks and blood vessels. If the rotation of the abomasum is 180° or less, it will usually correct itself when the contents have been drained by gastrocentesis. If the volvulus is more severe, it must be corrected manually after drainage. To determine the direction of rotation it is necessary to palpate along the pyloric part of the abomasum to the pylorus. In a 360° counterclockwise volvulus, the pylorus will be found cranially on the right side with the duodenum passing cranially, medially, and ventrally around the neck of the omasum. Its further course is out of reach, but it continues on the medial side of the neck of the omasum, then between the displaced reticulum and the rumen to the hepatoduodenal ligament. The duodenum is freed from the omasum by retracting the latter caudoventrally and pushing the duodenum dorsocranially and then ventrally around the omasal curvature. The pylorus is pushed ventrally on the right and then to the left, ventral to the rest of the abomasum. This is the beginning of clockwise correction. It is usually completed spontaneously.[14] In some cattle, the omasum is not included in the volvulus, and the duodenum crosses the omasoabomasal junction, where a torsion in the stomach occurs. It is corrected in a similar manner. A 360° clockwise volvulus as viewed from the rear is less common. The pyloric part of the abomasum extends away from the right flank incision toward the median plane, and the pylorus should be pushed ventrally and to the left to begin the counterclockwise correction.[8]

The pathogenesis of atony, distention, and displacement of the abomasum varies with the conditions of husbandry, and many different causes have been reported. Only a few anatomical aspects will be discussed here. Pregnancy is a predisposing factor as shown in Figure 22–6. Intensive feeding of concentrates to dairy cattle disrupts the normal sequence of digestion in the compartments

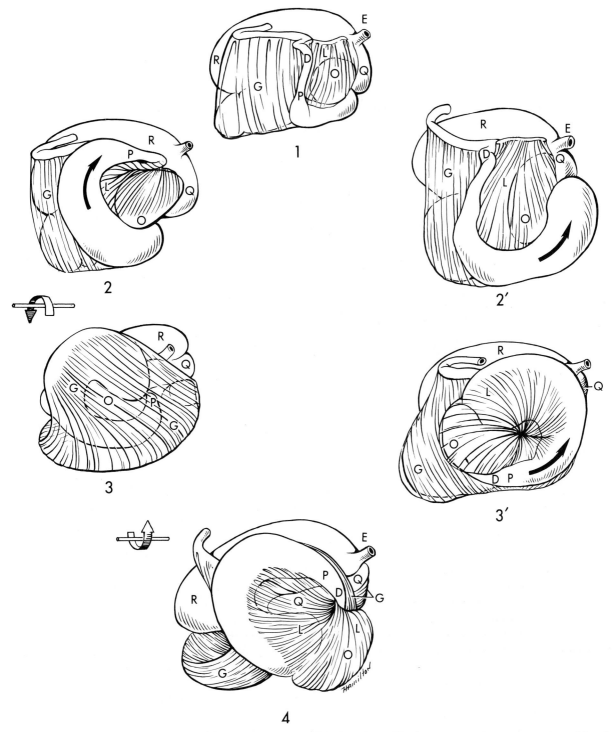

Figure 22–4. Diagrams showing two possible modes of rotation of the loop formed by the omasum, abomasum, and cranial part of the duodenum in volvulus. *1*, normal; *2*, simple dilatation and displacement on the right; *3*, 180° volvulus around the longitudinal axis of the lesser omentum, counterclockwise as seen from the rear; *2'*, 90° rotation of the abomasum in a sagittal plane, counterclockwise as seen from the right; *3'*, 180° rotation of the abomasum and omasum around the transverse axis of the lesser omentum, drawing the duodenum cranially, medial to the omasum; *4*, 360° counterclockwise volvulus, final stage resulting from either mode of rotation. Between *3* and *4* the greater omentum is forced cranial to the rotating abomasum. *D*, duodenum; *E*, esophagus; *G*, greater omentum; *L*, lesser omentum; *O*, omasum; *P*, pylorus; *Q*, reticulum; *R*, rumen.[14]

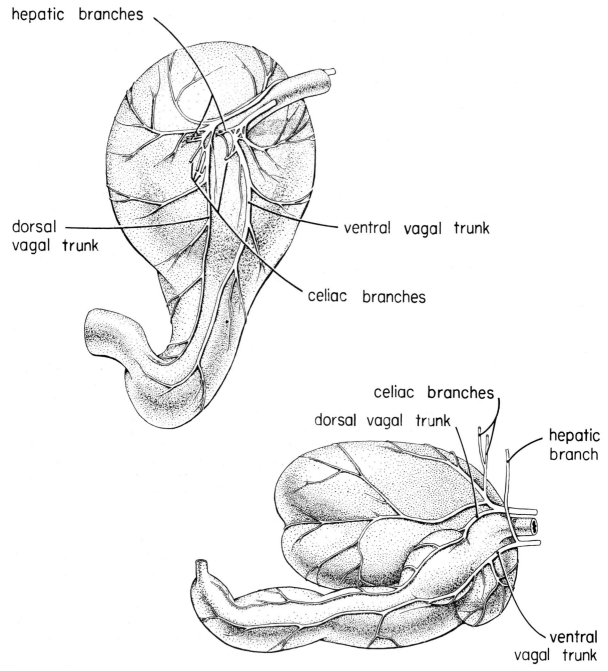

hepatic branches

dorsal
vagal trunk

ventral vagal trunk

celiac branches

celiac branches

dorsal vagal trunk

hepatic
branch

ventral
vagal trunk

Figure 22–5. The course of the dorsal and ventral vagal trunks along the lesser curvature of the canine stomach (above) and the fetal bovine stomach (below), viewed from the right. (Canine modified from N. J. Mizere: The anatomy of the autonomic nervous system in the dog. Am. J. Anat. *96* (1955): 285–318, and Bovine from H. Christ: Nervus vagus und die Nervengeflechte der Vormägen der Wiederkäuer. Zeitsch. Zellf. *11* (1930): 342–374.

of the ruminant stomach. On a natural diet of grass or dry roughage, the feed is coarse and light when first swallowed and therefore floats on the surface of the ingesta in the rumen. It stimulates mucosal receptors of the vagus, which reflexly increase motility. This coarse material floats at the proper level to enter the esophagus for regurgitation and rumination. When it is reswallowed, it is more finely comminuted and insalivated, has a higher specific gravity, and sinks below the surface in the constantly agitated contents of the ruminoreticulum. As the cellulose and other carbohydrates are fermented by microorganisms, the remaining fine particles filter down to the level of the reticulo-omasal orifice. When that opens, they are carried into the omasum and abdomasum as a fluid suspension. In the ruminoreticulum, the gas production from fermentation is eliminated by specialized eructation reflexes. When concentrates are fed, they sink rapidly to the level of the reticulo-omasal orifice. Fermentation and the rate of flow to the abomasum are increased; the abomasum is overloaded; its rate of contraction is decreased by a disputed mechanism;[2, 37] and gas production is increased. Gas accumulates in the fundus, raising it above the omaso-abomasal orifice, where gas normally escapes.

A few cases of abomasal atony, distention, and dislocation have been attributed to vagal paresis resulting from a lesion on the vagus nerve. This is one form of vagal indigestion. The vagus contains both afferent and efferent fibers that mediate the gastric reflexes through centers in the medulla, which are in turn influenced by the cerebral cortex and the hypothalamus. The gastric branches of the dorsal and ventral vagal trunks are distributed in essentially the same manner as in the simple stomach (Fig. 22–5). Both trunks run along the lesser curvature; the dorsal trunk supplies the visceral surface, and the ventral trunk supplies the parietal surface. The efferent fibers synapse with ganglion cells in the myenteric plexus and, in the abomasum, also in the submucosal plexus. There is strong evidence for association neurons in the myenteric plexus. The postganglionic axons innervate muscle and, in the abomasum, also glands. This system is vulnerable at any point from the receptors in the mucous membrane, up the vagus, through the centers in the brain, down the vagus, and through the plexuses in the stomach wall to the muscle or gland. Any element could conceivably be destroyed or irritated by a lesion, and both afferent and efferent neurons can be either inhibitory or stimulatory. Thus it is possible to take a simple abscess on or near a vagal trunk and interpret it to account for almost any gastric dysfunction.

The functions regulated by the vagus are: (1) the ruminoreticular contraction cycle; (2) the omasal cycle, required for the transport of ingesta from the reticulum to the abomasum, a vital function; (3) eructation, another vital function; (4) regurgitation for rumination; (5) reflex closure of the reticular groove in the suckling, also elicited in the adult; (6) abomasal motility, to a limited extent, increasing or decreasing the tonus and frequency; (7) abomasal secretion, but the influence is slight because the secretion of gastric juice in ruminants is almost continuous.

The concept of vagal indigestion was developed largely from the experimental sectioning of the vagal trunks and their branches at various points and observing syndromes like those of spontaneous diseases.[13] Section of the dorsal and ventral trunks on the terminal esophagus was fatal in 20 to 30 days. The rumen cannot be heard or seen to contract, but the animal continues to eat and the ruminoreticulum becomes distended. Eructation and rumination cease and mild bloat occurs. The reticular groove reflex is abolished. The abomasum can slowly empty itself, and sheep, at least, can be maintained by feeding through an abomasal fistula. There is, therefore, no pyloric stenosis. The elimination of vagal impulses does not result in spasm of the orifices from unopposed sympathetic stimuli. Splanchnotomy does not prevent the effects of vagotomy, which are paretic, not spastic. The splanchnic nerves have an inhibitory effect on the motility of the stomach.

Dorsal vagotomy on the terminal esophagus stops the activity of the ruminoreticulum for a longer period than ventral vagotomy. The fact that the animal recovers from either operation indicates an important associative function of the ganglion cells of the myenteric plexus. The enteric nervous system is extremely complex, not well understood, and has extensive autonomous capability.

Section of both dorsal and ventral trunks just distal to the origin of the ruminal nerves causes fatal omasal paralysis. The ruminoreticulum is distended but continues to contract. The omasum and abomasum are practically empty at autopsy. Unfortunately, this condition, which also occurs spontaneously, has been called "functional reticulo-omasal stenosis." It is not a stenosis.

Section of both dorsal and ventral trunks on the omasum produces a fatal abomasal atony and distention. Ruminoreticular motility is retained and often increased.

Spontaneous vagal indigestion with signs like those described in the previous paragraphs has been attributed to a variety of lesions that could interrupt motor impulses in the vagus nerves. The most convincing are abscesses of the caudal mediastinal lymph nodes that involve the dorsal vagal trunk on the esophagus and abscesses from penetrating foreign bodies that involve the vagal trunks along the gastric groove. Only in rare cases, however, have such lesions been shown to produce significant degeneration of nerve fibers. Many cases with the clinical syndrome have no lesion at autopsy that involves a vagal trunk.

The afferent neurons of excitatory and inhibitory gastric reflexes are important in disorders of gastric motility.[18, 19] The low-threshold tension receptors in the wall of the reticulum that stimulate contractions could be blocked by the changes of traumatic reticulitis. The acid receptors in the abomasum that excite forestomach motility could be damaged by stretching or disease of the wall. Inhibitory afferents demonstrated are: high-threshold tension receptors that slow the contractions of the ruminoreticulum when it is overloaded, tension receptors in the abomasum that slow the ruminoreticulum, and receptors anywhere in the body that evoke pain. Thus in some cases vagal inhibition of gastric function may be a normal protective reflex elicited by the pain of traumatic peritonitis. Some feel that the most effective treatment of "vagal indigestion" is the surgical removal of a penetrating foreign body.[5]

A theory of irritative as well as destructive vagal lesions has evolved to account for certain side reactions. Occasionally cattle with so-called vagal indigestion have bradycardia.[9, 26, 28] This is explained as an irritating lesion of the vagal afferent neurons in the abdomen that causes reflex activity of the parasympathetic vagal motor neurons in the medulla. This may result in bradycardia and an increased rate of ruminal contractions. The latter are usually less effective than normal contractions, and the rumen is distended, causing a visible abdominal enlargement. The bradycardia can be eliminated by atropine.

There are several diagnostic measures in addition to the atropine test that can be used to evaluate the vagus.[5] If the reticular groove reflex is elicited by a 10 percent solution of sodium sulfate administered in the oral vestibule, the sound of the solution splashing into the abomasum can be heard with a stethoscope. This is normal in adult cattle and indicates integrity of the vagus as far distally as the reticular groove. If the sodium sulfate is added to a contrast medium, radiographic studies of the motility of the gastric groove, omasum, and abomasum are possible in cattle. The clinical significance of this reflex in the adult should not be overlooked. Many pharmaceutical products intended to act in the rumen have been shown to elicit the reticular groove reflex if given by mouth. They must be placed in the rumen by stomach tube.

The omasal canal and part of the abomasum can be explored during rumenotomy by passing the left hand through the reticulo-omasal orifice.[5, 7] In some cases of digestive disease the orifice is open, but normally it is only passable for one to three fingers. Dilatation is facilitated by eliciting the reticular groove reflex.

22c. DISSECTION, THORAX, ABDOMEN, NEWBORN CALF

Identify the following structures: diaphragm, lungs, aorta, esophagus, caudal vena cava, liver. Observe the relation of the caudal mediastinal lymph node to the right dorsal surface of the esophagus. Abscesses of the node can cause bloat by compression of the esophagus. They may also injure the dorsal vagal trunk and disturb the motility of the stomach. Identify the reticulum and the fundus of the abomasum ventral to it. Attached to the left side of the rumen is the spleen, disassociated from the greater omentum by the development of the rumen. Find the omasum, abomasum, pylorus, duodenum, and jejunum and the umbilical vein entering the liver.

22d. LIVE COW

Rumen

Palpation. The rumen, palpated through the left paralumbar fossa, is normally resilient but yields to firm pressure. The ruminoreticular contraction cycle begins with a double contraction of the reticulum, followed immediately by a contraction of the rumen. The rumen contraction begins in the cranial sac and progresses to the dorsal sac and then to the ventral sac. A palpable swelling occurs in the paralumbar fossa when the wall of the dorsal sac is forced outward by ingesta that have been elevated by the contraction of the pillars and the wall of the dorsal sac.[21] After a pause of about 30 seconds, there is usually a second rumen contraction associated with eructation. This eructation contraction is not preceded by a contraction of the reticulum. Thus there are normally two palpable rumen contractions per minute. The rate is increased to about 2.8 contractions per minute while the animal is eating.

Percussion. The upper third gives a tympanitic sound, changing to dullness at the middle third.

Auscultation. A churning sound is heard at the time of each rumen contraction. The sound gradually reaches a peak, then recedes.

Reticulum

Palpation. The organ cannot be palpated. It is in contact with the left abdominal wall at the ventral ends of the sixth and seventh intercostal spaces. In traumatic gastritis, pain may be produced by deep pressure here or in the left xiphoid region (see Fig. 22–6; see also Plate II).

Auscultation. The double contraction is difficult to separate into two components. The sound of liquid and gas in motion can be heard at the ventral ends of the sixth and seventh intercostal spaces at intervals of about 1 minute, followed by a rumen contraction. Usually there are two palpable rumen contractions between contractions of the reticulum. Variations in the cycle are not necessarily pathological, nor is absence of sound in the reticulum. A grunt of pain may be associated with contraction of the reticulum in traumatic reticulitis.[39]

Omasum

Palpation. The organ is enclosed by the ribs but can be palpated through the wall of the rumen during rumenotomy. (See Getty, Figure 29–43.[10]) This should be done routinely when the rumen is explored. Enlargement indicates atony or paralysis of the omasum. In traumatic peritonitis involving the omasum, pain may be produced by deep pressure in the ventral part of the right seventh to ninth intercostal spaces and in the right xiphoid region (see Fig. 22–6).

Percussion. Dullness, indistinguishable from that of the liver dorsally.

Auscultation. The spaces mentioned above should be auscultated, although only slight noises are heard there normally. Liquid sounds are said to indicate a back-up of fluid accumulated as a result of atony of the abomasum. The dull transmitted roar of rumen contractions must be eliminated from consideration. If the stethoscope is placed too far caudally, the normal sounds of the pylorus may be heard.

Abomasum

The fundus is in the xiphoid region; the body lies on the midline, with more than half of it on the left in the Holstein and a smaller portion in the Jersey.[22] The pyloric part curves around to the right behind the omasum, with the greater curvature crossing the midline at the umbilicus or a few centimeters caudal to it. The pylorus is in the transverse plane of the 10th, 11th, or 12th rib and 10 to 20 cm. ventral to the costal arch (see Fig. 22–6).[22]

The site for puncture of the abomasum to sample its contents is on the midline, one-third of the distance from the ''nick'' to the umbilicus.[36] The nick is seen from the side of the standing cow as a break in the ventral contour between the horizontal sternal surface and the decline of the abdominal wall. It marks the junction of the xiphoid cartilage with the xiphoid process.

The position just described is that of the normal abomasum in a standing cow. The position varies with the relative size and weight of the rumen, omasum, and abomasum. In the sheep, goat, and calf, the omasum is small and rides high on the abomasum, allowing the latter to run parallel to the right costal arch. In the cow, the larger and heavier omasum forces the abomasum to the left. The pregnant uterus pressing forward on the pyloric part of the abomasum tends to accentuate the curvature and promote displacement to the left. Rolling a cow on her back for laparotomy or autopsy causes marked changes in the position of the abomasum.

The percussion note is normally a muffled resonance, which may become tympanitic in gastrointestinal disease of calves. The auscultation sound is a gurgle or tinkle resembling that of the intestine.

Displacement to the left is diagnosed by simultaneous percussion and auscultation of high-

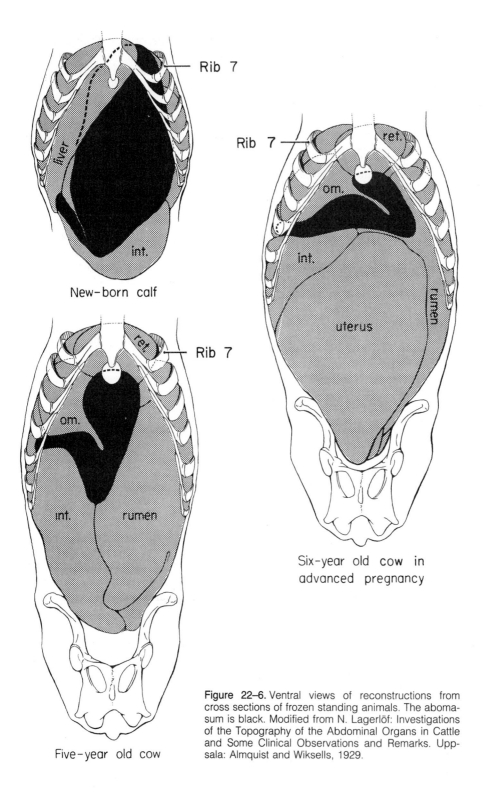

Rib 7

New-born calf

Rib 7

Five-year old cow

Rib 7

Six-year old cow in
advanced pregnancy

Figure 22–6. Ventral views of reconstructions from cross sections of frozen standing animals. The abomasum is black. Modified from N. Lagerlöf: Investigations of the Topography of the Abdominal Organs in Cattle and Some Clinical Observations and Remarks. Uppsala: Almquist and Wiksells, 1929.

pitched sounds high on the left side in the 11th intercostal space. Distention on the right causes elevation of the last rib. Splashing noises can be elicited in the right flank by movement of the animal or by ballottement. Percussion reveals a horizontal line between tympany in the upper part of the abomasum and fluid contents in the lower part. In simple distention, the area of liver dullness (see Chapter 24) is not reduced. In counterclockwise volvulus the abomasum moves in between the liver and the right abdominal wall, causing the disappearance of the area of liver dullness (see Fig.

22–3). Distention on the right side is palpable per rectum. It can be differentiated from distention of the cecum by the fact that only the left side of the distended abomasum can be felt, while the whole circumference of the distended cecum is palpable.

An important early step in the diagnosis of abdominal disease is to observe the outline of the abdomen from the rear.[12] Distention of the dorsal part of the left flank indicates acute bloat with free gas. Elevation of the last few ribs on the left is associated with displaced abomasum on the left. Distention and tympany of the whole left and ventral contour is a sign of foamy bloat. Enlargement of the whole left flank and the ventral part of the right flank without tympany is seen in engorgement of the rumen with fluid ingesta, resulting from a disturbance of motility of the forestomach. Elevation of the dorsal part of the right flank with tympany occurs with distention and volvulus of the abomasum on the right and with distention of the cecum.[34] Distention of the right ventral abdomen in calves is seen in chronic distention of the abomasum. In adult cows, it accompanies pregnancy. Bilateral ventral distention, the pear-shaped abdomen, is associated with dropsy, either ascitic or in the fetal membranes.[11, 31]

Radiography of the reticulodiaphragmatic region with the animal standing or in dorsal recumbency may identify a radiopaque foreign object within or passing through the wall of the reticulum. Dorsal recumbency causes gas to rise into the reticulum and permits better contrast to diagnose a penetrating foreign body.

Note the position of the superficial epigastric (mammary) veins on the ventral abdominal wall. These should be identified before the cow is put in dorsal recumbency for paramedian abdominal surgery, when they will be collapsed.

22e. RADIOGRAPHS, STOMACH, DOG AND CAT

Radiographs will show the stomach in various states of distention and contraction. The empty stomach is well within the costal arch, caudal to the liver between the planes of the ninth thoracic and first lumbar vertebrae (see Plate III). It usually parallels the tenth intercostal space. The ventral surface of the stomach is separated from the abdominal floor by coils of small intestine. The transverse colon is often just caudal to the stomach and filled with gas. When moderately filled, the stomach expands to the left, coming into contact with the diaphragm at the left of the liver but does not reach the abdominal floor. The greater curvature will parallel the left 12th rib. The filled stomach dilates caudoventrally so that the greater curvature may lie transversely on the floor of the abdomen midway between the xiphoid cartilage and the pubis.

The stomach is most readily recognized by the gas that is usually in it. This gas accumulates in the fundus, which is the most dorsal part of the stomach caudal to the left crus of the diaphragm. In some radiographs, a fluid level appears below the gas. In right lateral recumbency most of the gas accumulates in the fundus, whereas in left recumbency it may rise into the pyloric part. The opposite effect is observed on the fluid contents or barium in contrast studies. As a rule, there is less gas in the stomach and small intestine of the cat. The pylorus may be seen as a round dense structure in the ventral half of the abdomen caudal to the liver, superimposed on the body of the stomach. Do not mistake it for a foreign body. The fundus and body are usually twice the size of the pyloric part. In ventrodorsal radiographs the fundus and body are on the left, with the pyloric part on the right of the midline in the dog. In the cat, the entire stomach is usually on the left, with the pyloric part extending to the midline, and the angle between the body and pyloric part is more acute.[24] The fundus is adjacent to the left crus of the diaphragm; the pyloric part is next to the liver. In ventrodorsal radiographs the stomach gas is usually in the body and pyloric part. In dorsoventral radiographs it is in the fundus. The radiographic appearance of the stomach is influenced by the breed and by the shape of thorax and abdomen. Breeds with a wide thorax have a wider-appearing fundus and body and a more convex caudal border in both views. Those with a deep narrow thorax have a long, slender-appearing stomach with a more straight caudal border.

Enlargement of adjacent organs may be diagnosed by the displacement of the stomach. The stomach will be displaced caudally by a liver mass, cranially by a mass in the left lobe of the pancreas or secondary to liver atrophy or a diaphragmatic hernia, and cranially and to the right by a splenic mass.

The administration of a radiopaque suspension, usually barium sulfate, will outline the esophagus, which is normally not visible on plain radiographs. The barium will more accurately determine the position, size, and shape of the stomach as well as outline its mucosal pattern and will allow assessment of its ability to move the contrast agent into the small intestine.

Following the swallow of a paste preparation of barium sulfate, the esophagram of a normal dog will show linear streaks outlining the crypts between longitudinal folds of mucosa. The same will be observed in the cranial two-thirds of a cat's esophagus, but transverse and oblique striations will be apparent in the caudal third. Barium suspension will seek the lowest level in the stomach and therefore will fill and distend the fundus when the animal is in left lateral or dorsal recumbency. The pyloric part will be filled in right lateral and ventral recumbency.

22f. STOMACH, SPLEEN, AND OMENTUM, DOG

Orient the stomach as it would be seen after a paracostal incision. The fundus is on the dog's left, the pylorus on the right; the greater omentum extends caudally from the greater curvature. The parietal surface of the stomach is in contact with the liver in the standing position. The lesser curvature is attached to the liver by the lesser omentum. The spleen is attached to the greater omentum along the left part of the greater curvature of the stomach.

The main blood vessels of the stomach run along both curvatures. The greater curvature is supplied by the gastroepiploic arteries: the right from the gastroduodenal, a branch of the hepatic, and the left from the splenic artery. The left end of the greater curvature is supplied by the short gastric arteries from the splenic branches in the dorsal part of the hilus of the spleen. The lesser curvature is supplied by the right gastric artery from the hepatic and the left gastric artery from the celiac. The best site for gastrotomy is in the middle of the parietal surface.

Palpate the pylorus. The treatment for congenital pyloric stenosis is incision of the pyloric sphincter from the serosa down to the submucosa.

To understand the mechanics of volvulus, think of the stomach as a tubular organ with its two ends attached close together and the organ forming a loop, which extends caudoventrally on the abdominal floor.[38] The more the stomach is distended, the longer the loop becomes. Volvulus is a twist of this distended loop on the axis of the lesser omentum. Usually it turns clockwise as seen from the caudoventral aspect. The fixed attachments are the esophagus and the hepatoduodenal ligament at opposite sides of the lesser omentum. In clockwise volvulus, the fundus turns dorsally and to the right and then ventrally, passing through 270° so that the greater curvature of the body is on the ventral midline. This twists the cardiac end of the esophagus into a tight closure; inability to pass a stomach tube is a diagnostic sign. The pylorus, turning only 180°, moves from right to left and stretches the duodenum across the ventral surface of the esophagus.[25]

The dorsal end of the spleen is attached to the diaphragm by a part of the greater omentum—the phrenicosplenic ligament. The middle of the spleen is attached by the left gastroepiploic vessels and the gastrosplenic ligament to the greater curvature of the stomach. When the greater curvature moves to the right, the spleen is pulled into a V shape with the dorsal and ventral ends lagging. Constriction of the veins caused by the torsion results in congestion of the stomach and great enlargement of the spleen, which may be palpated through the abdominal wall. If the patient goes to autopsy, the volvulus of the stomach may be inadvertently reduced post mortem, but the coagulated blood in the spleen holds the tell-tale V shape.[16]

Lateral radiographs of the abdomen of a dog with gastric volvulus usually show a severely enlarged gas-filled stomach that appears to be oriented craniocaudally and has a fold cranially in the dorsal plane that partially divides it into dorsal and ventral compartments.[15] Usually the pyloric part of the stomach is dorsal and the fundic part is ventral. Gastric dilatation compresses the caudal vena cava as it passes dorsal to the stomach. Volvulus of the stomach causes torsion of the portal vein in the hepatoduodenal ligament. Both of these venous compressions result in decreased cardiac output and ineffective tissue perfusion and lead to hypovolemic shock.[20] Decompression of the gas-filled stomach can be performed by gastrocentesis in either the left or right paracostal area, where the distended stomach is most prominent. To reposition the stomach after exposure by a laparotomy, the pylorus should be located on the left side near the cardia. Simultaneously lift the pylorus toward the incision and push the fundus dorsally into the abdomen. This usually results in a rapid counterclockwise movement of the loop of stomach to its normal position.

Gastrostomy and placement of a tube through the abdominal wall into the stomach are done for feeding or for decompression and to create adhesions.[4] A tube for decompression is usually placed into the pyloric part through the cranial ventral abdominal wall in the angle between the xiphoid cartilage and right costal arch. For placement of a feeding tube the fundus is approached through the left dorsal paracostal area. The fibers of each abdominal muscle are separated parallel to their orientation.

References

1. Brawner, W. R., Jr. and J. E. Bartels: Contrast radiography of the digestive tract—indications, techniques, complications. Vet. Clin. North Am. *13* (1983):599–626.
2. Breukink, H. J. and T. de Ruyter: Abomasal displacement in cattle: influence of concentrates in the ration on fatty acid concentrations in ruminal, abomasal, and duodenal contents. Am. J. Vet. Res. *37* (1976):1181–1184.
3. Christ, H.: Nervus vagus und die Nervengeflechte der Vormägen der Wiederkäuer. Zeitschr. Zellf. *11* (1930):342–374.
4. Crane, S. W.: Placement and maintenance of a temporary feeding tube gastrostomy in the dog and cat. Comp. Cont. Ed. *11* (1980):770–776.
5. Dietz, O. et al.: Untersuchungen zur Vagusfunktion, zur Vagusbeeinflussung und zu Vagusausfällen am Verdauungsapparat des erwachsenen Rindes. Arch. Exp. Veterinärmed. *24* (1970):1385–1439.
6. Dirksen, G.: Die Erweiterung, Verlagerung und Drehung des Labmagens beim Rind. Zentralbl. Vet. Med. *8* (1961):977–1015.
7. Ducharme, N. G.: Surgical considerations in the treatment of traumatic reticuloperitonitis. Comp. Cont. Ed. *5* (1983):S213–S219.
8. Espersen, G.: Die rechtseitige Labmagenerweiterung und -verlagerung (Dilatatio abomasi cum dislocatione dextra) beim Rind. Deutsche Tierärztl. Wschr. *68* (1961):2–7.
9. Ferrante, P. L. and R. H. Whitlock: Chronic (vagus) indigestion in cattle. Comp. Cont. Ed. *3* (1981):S231–S237.
10. Getty, R. (ed.): Sisson and Grossman's The Anatomy of the Domestic Animals, 5th ed., Philadelphia: W. B. Saunders, 1975.
11. Gibbons, W. J.: Clinical Diagnosis of Diseases of Large Animals. Philadelphia: Lea & Febiger, 1966.
12. Grymer, J. and N. K. Ames: Bovine abdominal pings: clinical examination and differential diagnosis. Comp. Cont. Ed. *8* (1981):S311–S318.
13. Habel, R. E.: A study of the innervation of the ruminant stomach. Cornell Vet. *46* (1956):555–628.
14. Habel, R. E. and D. F. Smith: Volvulus of the bovine abomasum and omasum. JAVMA *179* (1981):447–455.
15. Kneller, S. K.: Radiographic interpretation of the gastric dilatation-volvulus complex in the dog. J. Am. Anim. Hosp. Assoc. *12* (1976):154–157.
16. Krook, L.: Department of Pathology, New York State College of Veterinary Medicine, Cornell University, Ithaca, N.Y. Personal communication, 1963.
17. Lagerlöf, N.: Investigations of the Topography of the Abdominal Organs in Cattle and Some Clinical Observations and Remarks. Uppsala: Almqvist and Wiksells, 1929.
18. Leek, B. F.: "Vagus indigestion" in cattle. Vet. Rec. *82* (1968):498–499.
19. Leek, B. F.: Reticulo-ruminal function and dysfunction. Vet. Rec. *84* (1969):238–243.
20. Matthiesen, D. T.: The gastric dilatation-volvulus complex: medical and surgical considerations. J. Am. Anim. Hosp. Assoc. *19* (1983):925–932.
21. McCarthy, P. H.: Surface rippling of the lower left flank of the cow: mirror of rumen motility. Am. J. Vet. Res. *42* (1981):225–228.
22. McCarthy, P. H.: Transruminal palpation and surface projection of the abomasum in the permanently fistulated dairy cow. Am. J. Vet. Res. *42* (1981):1927–1932.
23. Mizeres, N. J.: The anatomy of the autonomic nervous system in the dog. Am. J. Anat. *96* (1955):285–318.
24. Morgan, J. P.: The upper gastrointestinal examination in the cat: normal radiographic appearance using positive contrast medium. Vet. Rad. *22* (1981):159–169.
25. Morgan, R. V.: Acute gastric dilatation-volvulus syndrome. Comp. Cont. Ed. *4* (1982):677–682.
26. Neal, P. A. and G. B. Edwards: "Vagus indigestion" in cattle. Vet. Rec. *82* (1968):396–402.
27. O'Brien, T.: Radiographic Diagnosis of Abdominal Disorders in the Dog and Cat. Philadelphia: W. B. Saunders, 1978.
28. Rebhun, W. C.: Vagus indigestion in cattle. JAVMA *176* (1980):506–510.
29. Rebhun, W. C., S. G. Dill, and H. T. Power: Gastric ulcers in foals. JAVMA *180* (1982):404–407.
30. Rice, D. L.: Gastric torsion in dogs. Mod. Vet. Pract. *64* (1983):117–121.
31. Rosenberger, G.: Die klinische Untersuchung des Rindes. Berlin: Parey, 1964.
32. Sack, W. O.: Abdominal topography of a cow with left abomasal displacement. Am. J. Vet. Res. *8* (1968):1567–1576.
33. Smith, D. F.: Treatment of left displacement of the abomasum. Part I. Comp. Cont. Ed. *3* (1981):S415–S422.
34. Smith, D. F., H. N. Erb, K. M. Kalaher, et al.: The identification of structures and conditions responsible for right side tympanic resonance (ping) in adult cattle. Cornell Vet. *72.* (1982):180–199.
35. Stevens, C. E., A. F. Sellers, and F. A. Spurrell: Function of the bovine omasum in ingesta transfer. Am. J. Physiol. *198* (1960):449–455.
36. Stöber, M.: Die Technik der Labmageninjektion beim Rind. Deutsche Tierärztl. Wschr. *68* (1961):72–75.
37. Svendsen, P.: Abomasal displacement in cattle. Nord. Vet. Med. *22* (1970):571–577.
38. Van Kruiningen, H. J., K. Gregoire, and D. J. Meuten: Acute gastric dilation: a review of comparative aspects, by species, and a study in dogs and monkeys. J. Am. Anim. Hosp. Assoc. *10* (1974):294–324.
39. Williams, E. I.: A study of reticulo-ruminal motility. Vet. Rec. *67* (1955):907–911.

CHAPTER 23

INTESTINES

OBJECTIVES

1. To be able to trace the course of the intestines in each species with reference to the cranial mesenteric artery. This is useful at surgery and at autopsy.
2. To be able to follow the steps in the development of the loop of ascending colon in the pig, ruminant, and horse in order to understand its final placement.
3. To be able to locate each part of the intestinal tract by its position in the abdominal cavity in each species. The location of the ileocolic junction is especially important. This information is useful:
   a. In projecting the parts of the intestinal tract to the body wall for physical diagnosis by palpation, percussion, and auscultation.
   b. For recognition of the segments of the intestines in radiographs of small animals.
   c. For identification of intestines palpated per rectum.
   d. For identification of intestines palpated at laparotomy.
4. To be able to identify the parts of the intestines of the horse at autopsy, laparotomy, or rectal examination by palpation of the longitudinal bands and sacculations of the large intestine. These bands and sacculations are also present in the pig and man but not in carnivores or ruminants.
5. To be able to utilize certain peritoneal folds as landmarks: the duodenocolic, ileocecal, and cecocolic folds.
6. To understand the various displacements of the colon in the horse, including volvulus, and to know how to recognize them on rectal examination and exploratory laparotomy.
7. To know the points of intestinal obstruction in the horse and how to recognize these by the distention of bowel proximal to the obstruction and collapse of bowel caudal to it.
8. To be able to identify the arteries of the intestines, especially in the horse at autopsy in cases of arterial thrombosis.
9. To understand mesodiverticular bands of the mesentery and how these can be a cause of colic.
10. To be able to find the jejunal lymph nodes, which have a different location in the dog and horse from that of the pig and ruminants.

23a. INTESTINES, NEWBORN FOAL AND MODEL

Review the development of the intestines in animals that have a simple colon (man, dog, and cat; see Fig. 23–2). As a result of the clockwise twist of the umbilical loop, as seen from the dorsal aspect, the adult colon and duodenum are hooked into each other with the cranial mesenteric artery enclosed between them. The large colon of the horse develops as a loop of the ascending colon (see Fig. 23–2) between the cecum and the transverse colon. The loop grows cranially to the diaphragm, turns left, and grows caudally to the pelvic region, where the crest of the loop is called the pelvic flexure. The limbs of the loop are the ventral and dorsal colon. The bend in the ventral colon is the sternal flexure, that of the dorsal colon is the diaphragmatic flexure. Because the mesocolon extends all the way from the right side, attached to the apposed surfaces of the dorsal and ventral colon, the large colon is subject to volvulus around the mesocolic axis. In the horse, unlike any other domestic animal, the descending colon also undergoes great elongation and becomes the small colon.

Locate the proximal end of the cranial mesenteric artery and use it as a reference point. It is craniomedial to the base of the cecum. Orient the intestines so that the large colon and cecum are on the right and the small intestine and small colon are on the left. The cranial end of the duodenum lies on the right of the cranial mesenteric artery and cranial to the base of the cecum. The duodenum then passes along the right side of the base of the cecum and crosses from right to left behind it. The duodenojejunal junction is on the left of the cranial mesenteric artery and ventral to the origin of the small colon from the transverse colon. Note the duodenocolic fold at this point. The small intestine usually lies in the left dorsal part of the abdominal cavity and has no bands or sacculations. The lymph nodes of the small intestine are near the root of the mesentery in the horse and dog.

The ileum joins the lesser curvature of the base of the cecum on its medial side. Note the ileocecal fold, a means of identification, attaching the ileum to the dorsal band (tenia) of the cecum. The ileum is affected by various obstructive diseases. Function can be restored by removing the diseased ileum, suturing the stump, and anastomosing the sound ileum to the cecum.[8]

The bands and sacculations of the large intestine are valuable aids in identifying its parts per rectum, at autopsy, or in surgery (Fig. 23–1). The *cecum is sacculated and has four bands.* The dorsal and medial bands extend to the apex. The lateral band may or may not reach the apex. The ventral band joins the medial. The medial and lateral bands are accompanied by the medial and

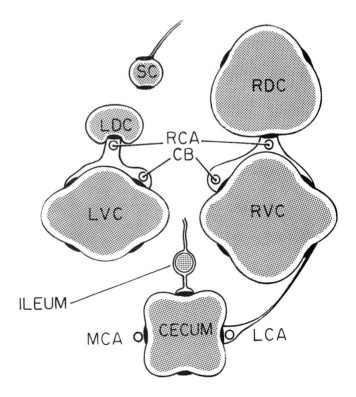

Figure 23–1. Schematic cross sections of the large intestine of the horse. The longitudinal bands of smooth muscle (teniae) are shown as dense black sections. *CB*, colic branch of the ileocolic artery; *LCA*, lateral cecal artery; *LDC*, left dorsal colon; *LVC*, left ventral colon; *MCA*, medial cecal artery; *RCA*, right colic artery; *RDC*, right dorsal colon; *RVC*, right ventral colon; *SC*, small colon. The mesocolon connects the mesocolic bands of the large colon and contains the blood vessels; it is also attached to the small colon. The ileocecal fold connects the ileum to the dorsal band of the cecum. The cecocolic fold connects the lateral band of the cecum to the lateral free band of the right ventral colon.

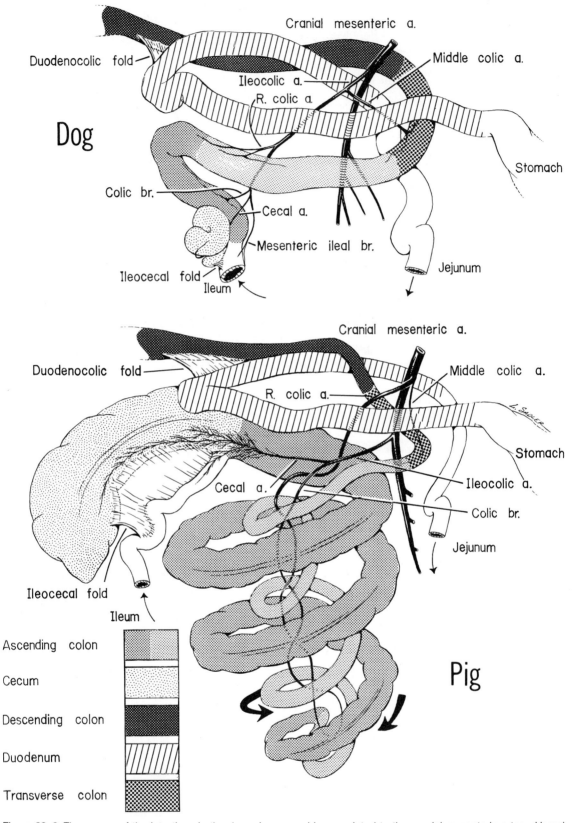

Figure 23–2. The course of the intestines in the dog, pig, ox, and horse related to the cranial mesenteric artery. Homologies indicated by shading.

Illustration continued on opposite page

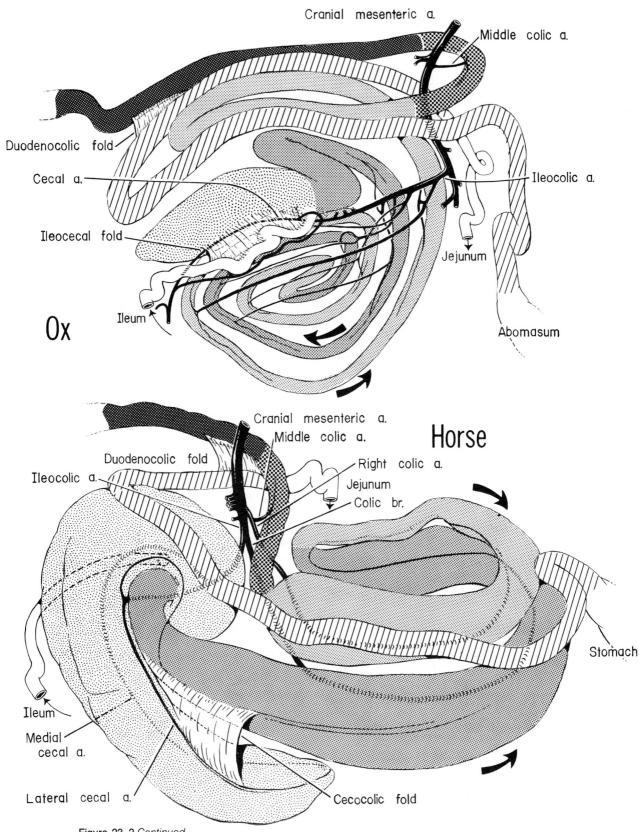

Cranial mesenteric a.

Middle colic a.

Duodenocolic fold

Cecal a.

Ileocolic a.

Ileocecal fold

Jejunum

Ileum

Abomasum

Ox

Cranial mesenteric a.

Middle colic a.

Horse

Duodenocolic fold

Right colic a.

Ileocolic a.

Jejunum

Colic br.

Stomach

Ileum

Medial
cecal a.

Lateral cecal a.

Cecocolic fold

Figure 23–2 *Continued.*

lateral cecal arteries. The cecocolic fold connects the lateral band of the cecum with the lateral free band of the right ventral colon.

The entire *ventral colon is sacculated and has four bands*. On the ventral surface are the lateral and medial free bands, i. e., free of mesocolon and exposed. On the dorsal surface are the lateral and medial mesocolic bands, which are concealed, but can be palpated. At the pelvic flexure only the medial mesocolic band is continued to the left dorsal colon, and the sacculations disappear. Therefore, the *left dorsal colon has only one band*, the mesocolic, *and no sacculations*. There is also a marked decrease in diameter in passing from the left ventral colon to the pelvic flexure, which is a common site for impaction to occur. Near the diaphragmatic flexure, the dorsal colon acquires two free (dorsal) bands so that the *diaphragmatic flexure and the right dorsal colon have three bands*. There are *no sacculations in the dorsal colon*, except some indistinct ones in the terminal part.

The right dorsal colon is the largest part. It turns to the left and decreases markedly in diameter, forming a point of impaction as it becomes the transverse colon. The latter crosses the cranial surface of the cranial mesenteric artery and is continued by the descending colon, which is called the small colon in the horse. The *small colon is sacculated and has two bands*, one of which is concealed in the mesocolic attachment. It is the only part that contains fecal balls.

The arteries of the large colon are the most frequent site of emboli causing colic. The emboli come from a thrombus in the cranial mesenteric artery in strongylosis. The right colic artery follows the mesocolic band of the dorsal colon to the pelvic flexure, where it anastomoses end-to-end with the colic branch of the ileocolic artery (see Fig. 23–2). The colic branch follows the medial mesocolic band of the ventral colon. In addition to the anastomosis at the pelvic flexure, these two arteries are connected by small anastomotic branches, which are most numerous proximally. Each large artery has many connections with an arterial network on the accompanying vein. The anastomoses and the arterial network may serve to by-pass many embolic obstructions.[7] A post-mortem diagnosis of embolism as the cause of colic requires the demonstration of a circulatory lesion in the wall of the intestine in the field supplied by the obstructed vessel. Total obstruction of the cranial mesenteric or ileocolic artery can occur gradually without causing clinical signs of colic.

In the embryo, the yolk (vitelline) sac is attached by its stalk to the intestinal loop where the distal jejunum will form. The yolk sac is supplied by the vitelline vessels that degenerate along with the yolk sac. The proximal right vitelline artery persists as the cranial mesenteric artery. If part of the yolk stalk or its vitelline arteries persist, this creates a fold or outgrowth of mesentery where the aberrant vessel courses around the jejunum to its ventral surface. These small aberrant outgrowths of mesentery have been called mesodiverticular bands.[13] Their free edge contains the aberrant artery. A pocket is formed where they attach to the normal mesentery. Occasionally a loop of jejunum moves into the pocket, wears a hole through the mesentery, passes through the rent, and becomes obstructed, or its vasculature is strangulated, causing colic.

23b. LIVE HORSE

Examine, by auscultation and percussion, the approximate areas of contact of the parts of the intestine with the abdominal walls.

Left side:
1. Dorsal half:
    a. The spleen extends from the dorsal ends of ribs 17 to 18 to the junction of the middle and ventral thirds of ribs 10 to 11.
    b. The small colon area is cranial to the tuber coxae.
    c. The small intestine occupies an area ventral to that of the small colon.
2. Ventral half: large colon (see Plate I)

Right side:
1. The base of the cecum is in contact with the paralumbar fossa. The cecum is trocarized here at a point equidistant from the last rib, lumbar transverse processes, and tuber coxae.
2. The body of the cecum occupies most of the caudal border of the lateral abdominal wall.

3. There may be an area of small intestinal contact behind the body of the cecum.
4. The right ventral colon is in contact with the cranioventral wall. The right dorsal colon is medial to the ribs.

Rectal palpation requires a knowledge of what organs can be reached by the hand in the colon and where they are located.[15, 34] These will be listed by organ systems. Under average conditions it is possible to reach the transverse plane of the first lumbar vertebra.

In the digestive system the first segment palpable is the caudal flexure of the duodenum, passing around the dorsocaudal surface of the base of the cecum at the pelvic inlet. It can be recognized only if distended. The jejunum, in the left ventral region, is clearly palpable only if distended by an obstruction. If the obstruction is a volvulus, it may be possible to palpate the twisted mesentery. The ileum can be palpated as it joins the medial side of the lesser curvature of the base of the cecum in the transverse plane of the left kidney. It can be recognized by its normally thick muscular wall. If the terminal ileum is obstructed, the preceding portion is distended and becomes palpable. If the cecum is distended by ingesta or gas, the medial and caudal surfaces of the base become resistant enough to be palpated in the right dorsal region. The pelvic flexure of the large colon is a frequent site of impaction. It may be in the left ventral region at the pelvis, or it may turn to the right. In volvulus of the left large colon the pelvic flexure is distended, and its veins are prominent. The left large colon may be displaced dorsally and trapped by the spleen, the phrenicosplenic ligament, and the body wall.[23] The right dorsal colon may be distended and palpable at arm's length in the median plane. The small colon, in the left dorsal region, may be obstructed.

The left kidney can be reached, and the ureters can be traced, if enlarged, to the neck of the bladder. The internal genital organs can be examined, as well as the vaginal and deep inguinal rings.

The arteries and lymph nodes of the pelvic region can be identified. Sometimes the aneurysm of the cranial mesenteric artery caused by strongylus larvae is large enough to palpate at arm's length in the median plane. The dorsocaudal border of the spleen may be palpable near the left kidney.

In the normal animal, it is not possible to palpate the stomach, liver, right kidney, transverse colon, or the last rib.

The following is a method of systematic examination of the abdomen of a horse through a linea alba celiotomy.[1] Identify the body and apex of the cecum on the midline. Exteriorize the cecum by reflecting the apex caudoventrally and to the right. Follow the cecocolic fold from the lateral band of the cecum to the ventrolateral band of the right ventral colon. Examination of small intestine: Identify the thinner ileocecal fold medial to the cecocolic fold and follow it from the dorsal band of the cecum to the antimesenteric side of the ileum. Exteriorize as much of the ileum as possible and follow it to the cecum at the ileocecal papilla. Examine the entire jejunum from the ileum toward the duodenum by progressively passing the jejunum through your hands. The part being handled and observed is first exteriorized, then returned to the abdomen. Note the arcuate nature of the mesenteric vessels. There are about 21 meters of intestine to examine. As the duodenum is approached, it will no longer be possible to exteriorize the jejunum. Follow the jejunum to the duodenocolic fold. Examination of the large intestine: Identify the cecocolic fold. Follow it to the right ventral colon and examine the entire ventral colon, including sternal and pelvic flexures. Note the normal narrowing of the bowel at the pelvic flexure. Exteriorize the entire colon. Turn it medially toward the midline to expose the dorsal colon. Examine the dorsal colon. By palpation, follow the right dorsal colon to the transverse colon in the abdomen. Examination of other organs: With the colon still exteriorized examine the cranial abdomen for these structures: the diaphragm and liver; the spleen with its attachments to the diaphragm, left kidney, and stomach; the stomach; the duodenum; and the epiploic foramen. Palpate the descending duodenum, caudal flexure, and ascending duodenum on the left side. Replace the colon by returning the sternal and diaphragmatic flexures first, followed by the pelvic flexure. Be sure the colon is not twisted by examining the cecocolic fold and following the lateral free band on the ventral colon to the pelvic flexure.[2] With the cecum still exteriorized, identify the small colon on the left by its firm fecal contents and large free band. Follow the small colon hand over hand from the transverse colon to the rectum. Except for the two ends, most of the small colon can be exteriorized during this examination. Examine the root of the mesentery. Note the mesenteric lymph nodes. Examine the kidneys on each side and the transverse colon cranial to the root of the mesentery. In the caudal abdomen examine the bladder, ureters, reproductive organs, vaginal and deep inguinal rings, and lumbar lymph nodes. Upon completion of this examination, replace the cecum.

Certain segments of the intestinal tract of the horse are anatomically predisposed to obstruction. The jejunum, left parts of the large colon, and the small colon are especially subject to volvulus because of their long mesenteries. The terminal ileum has a narrow lumen subject to impaction, intussusception, and stenotic muscular dysfunction. The cecum is frequently distended with ingesta because of its shape, position, and muscular and fermentative disorders. The pelvic flexure and the right dorsal colon undergo a marked reduction in diameter predisposing to impaction. The small colon is less frequently impacted. To find the site of obstruction the clinician must be able to identify the parts of the intestines that are distended and therefore proximal to the blockage and those that are less filled or collapsed and therefore distal to it.

Various displacements of the colon that initially do not strangulate the blood supply can occur.[17]

These cause mild to moderate colic that resembles an obstruction. Rectal examination will reveal gaseous distention of colonic segments but no impaction of feed. These displacements must be treated surgically before strangulation occurs, but they can usually be differentiated only at laparotomy. They include:

1. Volvulus of the entire loop of large colon on its mesocolic axis, beginning on the right side and including the sternal and diaphragmatic flexures. This causes a torsion of the right ventral colon. The direction is usually clockwise as the standing horse is viewed from behind.[2, 12] The correct direction must be diagnosed for surgical repair.

2. Volvulus of the right parts of the large colon and cecum on the base of the cecum, with the body of the cecum moving dorsally, medial to the right parts of the large colon over the dorsal surface of the right dorsal colon and ventrally on the right side.

3. Displacement of the left large colon to the right side between the body of the cecum, the right large colon, and the right abdominal wall by twisting at the sternal and diaphragmatic flexures.

4. Volvulus of the left parts of the large colon at the sternal and diaphragmatic flexures.

5. Cranial displacement of the pelvic flexure dorsal to the left dorsal colon, causing a fold in the left large colon.

6. Displacement of the left large colon dorsally along the left body wall and entrapment between the phrenicosplenic ligament and the left dorsolateral body wall.

Peritoneocentesis is usually performed at the most ventral aspect of the abdominal wall, between the xiphoid process and the umbilicus on the midline.[16] This is usually 10 to 14 cm. caudal to the xiphoid process. After a short incision through the skin and subcutaneous tissue is made, a blunt teat tube is thrust through the linea alba into the peritoneal cavity. In obese horses, a 10 to 14 cm. long tube will be needed to penetrate the fat in the transversalis fascia.

23c. INTESTINES, CALF, AND MODELS, RUMINANT AND PIG

Place the intestinal mass so that the duodenum and the proximal and distal loops of the colon are uppermost. The greater omentum remains attached to the duodenum. Trace the duodenum to the jejunum. The caudal flexure and ascending duodenum are attached to the descending colon by the duodenocolic fold. In the intestinal border of the mesentery, observe the large elongated lymph nodes and the arch of the cranial mesenteric artery.

The proximal end of the cranial mesenteric artery is caudal to the short transverse colon. The coiled colon is adhered to the left side of the mesentery. The coiled colon, like the large colon of the horse, is a loop of the ascending colon. In the ruminant embryo, it passes over the caudodorsal border of the mesentery containing the ileocolic artery, coils up, and flattens out against the left surface of the mesentery of the jejunum. Adhesion of the serous surfaces has led to the notion that the coiled colon is between the layers of the mesentery. This is a secondary relationship like the adhesion of the duodenum to the greater omentum. In the pig, the coiled colon is not flattened, but conical, with the apex directed cranially, ventrally, and to the left, and the cecum is drawn around behind the root of the mesentery into the left flank. Trace the colon from both ends. The proximal loop begins at the cecum and the distal loop ends at the transverse colon (see Fig. 23–2).

In cattle with colonic atresia or acquired obstruction, the distal ileum, cecum, proximal loop of the ascending colon, and the centripetal coils of the spiral colon can be by-passed for surgical correction.[28-30]

As in all domestic animals except the pig, the proximal part of the bovine cecum is located in the upper right flank. The elongated cecum is directed caudally but is freely movable, and the apex may be in the pelvis or turned to the left or ventrally. Cecal dilatation occurs in cattle and occasionally is accompanied by torsion of the cecum on its long axis. A relatively rare condition involves atony, distention, and volvulus of the cecum and proximal loop of the colon. This usually causes torsion of the proximal loop of the colon. The overloaded cecum sinks to the floor of the abdomen, and in most cases, a gas pocket buoys up the apex in the right paralumbar fossa. It may be outside the omentum, directed cranially, and readily visible as a bulge in the abdominal wall. Other displacements have been described,[6] but the treatment is the same—surgical evacuation of the cecum and proximal colon. Volvulus of the jejunum and colon around the mesenteric axis has been described.[18]

Cecal surgery requires an understanding of the blood supply to the cecum, terminal ileum, and proximal colon. These are supplied by the ileocolic and ileal arteries from the cranial mesenteric.[21] The cecum and ileum are attached by the ileocecal fold. The cecal artery enters this fold at the ileocecal junction where an arterial arch passes around the lateral side of the junction (see Fig. 23–2). The cecal artery runs caudally in the ileocecal fold supplying branches to both organs and terminating by anastomosis with the ileal artery from the cranial mesenteric. This ileal artery also anastomoses with the mesenteric ileal artery from the ileocolic. The ileum is highly vascularized. The extrinsic innervation of the cecum and ileum accompanies the arteries.[22]

23d. LIVE COW

Examine by percussion and auscultation the right abdominal wall caudal to the lung sounds. The upper half of the wall is the area for examination of the cecum and proximal loop of the colon.[31, 33] Normally there is a resonant gas pocket in the large intestine under the last two ribs. A high-pitched tympanitic "ping" from the eighth to thirteenth ribs is caused by distention of the abomasum. A similar percussion sound from the tenth rib to the tuber coxae indicates abnormal distention of the cecum. The presenting sign is distention, which may or may not be associated with torsion. When the cecum is emptied surgically, the torsion, if present, disappears. Probably the pathogenesis is the same as in abomasal atony, distention, and displacement.[33]

The lower half of the right side of the abdominal cavity is usually occupied by the small intestine. (The greater omentum intervenes between the wall and all of the intestines except the descending duodenum.) The relations are somewhat variable because of differences in the distention of the ventral sac of the rumen, which may encroach on the right side enough to displace the intestines caudodorsally.

The structures palpable per rectum in the cow are listed here in order of the organ systems. The transverse plane of the second lumbar to the last thoracic vertebra can be reached, depending on the length of the arm and the size of the cow. The caudal part of the rumen can be felt on the left. In atony and distention of the rumen, the ventral sac expands to the right and bulges upward, forming a horizontal shelf. No other part of the normal stomach is within reach. A distended abomasum on the right can be felt. The caudal flexure of the duodenum can be recognized dorsally at the pelvic inlet if distended. Distinct loops of jejunum can be felt only if made turgid by some obstruction. Intussusception can be recognized as a solid cylindrical structure with a mesenteric cord. The terminal ileum can be reached only if the forequarters are elevated.[27] The apex of the cecum can be felt in the pelvis or cranial to it. A distended cecum with the apex turned forward out of reach is very hard to differentiate from an abomasum displaced on the right. Loops of colon can be recognized only if distended. The caudal fold of the greater omentum can be palpated caudally on the right, ventral to the duodenum.

The left kidney is palpable, pushed over on the right by the rumen. If enlarged, the ureters can be traced to the bladder. The internal genital organs can be palpated, and the vaginal and deep inguinal rings should be examined in the bull.

The pelvic arteries and lymph nodes can be felt.

In the normal animal it is not possible to reach the liver, spleen, or the last rib.

23e. RADIOGRAPHS, INTESTINE, DOG AND CAT

Remember that the ability to define the borders of an organ requires a difference in radiographic density between adjacent structures.[3] All intra-abdominal organs are composed of fluid-density tissue. Their borders only become visible by the fat that separates them. Puppies and kittens and emaciated animals have no abdominal fat, and therefore it is very difficult to differentiate abdominal organs.

The stomach and intestines are in constant motion in the normal resting animal. Therefore, sequential radiographs, especially in contrast studies, will show variation in the shape of the stomach and shape and position of the small intestine. Each radiograph is a "stop-action" view of a dynamic system.

On a lateral view of a plain radiograph of the abdomen, the duodenum is not readily apparent. The jejunum is visible as a mass of small-diameter bowel in the ventral half between the bladder caudally and the spleen, if visible, and liver cranially. The jejunum is readily displaced by large abdominal masses: caudally by a liver mass; dorsally, cranially, and caudally by a splenic mass; dorsally by a pregnant or infected uterus; and cranially by a prostatic mass and full bladder. As a rule, the diameter of the lumen is no larger than 2.5 times the width of the last rib. Portions of the jejunum often contain a small amount of gas. Excessive dilation with gas or fluid indicates stasis.[9] If the cecum is gas-filled, it will be visible in the center of the abdomen by its partially circular shape. Frequently the transverse colon will be gas-filled and visible in the middle of the abdomen or more dorsal, caudal to the body of the stomach. The descending colon is usually evident in the same plane, coursing caudally to the pelvis. Its larger size and more dense fecal contents are apparent. On ventrodorsal view the jejunum will be visible on both sides in the middle and caudal abdomen. The cecum will be on the right side and the descending colon on the left.

The components of the intestines can all be identified after the ingestion of a suspension of barium sulfate. Rectal administration of the barium will outline the colon. In the cat, regular segmental bands of contraction in the descending duodenum will give it the appearance of a "string of pearls" for a short time after barium enters the duodenum.[24] In the dog, the barium may outline normal depressions in the duodenal mucosa where it is thin over submucosal lymphoid follicles. The cecum in the dog appears partially coiled or twisted. In the cat, it is short and relatively straight. Its distal end is pointed. Proximally it blends with the colon without any narrowing.

23f. INTESTINES AND MODEL, DOG

The intestines should be arranged as in a ventral view of the animal, with the cecum on the dog's right. Note the course of the duodenum from the pylorus caudally along the lateral side of the ascending colon and cecum. It then returns abruptly cranially and runs along the left side of the root of the mesentery to the beginning of the jejunum. Note the large elongated jejunal lymph node on the cranial mesenteric artery in the root of the mesentery. This may be pathologically enlarged enough to palpate.

In surgery of the small intestine it may be of interest to know which end of an exposed loop is oral and which is aboral. To determine this, the loop is held in a sagittal plane. The thumb and forefinger encircle one limb of the loop, and the mesentery is palpated dorsally to the root. If a twist in the mesentery is felt, the loop is rotated to correct it. When the mesentery is no longer twisted and the loop is in a sagittal plane, the cranial limb of the loop is the oral limb.

The ileum approaches the cecum from the left and joins the cecocolic junction. The cecum is usually ventral to the second and third lumbar vertebrae and is in the middle of the right half of the abdomen. The position is quite variable craniocaudally, however. In operations on the cecum, the surgeon should know that the largest artery is hidden on the dorsal surface. The ileocolic artery gives off the colic branch and the mesenteric ileal branch and is continued as the cecal artery (see Fig. 23–2). This runs across the dorsal surface of the ileocolic junction and turns caudally between the ileum and cecum, supplying branches to both, and terminating as the antimesenteric ileal branch.

Observe that the transverse colon crosses from right to left cranial to the cranial mesenteric artery and caudal to the celiac artery. The duodenal and colic loops are hooked into each other (see Fig. 23–2).

23g. LIVE DOG

If the abdominal muscles are sufficiently relaxed, it may be possible to palpate on the right the descending duodenum. This is done by pressing it dorsally against the sublumbar muscles and rolling it from medial to lateral. The descending colon on the left is more readily palpated, especially if the dog is constipated. The jejunum is palpable in the ventral abdomen. In the cat, the ileocolic junction may be palpable and should not be mistaken for a foreign body. Intussusception occurs here, as well as lymphosarcoma. Both are palpable.[26]

A method of systematic surgical exploration of the abdomen of the dog through the linea alba includes:[5]

1. Elevate the xiphoid process and retract the liver caudally to inspect and palpate the attachments and hiatuses of the diaphragm. Inspect the liver.

2. Replace the liver against the diaphragm and retract the stomach caudally. On the right side between the pylorus and liver place a finger in the epiploic foramen dorsal to the pylorus and cranial duodenum and palpate the hepatoduodenal ligament containing the hepatic artery, hepatic ducts, bile duct, and portal vein. Gently express the gallbladder. Place the stomach between your hands and palpate it.

3. Reflect the greater curvature of the stomach cranially with its attached greater omentum. Inspect the spleen as it is reflected with the stomach. This exposes the root of the mesentery with the cranial mesenteric artery and its branches, the jejunal lymph node, the aorta, caudal vena cava, kidneys, and left lobe of the pancreas. The celiac artery and its branches are visible cranial to the cranial mesenteric artery.

4. Replace the stomach but keep the greater omentum reflected cranially. Examine by palpation the entire intestine from pylorus to rectum. When palpating the descending duodenum, inspect the right lobe of the pancreas in the mesoduodenum. As the jejunum is palpated, pull it ventrally to expose the vasculature in the mesentery. Identify the ileum by its antimesenteric ileocecal fold and vessels. Examine the colic lymph nodes in the cecocolic area.

5. Pull the descending duodenum and its mesoduodenum ventrally to the left to reflect the rest of the viscera away from the right body wall. Do the same procedure on the left using the descending colon and its mesocolon to inspect the left side of the abdomen. This exposes the aorta, caudal vena cava, their major branches, the adrenals, kidneys and ureters, and ovaries and uterus. This is a useful procedure to find the bleeding stump of an ovarian artery that has not been ligated properly. In the male, the vaginal ring and ductus deferens can be inspected in the caudal abdomen and the ductus can be followed to the urethra. Trace the ureters to the bladder. Examine the bladder and proximal urethra, the prostate in the male, and the body and cervix of the uterus in the female. Be sure to examine the stump of the uterus in the spayed female.

References

1. Adams, S. B.: Surgical approaches to the exploration of the equine abdomen. Vet. Clin. North Am. (Large Anim. Pract.) 4 (1982):89–104.

2. Barclay, W. P., J. J. Foerner, and T. N. Phillips: Volvulus of the large colon in the horse. JAVMA 177 (1980):629–630.

3. Brawner, W. R., Jr. and J. E. Bartels: Contrast radiography of the digestive tract. Indications, techniques and complications. Vet. Clin. North Am. (Small Anim. Pract.) 13 (1983):599–626.

4. Byars, T. D., L. W. George, and D. S. Beisel: A laboratory technique for teaching rectal palpation in the horse. J. Vet. Med. Ed. 7 (1980):80–82.

5. Crane, S. W.: Exploratory celiotomy in the diagnosis of gastrointestinal diseases. Vet. Clin. North Am. (Small Anim. Pract.) 13 (1983):477–483.

6. Dirksen, J.: Die Blinddarmerweiterung und Drehung beim Rind. Deutsche Tierärztl. Wschr. 69 (1962):409–416.

7. Dobberstein, J. and H. Hartmann: Über die Anastomo-

senbildung im Bereich der Blind- und Grimmdarmarterien des Pferdes und ihre Bedeutung für die Entstehung der embolischen Kolik. Berl. Tierärztl. Wochenschr. *48* (1932):397–402.

8. Donawick, W. J., B. A. Christie, and J. V. Stewart: Resection of diseased ileum in the horse. JAVMA *159* (1971):1146–1149.

9. Douglas, S. W. and H. D. Williamson: Veterinary Radiological Interpretation. Philadelphia: Lea & Febiger, 1970.

10. Espersen, G.: Cecal dilatation and dislocation. Mod. Vet. Pract. *42/16* (1961):25–27.

11. Evans, H. E. and G. C. Christensen: Miller's Anatomy of the Dog, 2nd ed. Philadelphia: W. B. Saunders, 1979.

12. Foerner, J. J.: Diseases of the large intestine. Vet. Clin. North Am. (Large Anim. Pract.) *4* (1982):129–146.

13. Freeman, D. E., D. B. Koch, and C. L. Boles: Mesodiverticular bands as a cause of small intestinal strangulation and volvulus in the horse. JAVMA *175* (1979):1089–1094.

14. Gibbons, W. J.: Clinical Diagnosis of Diseases of Large Animals. Philadelphia: Lea & Febiger, 1966.

15. Greatorex, J. C.: Rectal exploration as an aid to the diagnosis of some medical conditions in the horse. Equine Vet. J. *1* (1968):26–30.

16. Hackett, R. P.: Management of acute abdominal disease in the horse. 73rd Annual Conf. New York State College of Veterinary Medicine (1981).

17. Hackett, R. P.: Nonstrangulated colonic displacement in horses. JAVMA *182* (1983):235–240.

18. Huskamp, B.: Zur Torsio intestini des erwachsenen Rindes. Berl. Münch. Tierärztl. Wochenschr. *82* (1969):101–102.

19. Kadletz, M.: Anatomische Grundlagen der rektalen Untersuchung beim Pferd. Wien. Tierärztl. Mnschr. *17* (1930):765.

20. Kadletz, M.: Anatomische Grundlagen der rektalen Untersuchung beim Rind. Deutsche Tierärztl. Wschr. *39* (1931):665.

21. Maala, C. P. and W. O. Sack: The arterial supply to the ileum, cecum, and proximal loop of the ascending colon in the ox. Zentralbl. Vet. Med. C. *10* (1981):130–146.

22. Maala, C. P. and W. O. Sack: Nerves to the cecum, ileum, and proximal loop of the ascending colon in cattle. Am. J. Vet. Res. *43* (1982):1566–1572.

23. Milne, D. W., M. J. Tarr, R. K. Lochner, et al.: Left dorsal displacement of the colon in the horse. J. Eq. Med. Surg. *1* (1977):47–52.

24. Morgan, J. P.: The upper gastrointestinal examination in the cat: normal radiographic appearance using positive contrast medium. Vet. Radiol. *22* (1981):159–169.

25. Müller, W.: Blinddarmerweiterung und -drehung beim Rind. Schweiz. Arch. Tierheilkd. *112* (1970):117–124.

26. Nielsen, S. W.: Neoplastic diseases. *In* Catcott, E. J. (ed.) Feline Medicine and Surgery. Wheaton Ill.: Am. Vet. Public., pp. 156–176, 1964.

27. Schreiber, J.: Topographisch-anatomischer Beitrag zur klinischen Untersuchung der Rumpfeingeweide des Rindes. Wien. Tierärztl. Mnschr. *40* (1953):131–144.

28. Smith, D. F. and W. J. Donawick: Obstruction of the ascending colon in cattle: I. Clinical presentation and surgical management. Vet. Surg. *8* (1979):93–97.

29. Smith, D. F. and W. J. Donawick: Obstruction of the ascending colon in cattle: II. An experimental model of partial by-pass of the large intestine. Vet. Surg. *8* (1979):98–104.

30. Smith, D. F.: Atresia of the colon in a newborn calf. Comp. Cont. Ed. *4* (1982):S441–S445.

31. Smith, D. F., H. N. Erb, K. M. Kalaher, et al.: The identification of structures and conditions responsible for right side tympanic resonance (ping) in adult cattle. Cornell Vet. *72* (1982):180–199.

32. Udall, D. H.: The Practice of Veterinary Medicine, 6th ed. Ithaca, N.Y.: Udall, 1954.

33. Whitlock, R. H.: What's new in the lower digestive tract? Am. Assoc. Bov. Pract., Proc. *4* (1971):38–43.

34. Witherspoon, D. M.: Exploration of the abdominal cavity by digital manipulation. Am. Ass. Eq. Pract. Proc. *23* (1977):15–24.

CHAPTER 24

LIVER, PANCREAS, SPLEEN, URINARY ORGANS, AND UTERINE ARTERY

OBJECTIVES

1. To be able to project the liver on the surface of the body in relation to skeletal landmarks, to detect enlargement or displacement by percussion or palpation, to elicit pain by palpation, to perform biopsy, and to recognize the liver in radiographs.
2. To be able to distinguish the portal and hepatic veins and the bile ducts in the liver at autopsy. To be able to find the hepatic lymph nodes.
3. To know the tributaries to the portal vein and its branches in the liver to be able to diagnose a portosystemic shunt on venography and locate it at surgery.
4. To understand the relations of the pancreas, its blood supply, and ducts and where to palpate the abdomen for pain associated with pancreatitis.
5. To be able to project the kidneys on the surface of the body in relation to the ribs and transverse processes of the lumbar vertebrae for palpation, biopsy, and radiology.
6. To be able to trace the course of the ureters by rectal palpation in large animals and to recognize them in small animal surgery so as to avoid them in ovariohysterectomy.
7. To appreciate the extent of the filled bladder and the danger of cutting into it with an incision of the abdominal wall.
8. To be able to recognize the normal urinary organs in a series of urograms.
9. To be able to palpate the uterine artery in the cow as a part of the examination for pregnancy.
10. To be able to find the renal, lumbar, and iliac lymph nodes at autopsy and to palpate per rectum the node that receives lymph from the superficial inguinal (mammary) node in the cow.
11. To be able to project the spleen on the surface of the body for biopsy in large animals and to be able to palpate and recognize it in radiographs in the dog.

The liver of carnivores and the pig is oriented transversely in the abdomen and the lobes on each side are named appropriately by their position on the left or right. In the horse, the liver is positioned obliquely with the left lobes located ventrally near the seventh to tenth intercostal spaces and the right lobes more dorsally opposite the tenth to fifteenth intercostal spaces. In ruminants, because of the greater development of the stomach on the left, the liver is displaced to the right and rotated so that the left lobe is ventral and the right lobe is dorsal. The liver therefore is accessible only on the right side. These variations are important in knowing where to examine the animal for liver enlargement and liver pain and for obtaining biopsy specimens. In all species, the caudate lobe is located on the visceral surface between the portal vein ventrally and caudal vena cava dorsally.

24a. LIVE HORSE

The purpose of locating the liver on the lateral body wall is to detect enlargement or to perform biopsy. Percuss lightly the right tenth to fifteenth and the left seventh to tenth intercostal spaces. There is usually a narrow zone of relative dullness between the lung resonance and the intestinal resonance on the right side only. Absolute dullness in right or left zones indicates pathological enlargement of the liver in the adult. Marked enlargements of the liver may also be detected by palpation of the liver below the costal arch and by rectal palpation of the caudate process.

Liver biopsy is difficult in the horse because of the great expanse of the lung. The usual site is in the 12th intercostal space on the right, on a line from the tuber coxae to the point of the shoulder.[11] This method requires penetration of a considerable thickness of lung, and also has the disadvantage that the right lobe of the liver is often atrophied in old horses. The left lobe (see Plate I) can be sampled by inserting a 20 cm. needle in the left eighth intercostal space at the level of the deltoid tuberosity.[19] It is advanced during expiration, to avoid the border of the lung, in a dorsal, medial, and cranial direction.

The spleen in the horse is not normally palpable through the abdominal wall. The dorsal end may be palpated per rectum lateral to the left kidney. The ventral end extends to the ventral third of ribs 10 and 11 (see Plate I).

The left kidney lies ventral to the last rib and first two or three lumbar transverse processes. The right kidney is ventral to the 16th to 18th ribs and the first lumbar transverse process and cannot normally be reached on rectal examination. For biopsy, the left kidney can be pushed against the left flank by a hand in the rectum while the needle is passed through the skin (see Plate I).[26]

24b. DISSECTION, SUBLUMBAR REGION, COW

Observe the termination of the aorta. Seven branches are visible in the ventral view (Fig. 24–1). The small paired cranial arteries are the ovarian. The unpaired artery at the same level as the external iliacs is the caudal mesenteric. The two large terminal arteries are the internal iliacs. They originate 5 cm. cranial to the sacral promontory.

About 4 cm. from its origin, the internal iliac gives off the common trunk of the uterine and umbilical arteries. The internal iliac continues caudally. The uterine artery may be traced in the broad ligament to the horn of the uterus. The umbilical artery in the adult is a fibrous cord with a very small lumen. It passes through the parietal attachment of the broad ligament of the uterus and continues in the free edge of the lateral ligament of the bladder. It is called the round ligament of the bladder.

The uterine is the only large pulsating artery, ventrolateral to the rectum, that can be picked up in the fingers and moved. If the fingertips are drawn back along the lateral pelvic wall, the first large artery encountered is the external iliac, which lies on the abdominal side of the shaft of the ilium and is fixed in position. Caudal to the external iliac is the mobile uterine artery. The artery to the pregnant horn becomes enlarged and develops a characteristic vibration (thrill, fremitus) in addition to the pulse. In the early stages of pregnancy this is of little practical interest because it is easier to palpate the uterus. In the fifth to sixth month, when the uterus is drawn downward and forward out of reach, the enlargement of the uterine artery is a useful sign. In a nonpregnant cow that has

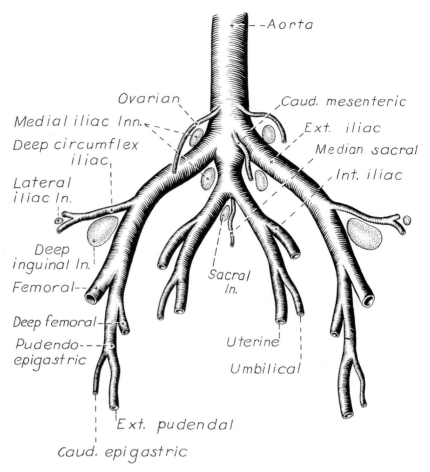

Figure 24–1. Termination of the bovine aorta, origin of the uterine artery, and the associated lymph nodes, ventral aspect.

calved before, the artery is about 5 mm. in diameter, and it runs downward and backward. It is smaller in the heifer. By the fifth or sixth month of gestation, it is 10 mm. in diameter and runs downward and forward. If both arteries are enlarged, it is probably a bicornual twin pregnancy.[29]

The lobation of the left kidney is normally palpable per rectum. In pyelonephritis the lobation may be obliterated. The right kidney is ventral to the last rib and first two or three lumbar transverse processes, usually too far forward to palpate. The left kidney is pushed to the right of the median plane by the rumen and lies ventral to the second to fifth lumbar vertebrae. A biopsy can be done percutaneously on the left kidney by pushing it against the right flank with the hand in the rectum.[26]

Note the course of the right ureter from the kidney caudally along the right side of the caudal vena cava. Both ureters cross the ventral surfaces of all the vessels except the ovarian (or testicular), and the right ureter can be palpated as it crosses the external iliac artery.[7] The left ureter runs across the dorsal surface of the caudal half of the left kidney and takes an oblique course to the left, ventral to the termination of the aorta. It can be palpated against the sacrum, caudal to the promontory. In the pelvis the ureters continue caudally in the dorsolateral part of the broad ligament, turn medially, and enter the neck of the bladder. The termination of the ureter is best palpated per vaginum. The course of the ureters is palpated for evidence of pyelonephritis, in which they are enlarged, firm, and thick-walled. They are enlarged, thin-walled, and fluctuating when obstructed by ureteral calculi. The stones can sometimes be massaged into the bladder under proper medication.[7]

The lumbar lymph nodes are small and scattered along the caudal vena cava and aorta. The renal node is located dorsal to the renal vein on both sides. The medial iliac nodes are clustered around the termination of the aorta (Fig. 24–1). The large node in the angle between the circumflex iliac artery and the external iliac artery is the deep inguinal. It receives lymph from the superficial inguinal nodes and is often greatly swollen in mastitis. This should not be confused with lymphosar-coma.

24c. LIVER, OX

The bovine liver is not obviously divided into lobes, but lobation is more distinct in the sheep and goat. The comparative terms of direction based on the transverse position of the liver common to most species will be used in the following description. On the visceral surface a line from the notch for the round ligament to the esophageal impression marks the division between the left lobe and the caudate and quadrate lobes. The caudate lobe is dorsal between the caudal vena cava and the left (intrahepatic) branch of the portal vein. The quadrate lobe is ventral to the left branch, between the notch for the round ligament and the gall bladder fossa. A line from the latter through the porta (where the portal vein enters) to the caudal vena cava demarcates the right lobe. The caudate lobe has two processes, the smaller and variable papillary process, which overlaps the left branch of the portal vein, and the long caudate process, which extends along the caudal vena cava on the visceral surface of the right lobe to the right kidney. On the diaphragmatic surface the left lobe is marked off by the line of attachment of the falciform ligament. There are no other visible interlobar boundaries on this surface.

On the visceral surface find the portal vein and the hepatic (portal) lymph nodes. The bile ducts are examined routinely for signs of fluke infection in meat inspection, and the left hepatic duct is a good place to start. Insert a finger from the portal vein into its left branch, which passes deep to the papillary process. Pull up and slice the papillary process and hepatic lymph nodes until the left hepatic duct is recognized. It is green if normal; distended and brown if infected. Slit it open toward the left lobe and back to the right and common hepatic ducts. The cystic duct should be left intact to avoid bile spillage from the gall bladder.

Find the openings of the hepatic veins into the caudal vena cava. A convenient way to handle a slippery fresh liver is to hook a finger into the right hepatic vein (see Fig. 19–1).

Post-mortem examination occasionally shows lesions restricted mainly to the right or left lobe of the liver. This finding has been attributed to laminar flow in the portal vein, whereby blood from the intestines might go to the right lobe, and blood from the stomach and spleen to the left lobe. Research on the cow,[39] sheep,[16] cat and rabbit,[17] and man[15] provides no evidence that laminar flow could account for preferential localization of metastases in the right or left lobes. Two anatomical reasons for skepticism about laminar flow in the ruminant are: (1) The splenic vein does not join the portal vein in a V pointed toward the liver but enters at a right angle, or even in the retrograde direction, depending on the fullness of the rumen. This causes turbulence and mixing. (2) The right and left lobes in ruminants are actually dorsal and ventral, so that the main branches of the portal vein in the liver are rotated 90° from the plane of junction of the splenic and portal veins.

24d. LIVE COW

Palpate the last four right intercostal spaces for evidence of pain (liver abscess). Attempt to palpate the liver in the cranial angle of the right paralumbar fossa. This is possible only if the liver is enlarged. The right kidney may be palpable here.

Percuss with a light stroke the last four right intercostal spaces caudal to the border of the lung. Heavy percussion evokes resonance from the intestine deep to the liver, and is to be avoided. Liver dullness is normal in the ox in a narrow zone along the dorsal third of the basal border of the lung. In enlargement of the liver, dullness expands caudoventrally toward the costal arch. In distention and volvulus of the abomasum on the right side, the area of liver dullness may be reduced or absent.

Liver biopsy is performed in the adult cow in the right 10th or 11th intercostal space, one fourth of the length of the bony rib ventral to the vertebra.[38]

Alternative: if the ventral boundary of the right paralumbar fossa is prominent, estimate the center of the fossa and draw a horizontal line cranially to the 10th or 11th intercostal space. Biopsy at this intersection. The needle must traverse the pleural cavity and diaphragm.

The liver is much larger in calves and may be reached from behind the last rib in the first 4 weeks. In older calves the liver can be sampled either in the 12th intercostal space 11 to 14 cm. from the ventral midline or through the dorsal end of the 11th intercostal space.[22]

The spleen is not palpable unless grossly enlarged. Splenic puncture is performed in the left 12th intercostal space at the level of the tuber coxae (see Plate II).

Fascioliasis causes enlargement of the liver and obstruction of the common bile duct, with signs of colic. Many affected animals can be made fit for slaughter by performing a laparotomy and massaging the debris into the duodenum. Although the gall bladder is normally at the ventral end of the 10th or 11th rib, the enlargement of the diseased liver brings the gall bladder back to the last costal cartilage. As a last resort if the common bile duct cannot be cleared, the gall bladder can be anastomosed to the duodenum.[35]

24e. DISSECTION, ABDOMEN, DOG

The pancreas lies in the craniodorsal part of the abdominal cavity with the right lobe enclosed in the mesoduodenum along the medial side of the descending duodenum; the body is in contact with the pylorus, and the left lobe is in the dorsal attachment of the greater omentum, craniodorsal to the transverse colon and caudodorsal to the stomach. Medioventral to the right lobe are the cecum and ascending colon; dorsal to the right lobe are the dorsal abdominal wall, right kidney, and caudate process of the liver. The left lobe is ventral to the caudate process of the liver, portal vein, aorta, left adrenal, and the cranial end of the left kidney. The left lobe lies caudal to the branches of the celiac artery and cranial to the cranial mesenteric artery.

The ducts of the pancreas are named from their relative importance in man: pancreatic duct and accessory pancreatic duct. The pancreatic duct develops from the ventral pancreatic bud, just caudal to the bile duct, while the accessory duct belongs to the dorsal pancreatic bud. When the stomach and duodenum rotate, the two pancreatic buds come together and fuse, and their ducts cross and usually anastomose. The left lobe and the body are from the dorsal bud and the right lobe is from the ventral bud. The pancreatic duct opens on the greater duodenal papilla with the bile duct; the accessory pancreatic duct opens on the lesser duodenal papilla. These names are appropriate in man, horse, and cat, but are paradoxical in the ox, pig, and dog, in which the accessory pancreatic duct is the main one. The sheep and goat have only the pancreatic duct, which joins the bile duct before it reaches the duodenum. In the dog, the pancreatic duct is small and occasionally absent. The orifice is close to that of the bile duct, but there is no common ampulla; therefore, an inflow of bile up the pancreatic duct cannot be a cause of pancreatitis in the dog, as it is said to be in man.[24] The accessory pancreatic duct opens about 3 cm. caudal to the greater duodenal papilla in the average dog. It is small and sometimes absent in the cat. Many variations of these pancreatic ducts occur in the dog either within the pancreas or in the entrance to the duodenum or both. Therefore, in removing one lobe or part of a lobe, one should find its axial duct and ligate it. It is not advisable to divide the pancreas between the pancreatic duct and the accessory duct as this may sever the duct of the remaining lobe and cause atrophy.[6]

Knowledge of the blood supply to the pancreas is critical when considering its surgical removal. The right lobe of the pancreas is supplied by the cranial and caudal pancreaticoduodenal arteries, which also supply the adjacent descending duodenum. The amount of the right lobe and descending duodenum supplied by these vessels varies. In one study the cranial vessel supplied all of the descending duodenum and the attached part of the right lobe in 30 percent of dogs, the cranial half of these structures in 60 percent, and the cranial third in 10 percent. The caudal end of the right lobe that turns to the left was always supplied by the caudal pancreaticoduodenal artery.[13] In removal of the right lobe, these blood vessels must be preserved to avoid ischemic necrosis of the descending duodenum. The pancreas must be bluntly dissected off these vessels. Gauze sponges may be useful in this process.[1, 40] The left lobe of the pancreas is supplied by pancreatic branches of the celiac, hepatic, and splenic arteries and occasionally by a proximal branch from the cranial mesenteric artery. These branches may be ligated where they enter the left lobe.

When the condition of the patient makes laparotomy under general anesthesia hazardous, the pancreas can be inspected and a biopsy performed through an infant-sized proctoscope. A 2 cm. incision is made in the right flank under local anesthesia. The right lobe and part of the left can be seen.[3] The biopsy should be done with care to avoid the duct running in the middle of the lobe and the vessels on the duodenal border. If endocrine function is in question, one must be aware of the normal absence of A-cells in the caudal half of the right lobe.[2] The right lateral lobe of the liver can be reached for biopsy by the same method.

A simpler method of liver biopsy, which can also be done under local anesthesia, employs a midventral incision. A finger is inserted to fix the most ventral left lobe against the abdominal wall, and the needle is inserted through a separate stab incision.[27]

Alternatively, a paramedian incision can be made between the xiphoid cartilage and the left costal arch, and an otoscope can be inserted to visualize the liver. The sample can be obtained through the otoscope. To avoid abdominal incision, local anesthetic can be infiltrated at this same site, and the dog can be held up, so that all its support is on the pelvic limbs, which allows the liver to drop caudally. The needle is passed through the skin and abdominal wall and directed toward the left shoulder to enter the liver.

Note on the Nomenclature of the Bile Ducts. In most animals, the hepatic ducts from each lobe join to form the left and right hepatic ducts. These unite in the common hepatic duct, which joins the cystic duct to form the (common) bile duct (ductus choledochus). In the dog, the hepatic ducts do not unite to form a common hepatic duct, but three to five of them empty directly into the cystic duct, which then becomes the (common) bile duct.

The bile ducts are subject to traumatic rupture, and the treatment depends on the location of the defect. If it is in the (common) bile duct, the duct can be ligated and the fundus of the gall bladder anastomosed to the duodenum. More often, one of the hepatic ducts is torn from its junction with the cystic duct, and the hole must be closed by sutures. The detached duct should be ligated if it can be found.[34]

The ureters can be traced on either side of the aorta and caudal vena cava. The bladder is capable of distention as far cranially as the umbilicus. Three peritoneal ligaments extend from the body wall to the bladder. The lateral ligaments enclose the round ligaments (umbilical arteries) in their free borders. The median ligament attaches the ventral surface of the bladder to the midventral abdominal wall.

Examine the adrenal glands. They may be removed for the treatment of Cushing's syndrome.[33] A paracostal incision is made for each gland. On the right the kidney is retracted caudally after severing the hepatorenal ligament. The adrenal gland is exposed with the phrenicoabdominal vein crossing its ventral surface. The caudal vena cava covers the medial border and must be carefully retracted. The phrenicoabdominal vein is ligated medial and lateral to the gland. The caudal part of the adrenal gland is supplied by arteries from the aorta and the renal and cranial mesenteric arteries, and the cranial part from the phrenicoabdominal. The left adrenal is removed in the same manner, except that the hazard of injury to the caudal vena cava is replaced by the danger of traumatic pancreatitis from injury to the left lobe of the pancreas and the proximity of the aorta. Dorsal to the adrenal gland on each side is the adrenal plexus, where the splanchnic nerves, on their way to the adjacent celiac plexus, give off branches to the adrenal ganglia. The nerves to the adrenal medulla must be severed in the operation, but one should avoid cutting the splanchnic nerves. A retroperitoneal approach has also been described.[20]

Note the position of the spleen, caudoventral to the left costal arch, and examine its blood vessels. The spleen is attached along its hilus to the left side of the greater omentum. The part of the omentum between the spleen and the greater curvature of the stomach is the gastrosplenic ligament. The dorsal end of the spleen is attached to the left crus of the diaphragm between the fundus of the stomach and the left kidney by the short phrenicosplenic (suspensory) ligament, which is a part of the deep wall of the greater omentum. The ventral end of the spleen has great freedom of movement due to the ventral expansion of the gastrosplenic ligament.

The splenic artery runs to the left from the celiac artery along the dorsocranial surface of the left lobe of the pancreas. It can be exposed by opening the omental bursa and retracting the cranial border of the left lobe of the pancreas, which is enclosed with the artery and vein in the deep wall of the greater omentum. The artery gives branches to the pancreas and usually gives off two large splenic branches, one dorsal and one ventral, and a smaller intermediate branch. The dorsal branch may originate close to the celiac artery. It divides twice, resulting in four small branches, which give off the short gastric arteries and enter the hilus of the spleen. The short gastric arteries pass in the gastrosplenic ligament to the dorsal part of the greater curvature of the stomach. After giving off the ventral splenic branch, the splenic artery is continued by the left gastroepiploic artery, which turns back in the gastrosplenic ligament to the greater curvature of the stomach. The ventral and intermediate branches divide into many small splenic branches. Many branches are given off to the omentum.

In splenectomy, the numerous splenic vessels are ligated and divided in the omental pedicle near the spleen. This should be done between ligatures because the capsule and trabeculae of the spleen contain smooth muscle that contracts and expels venous blood. The short gastric vessels should also be ligated. Ligation of the splenic artery, as some have advocated, would deprive the large left gastroepiploic artery of its blood supply.[18]

If a partial splenectomy is indicated, this can be performed by taking advantage of the fact that the spleen consists of segments supplied by end-arteries.[4] The blood vessels in the pedicle of the part of the spleen to be removed are ligated and cut as close to the spleen as possible. This causes ischemia of the part to be removed. The spleen is squeezed flat in a strip at the margin of the ischemic area, clamped, and transected. The cut edge is covered by suturing the capsule.

24f. RADIOGRAPHS, DOG AND CAT

The liver is seen as a density caudal to the diaphragm and on the ventral abdominal wall as far back as the transverse plane of the 12th rib. The left lateral lobe extends the farthest caudally in the ventral abdomen. Caudal to this an oblique section of the ventral end of the spleen may be seen on the floor of the abdomen in the lateral view (see Plate III), especially if the dog is in right lateral recumbency. In the dorsoventral view the spleen is often visible between the stomach and the left abdominal wall.[30, 31]

Portal venography is commonly done to identify anomalous portosystemic shunts. In the normal carnivore immediately following the injection of radiopaque dye into a jejunal vein, the portal vein and its main branches in the liver are opacified. These usually include a right branch that passes dorsally and to the right to supply the caudate process of the caudate lobe and the right lateral lobe. A long left branch inclines ventrally to the left. It gives off the right ventral branch to the right medial lobe. Branches supply the caudate lobe, including the papillary process, and the quadrate lobe. The left branch terminates in the left medial and lateral lobes. Anomalous protosystemic shunts include an intrahepatic persistent ductus venosus to the caudal vena cava and extrahepatic shunts to the caudal vena cava or azygous vein. A common extrahepatic shunt to the caudal vena cava involves an anastomosis of the left gastric vein with the caudal vena cava at the diaphragm. Numerous portosystemic venous communications will develop if portal hypertension occurs due to anomalous liver vasculature or liver lesions that restrict its blood flow. These communications develop between the branches of the portal vein and primarily the gonadal, renal, and phrenicoabdominal branches of the caudal vena cava. The left gastric vein may communicate with esophageal branches of the azygous vein at the diaphragm. The numerous variations of the branching pattern of the hepatic arteries that supply the liver have been described.[32]

Inflammation or neoplasia of the pancreas may cause an ill-defined increase in density in the right cranial part of the abdomen, or chronic disease may result in granular calcification, but radiological evidence of pancreatic disease is mostly indirect and based on the displacement of other organs in barium studies.[12, 23, 36] The descending duodenum is often pushed to the right and ventrally, so that it and the caudal flexure form a C rather than the normal reversed J as viewed ventrodorsally. The descending duodenum may show dilation and constriction or a filling defect. Serial studies reveal delayed transit through the duodenum. A barium enema may show caudal displacement of the transverse colon with a dense area between it and the stomach.

The kidneys are visible behind the fundus of the stomach. They are easier to see in obese dogs with perirenal fat. In the dog, the right kidney is ventral to the first to third lumbar vertebrae, and the left kidney is ventral to the second to fourth. Their positions vary with the posture of the dog and the stage of respiration. The best position for a single lateral radiograph of both kidneys is right lateral recumbency, because the lower (right) kidney moves cranially, reducing the amount of overlap. If the main interest is the right kidney, the best position is left lateral recumbency, because the upper kidney rotates on its long axis, exposing the flat surface and the hilus.[14] In the cat, the kidneys are more mobile and farther caudal: the right is ventral to L 2–4 and the left is ventral to L 3–5. As a rule, the length of the kidneys in the dog is about 2.5 to 3.5 times the length of the body of L 2. The kidneys in cats are slightly smaller relative to L 2 (2 to 2.5 times).

The urinary system can be delineated by intravenous urography.[8, 21] The excretory urogram that is produced has an initial nephrogram phase in which the cortex and medulla of the kidneys are opacified in 5 to 20 seconds. By 1 to 3 minutes the renal pelvis, its recesses, and the ureter will be opacified. This is the pyelogram phase. A cystogram is produced when the bladder fills with the radiopaque dye within 30 to 40 minutes. The ureters will be seen to bend ventromedially just before they enter the neck of the bladder. Normal peristaltic contractions of the ureters may produce non-opacified sections of the ureter that should not be interpreted as obstructive lesions.

The bladder and the urethra can also be demonstrated by inflation with air (pneumocystography) or contrast material (urethrography, cystography) or both (double contrast cystography). These procedures will outline changes in the wall of these organs and usually identify calculi. Note the cranial extent of the distended bladder on the ventral abdominal wall. Urine should be evacuated before laparotomy to avoid incising the bladder when the abdomen is opened. In the cat, the neck of the bladder is normally a few centimeters cranial to the pubis due to the long preprostatic urethra. In the dog, the neck of the bladder is usually at the pubis. A common cause of cranial displacement in the dog is enlargement of the prostate. In the male cat, the normal prostatic part of the urethra may be slightly narrowed. The urethra is widest at the ischial arch and progressively becomes more narrow toward the external urethral orifice, where calculi often accumulate. In the female cat, the urethra has a uniform diameter throughout its length. In the male dog, the normal urethra often appears more narrow at the ischial arch. This narrowing is gradual, with a tapered appearance, in contrast with the abrupt narrowing of a stricture. The prostatic part of the canine urethra may be wider when the bladder is distended. Frequently, the urethra just caudal to the prostate is wider than the prostatic urethra.

Occasionally, a small pouch persists at the apex of the bladder where the urachus is connected with the bladder in the fetus. This can be a site of chronic infection.

24g. LIVE DOG

Attempt to palpate the liver by pressing the fingertips gently inward and forward around the costal arch on either side. The liver is not palpable in normal dogs. A number of diseases cause it to be enlarged enough to palpate caudal to the costal arch. Although the normal liver extends beyond the costal arch ventrally, the rectus abdominis muscle prevents palpation in this area in most dogs.

The normal area of liver dullness to percussion forms a zone along the entire basal border of the right lung. Only cranially, at the ventral ends of the seventh to ninth ribs does it extend below the costal arch. On the left side there is a small area of dullness in the seventh to ninth spaces, caudal to the cardiac dullness.

The spleen may be palpable behind the left costal cartilages.

The kidneys are palpable in some dogs. The right kidney is more difficult to feel. Biopsy of the kidney can be performed under sedation and local anesthesia. The incision is oblique, bisecting the craniodorsal angle of the paralumbar fossa. A finger is inserted to fix the kidney against the lateral abdominal wall while the needle is inserted through a separate puncture. The needle is directed at the caudal end, away from the hilus.[28] The right kidney is preferred because it is more fixed in position.

The bladder can readily be palpated in dogs and cats and often is evacuated by manual compression. Be aware that this is often accompanied by reflux of urine into the ureters—vesicoureteral reflux. This is especially common when the compression is prolonged to initiate urination.[9] If cystitis is present, this can be a source of pyelonephritis.

24h. LIVE CAT

Palpate the liver. It should be possible to pass the fingertips around the costal arch and between the liver and the diaphragm, and also to palpate the visceral surface of the liver.

The kidneys of the cat are normally pendulous enough to palpate through the abdominal wall. They may be held for biopsy without an incision.[28] The kidneys are often affected in cases of lymphosarcoma, and the lesion can be palpated.[25] Normal kidneys should not be diagnosed as neoplasms or fetuses in the cat.

References

1. Archibald, J. (ed.): Canine Surgery, 2nd ed. Wheaton, Ill.: Am. Vet. Public., 1974.
2. Bencosme, S. A., E. Liepa, and S. S. Lazarus: Glucagon content of pancreatic tissue devoid of alpha cells. Proc. Soc. Exp. Biol. Med. *90* (1955):387–392.
3. Dalton, J. R. F. and F. W. G. Hill: A procedure for the examination of the liver and pancreas in dogs. J. Small Anim. Pract. *13* (1972):527–530.
4. deBoer, J. and H. G. Downie: Partial splenectomy in dogs: an experimental tool for studies of the spleen. Can. J. Physiol. Pharmacol. *49* (1971):1110–1112.
5. Denny, H. R. and J. N. Lucke: A case of acute pancreatic necrosis in the dog. J. Small Anim. Pract. *13* (1972):545–551.
6. Dingwall, J. S. and W. McDonnell: Partial pancreatectomy in the dog. J. Am. Anim. Hosp. Assoc. *8* (1972):86–92.
7. Fabisch, H.: Bericht über die operative Entfernung von Harnleitersteinen bei Kühen. Wien. Tierärztl. Mschr. *55* (1968):409–411.
8. Feeney, D. A., D. L. Barber, G. R. Johnston, and C. A. Osborne: The excretory urogram: Part I. Techniques, normal radiographic appearance, and misinterpretation. Comp. Cont. Ed. *4* (1982):233–240.
9. Feeney, D. A., C. A. Osborne, and G. R. Johnston: Vesicoureteral reflux induced by manual compression of the urinary bladder of dogs and cats. JAVMA *182* (1983):795–797.
10. Feldman, E. C. and S. J. Ettinger: Percutaneous transthoracic liver biopsy in the dog. JAVMA *169* (1976):805–810.
11. Gibbons, W. J.: Clinical Diagnosis of Diseases of Large Animals. Philadelphia: Lea & Febiger, 1966.
12. Gibbs, C., H. R. Denny, H. M. Minter, et al.: Radiological features of inflammatory conditions of the canine pancreas. J. Small Anim. Pract. *13* (1972):531–544.
13. Gomercic, H. and K. Babic: A contribution to the knowledge of variations of the arterial supply of the duodenum and pancreas in the dog (*Canis familiaris*). Anat. Anz. *132* (1972):281–288.
14. Grandage, J.: Some effects of posture on the radiographic appearance of the kidneys of the dog. JAVMA *166* (1975):165–166.
15. Groszmann, R. J., B. Kotelanski, and J. N. Cohn: Hepatic lobar distribution of splenic and mesenteric blood flow in man. Gastroenterology *60* (1971):1047–1052.
16. Heath, T.: Origin and distribution of portal blood in the sheep. Am. J. Anat. *122* (1968):95–106.
17. Heath, T. and B. House: Origin and distribution of portal blood in the cat and rabbit. Am. J. Anat. *127* (1970):71–80.
18. Hifny, A. and N. A. Misk: A modified simplified technique for partial and complete splenectomy in the dog. Assiut. Vet. Med. J. *7* (1980):215–220.
19. Hütten, H. and H. Wilkens: Zur Technik der diagnostischen Leberpunktion beim Pferd unter besonderer Berücksichtigung ihrer anatomischen Grundlagen. Berl. Münch. Tierärztl. Wochenschr. *70* (1957):401–405.
20. Johnston, D. E.: Adrenalectomy via retroperitoneal approach in dogs. JAVMA *170* (1977):1092–1095.
21. Johnston, G. R., D. A. Feeney, and C. A. Osborne: Urethrography and cystography in cats. Part 1. Techniques, normal radiographic anatomy and artefacts. Comp. Cont. Ed. *4* (1982):823–835.
22. Kaman, J. and H. Černý: The anatomical basis and the technique of liver biopsy in calves up to 2 1/2 months of age. Vet. Med. (Prague) *12* (1967):667–677.
23. Klein, L. J. and W. E. Hornbuckle: Acute pancreatitis: the radiographic findings in 182 dogs. J. Am. Vet. Radiol. Soc. *19* (1978):102–106.
24. Nielsen, S. W. and E. J. Bishop: The duct system of the canine pancreas. Am. J. Vet. Res. *15* (1954):266–271.
25. Nielsen, S. W.: Neoplastic Diseases. *In* E. J. Catcott (ed.): Feline Medicine and Surgery. Wheaton, Ill.: Am. Vet. Public., 1964., pp. 156–176.
26. Osborne, C. A., M. L. Fahning, R. H. Schultz, et al.: Percutaneous renal biopsy in the cow and horse. JAVMA *153* (1968):563–570.
27. Osborne, C. A., J. B. Stevens, and V. Perman: Needle biopsy of the liver. JAVMA *155* (1969):1605–1620.
28. Osborne, C. A.: Clinical evaluation of needle biopsy of the kidney and its complications in the dog and cat. JAVMA *158* (1971):1213–1228.
29. Roberts, S. J.: Veterinary Obstetrics and Genital Diseases. 2nd ed. Ithaca, N. Y. Roberts. Distrib. by Edwards Bros., Ann Arbor, Mich., 1971.
30. Root, C. R.: Abdominal masses: the radiographic differential diagnosis. J. Am. Vet. Radiol. Soc. *15* (1974):26–43.
31. Root, C. R.: Interpretation of abdominal survey radiographs. Vet. Clin. of North Am. (Small Anim. Pract.) *4* (1974):763–803.
32. Schmidt, S., C. L. Lohse, and P. F. Suter: Branching patterns of the hepatic artery in the dog: arteriographic and anatomic study. Am. J. Vet. Res. *41* (1980):1090–1097.
33. Siegel, E. T., D. F. Kelly, and P. Berg: Cushing's syndrome in the dog. JAVMA *157* (1970):2081–2090.
34. Slappendel, R. J. and A. Rijnberk: Traumatic bile duct rupture in dogs and its surgical treatment. Tijdschr. Diergeneeskd. *95* (1970):392–400.
35. Stöber, M.: Die operative Behandlung der Gallenkolik des Rindes durch die Cholezystoduodenostomie nach Hofmeyer. Deutsche Tierärztl. Wochenschr. *75* (1968): 532–537.
36. Suter, P. F. and R. Lowe: Acute pancreatitis in the dog. A clinical study with emphasis on radiographic diagnosis. Acta Radiol. (Suppl.) *319* (1972):195–208.
37. Ticer, J. W., C. P. Spencer, and N. Ackerman: Positive contrast retrograde urethrography: A useful procedure for evaluating urethral disorders in the dog. Vet. Radiol. *21* (1980):2–11.
38. Udall, R. H., R. G. Warner, and S. E. Smith: A liver biopsy technique for cattle. Cornell Vet. *42* (1952):25–27.
39. Williamson, M. E.: The venous and biliary systems of the bovine liver. Master's Thesis, Cornell University, 1967.
40. Wilson, J. W., and D. D. Caywood: Functional tumors of the pancreatic beta cells. Comp. Cont. Ed. *3* (1981):458–465.

CHAPTER 25

VESTIBULE, VULVA, VAGINA, AND PERINEUM

OBJECTIVES

1. To understand the surgical anatomy involved in episiotomy and the repair of perineal laceration in the mare and cow. This includes the muscles, vessels, and nerves of the region.
2. To be able to block the superficial perineal nerves in the mare ventrolateral to the anus to anesthetize the labia.
3. To be able to block the pudendal and caudal rectal nerves in the pelvis in the cow.
4. To be able to avoid the suburethral diverticulum in catheterizing the cow.
5. To be able to palpate the urethral tubercle to catheterize the bitch and to avoid the fossa clitoridis in the process.
6. To be able to distinguish by their location a cystic vestigial ductus deferens (duct of Gartner) from an enlarged vestibular gland in the cow.
7. To know that a swelling in the lateral wall of the vestibule in the mare and the bitch is normal erectile tissue—the vestibular bulb.

25a. DISSECTION, PERINEUM, MARE

The perineum is the region that surrounds the anus and urogenital tract at the pelvic outlet. It is bounded dorsally by the base of the tail and laterally by the semimembranosus muscles. Ventrally the boundary is the caudal attachment of the udder. The fibromuscular mass between the anus and the urogenital tract is the perineal body.

The sphincter ani externus has three parts. The caudal superficial part encircles the anus and is continuous with the constrictor vulvae—the muscle of the labia (Fig. 25–1). The cranial superficial part and the deep part form loops ventral to the anus.

The constrictor vestibuli is the thin sheet of striated muscle on the lateral and ventral surfaces of the vestibule. The boundary between vagina and vestibule is marked externally by the junction of the urethra with the genital tract.

The levator ani originates from the ischiatic spine inside the sacrosciatic ligament and runs back to the anus, where it has a complex insertion. One slip terminates in the wall of the anus. A middle slip forms a loop ventral to the anus. The third part terminates on a fascial septum in the perineal body (Fig. 25–1).

The rectal part of the retractor penis or retractor clitoridis in the horse is a band of smooth muscle that originates from the first or second caudal vertebra and passes around the rectum deep to the levator. Unlike the retractor clitoridis in other domestic animals, it meets its mate under the

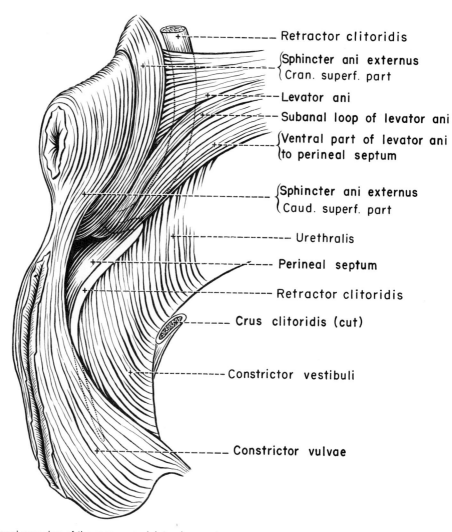

Figure 25–1. Perineal muscles of the mare, caudolateral aspect.

anus in a strong loop and a decussation. In the mare, the clitoral part of the retractor, which runs from the decussation into the labium for a variable distance, is rudimentary.

The components of the perineal body, shown in Figure 25–2,[13] are:

1. The skin
2. The column of muscle running between the external sphincter of the anus and the constrictor vulvae
3. The parts of the sphincter that pass ventral to the anus
4. The loop of the levator ventral to the anus

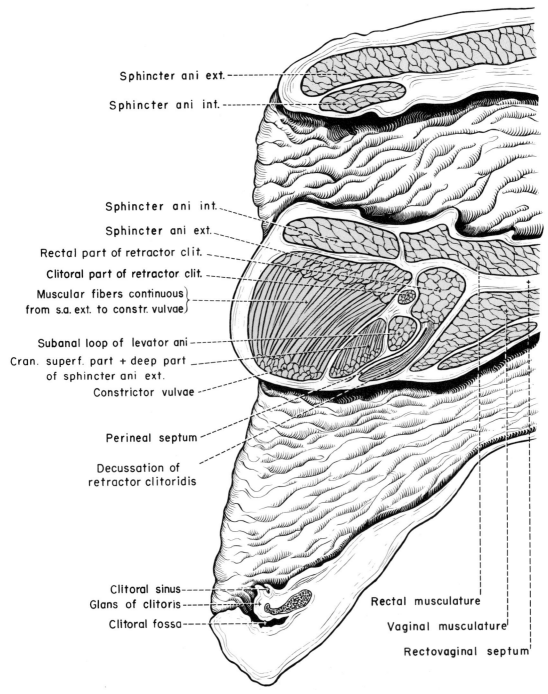

Sphincter ani ext.

Sphincter ani int.

Sphincter ani int.

Sphincter ani ext.

Rectal part of retractor clit.

Clitoral part of retractor clit.

Muscular fibers continuous } from s.a. ext. to constr. vulvae

Subanal loop of levator ani

Cran. superf. part + deep part of sphincter ani ext.

Constrictor vulvae

Perineal septum

Decussation of retractor clitoridis

Clitoral sinus

Glans of clitoris

Clitoral fossa

Rectal musculature

Vaginal musculature

Rectovaginal septum

Figure 25–2. Median section through the anus, perineal body, and vestibule of the mare.

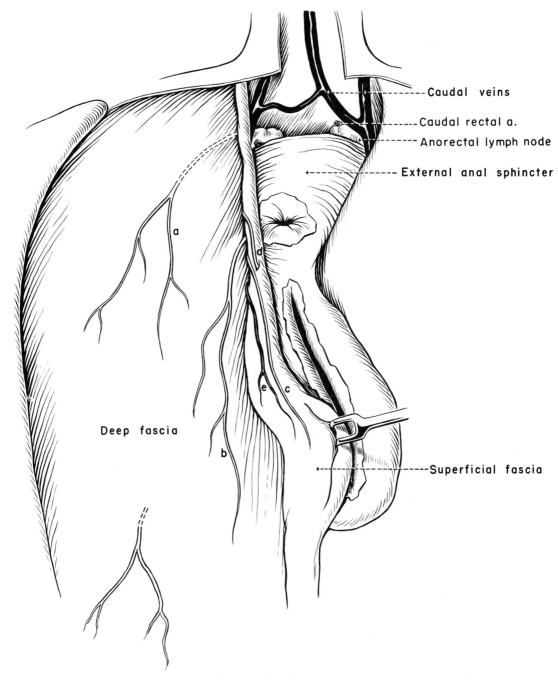

Figures 25–3. Perineal vessels and nerves, mare. *a,* ventral branch of fourth sacral nerve; *b, c, d,* superficial perineal nerves; *e,* labial branch of perineal artery. (Reprinted with permission from Sack, W. O., and R. E. Habel: Rooney's Guide to the Dissection of the Horse. Ithaca, N.Y.: Veterinary Textbooks, 1982.)

5. The loop and decussation of the rectal part of the retractor clitoridis
6. The perineal septum on which the ventral slips of the levator terminate and which is attached to most of the other components of the perineal body and to the perineal fascia
7. The smooth muscle of the internal anal sphincter.

When the perineal body is ruptured in foaling, the result is a third degree perineal laceration. The sphincters draw the parts of the perineal body laterally and the ventral branches of the levators draw them cranially. The result is a gaping common rectovaginal opening. The right and left parts of the perineal body should be reunited to effect repairs.[1,2,6]

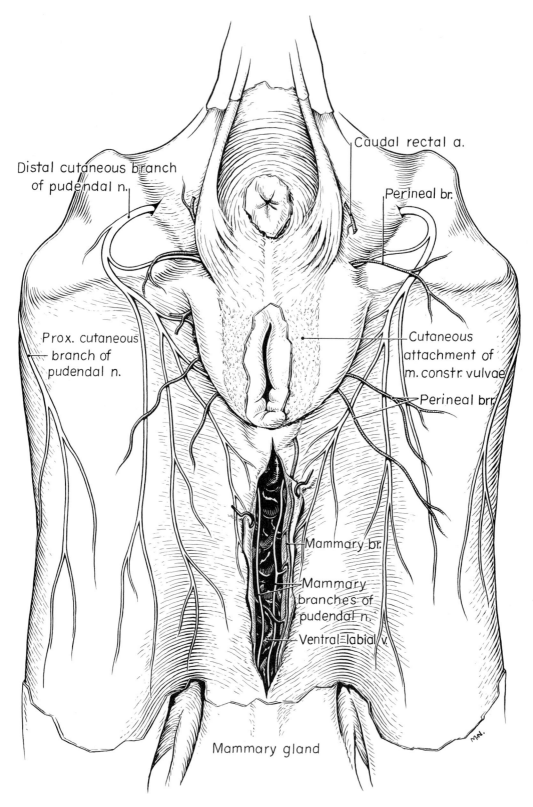

Figure 25–4. Perineum, cow, superficial dissection (Reprinted by permission from Habel, R. E.: Guide to the Dissection of Domestic Ruminants, 3rd. ed. Ithaca, N.Y.: published by author, 1983.)

The pudendal and caudal rectal nerves innervate the muscles and skin of the perineum. They both contribute fibers to the superficial perineal nerves, which emerge ventrolateral to the anus and supply the labia. The superficial perineal nerves can be blocked subcutaneously and subfascially on each side (see Fig. 25–3).[13] The pudendal nerve runs caudally on the floor of the pelvis and is continued as the nerve of the clitoris.

The internal pudendal artery gives off a variable vestibular branch at the lesser sciatic foramen and runs back to a point just inside the caudal border of the sacrosciatic ligament, where it gives off the ventral perineal artery. This immediately gives rise to a dorsal branch, the caudal rectal artery, supplies the ventrolateral part of the anus, and gives origin to the dorsal labial branches. The internal pudendal terminates as the artery of the vestibular bulb. The bulb is a mass of venous sinuses deep to the constrictor vestibuli in the mare and bitch.

The clitoris and ventral commissure are usually supplied by the obturator artery, but the vestibular branch may supply the ventral commissure.

Examine the glans of the clitoris. In the mare it is almost completely surrounded by the clitoral fossa (preputial cavity). The prepuce of the clitoris is formed by the ventral commissure of the labia and by a transverse fold of vestibular mucous membrane, to which the frenulum of the clitoris is attached. In the mare the frenulum is an area of adhesion between the glans and the vestibular wall

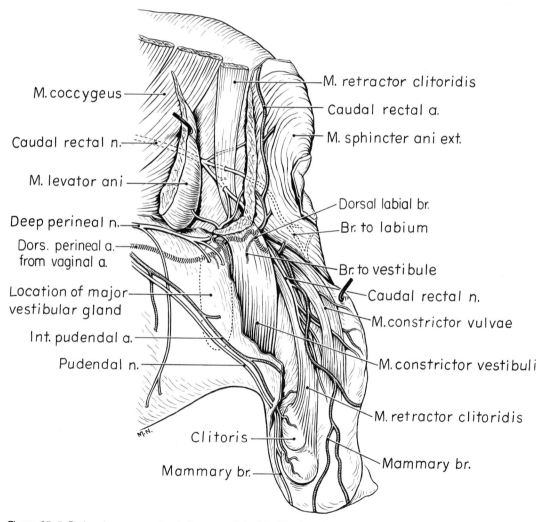

Figure 25–5. Perineal nerves and arteries, cow, left side. The levator ani is reflected to show the relation of the caudal rectal and deep perineal nerves. The arterial pattern shown here, in which the vaginal artery supplies the region lateral and ventral to the vulva, is less common than the one shown in Figure 25–6. (Reprinted by permission from Habel, R. E.: Guide to the Dissection of Domestic Ruminants. Ithaca, N.Y.: published by author, 1983.)

of the clitoral fossa. The frenulum is invaded by one to three clitoral sinuses, whose narrow openings are best seen when the glans is partially extruded and drawn ventrally. The median sinus is the most constant and often contains smegma. Other sinuses may be present in the crevice between the glans and the prepuce laterally and ventrally. The clitoral sinuses harbor the causative organism of contagious equine metritis and are swabbed for the diagnosis of that disease.[12] They are also surgically removed to eliminate the carrier state. The median sinus is seen in section in Figure 25–2.

Note the large diameter of the urethra. Cystic calculi can be removed by inserting forceps through the urethra. The bladder can prolapse through the urethra.

25b. NERVES OF THE PERINEUM, COW

The perineal region is bounded dorsally by the ventral caudal muscles; ventrally by the caudal attachment of the udder; and laterally by the sacrotuberous ligament, tuber ischiadicum, and a sagittal line from the tuber to the ventral boundary (Fig. 25–4 to 25–7).

The distal cutaneous branch of the pudendal nerve emerges from the ischiorectal fossa along the medial surface of the tuber ischiadicum, where it can be palpated and blocked. It sends branches to the labium and to the perineal region lateral and ventral to the vulva. The pudendal nerve ends

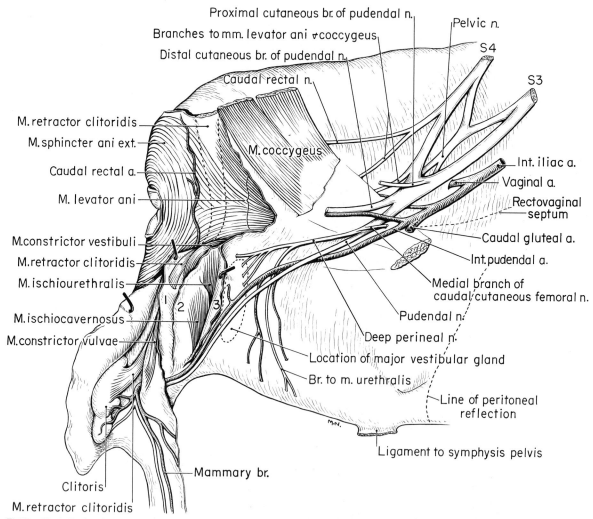

Figure 25–6. Perineal nerves and arteries, cow, right side. *1,* external layer of deep perineal fascia; *2,* perineal membrane; *3,* parietal pelvic fascia. The arterial pattern illustrated is the more common one, in which the internal pudendal artery supplies the region lateral and ventral to the vulva. Compare with Figure 25–5. (Reprinted by permission from Habel, R. E.: Guide to the Dissection of Domestic Ruminants. Ithaca, N.Y.: published by author, 1983.)

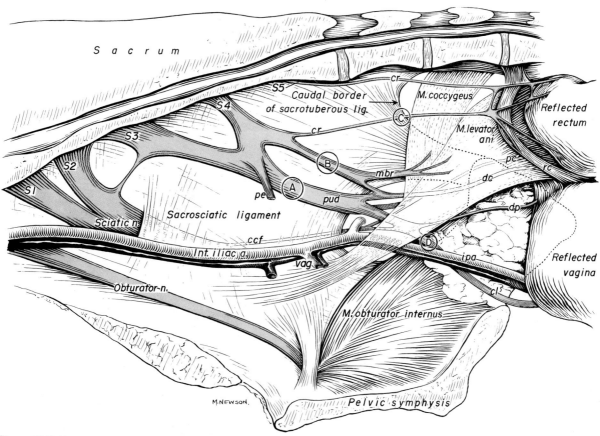

Figure 25–7. Nerves on the medial surface of the right pelvic wall of a cow: *A, B, C,* points of injection recommended by Larson; *D,* additional point; *ccf,* caudal cutaneous femoral n.; *cl,* continuation of pudendal n. to clitoris and mammary gland; *cr,* caudal rectal nn.; *dc,* distal cutaneous branch of pudendal n.; *dp,* deep perineal n.; *ipa,* internal pudendal a.; *mbr,* muscular branch; *pc,* proximal cutaneous branch of pudendal n.; *pe,* pelvic n.; *pud,* pudendal n.; *rc,* retractor clitoridis; *S 1–5,* sacral nn.; *vag,* vaginal a.

by dividing into the nerve of the clitoris and the mammary branch, which runs ventrally with the mammary vein. The caudal rectal nerve supplies the anal region and deep structures of the perineum and vulva. It communicates with a branch of the pudendal—the deep perineal, a motor nerve to the perineal muscles (Figs. 25–5, 25–6). These nerves may be blocked in the pelvis by a technique developed by Larson for the bull (Fig. 25–7; see also Chapter 28). The needle is inserted medial to the sacrotuberous ligament at C and guided to the main point of injection, A, by the hand in the rectum. Important landmarks are the internal iliac artery and the cranial border of the lesser sciatic foramen. The pudundal nerve itself is palpable through the rectal wall. As the needle is withdrawn, anesthetic is distributed along the line ABC to block the caudal rectal nerves and other sensory branches. The sacral plexus is variable. The needle should be redirected to D to block the pudendal nerve distal to its communication with the sciatic (ccf).

Note the course of the obturator nerve.

25c. DISSECTION, VAGINA, VESTIBULE, AND VULVA, COW

The most prominent feature of the floor of the vestibule is the orifice of the suburethral diverticulum. The urethral orifice is a small slit in the cranial side of the neck of the diverticulum. A catheter passed along the floor of the vestibule enters the diverticulum, not the urethra. The eminence of the mucosa cranial to the urethral orifice is the rudimentary hymen, marking the boundary between vagina and vestibule.

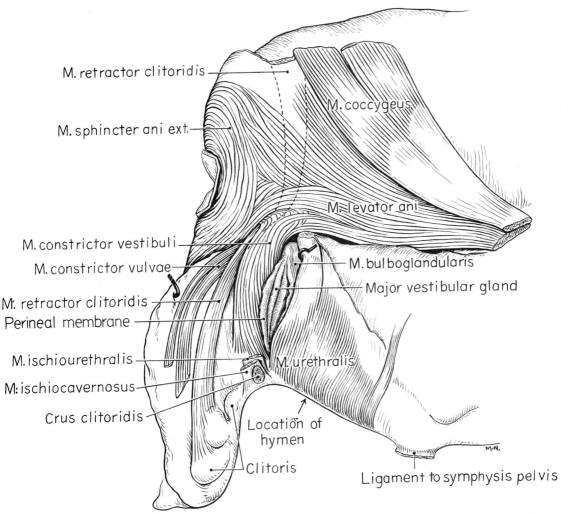

Figure 25–8. Perineal muscles of a cow, lateral view. The labium is drawn back, and the deep bands of the constrictor vulvae have been severed from their insertions on the fascia below the ischial arch. Most of the perineal membrane has been removed, as well as the visceral pelvic fascia on the urethral muscle. (Reprinted by permission from Habel, R. E.: Guide to the Dissection of Domestic Ruminants. Ithaca, N.Y.: published by author, 1983.)

Lateral to the hymenal eminence are the openings of the vestigial deferent ducts (Gartner's ducts). They extend cranially under the mucosa for variable distances. These are vestiges of the mesonephric ducts. They sometimes form cysts in the wall of the vagina.

The secretory sacs of the major vestibular glands (Bartholin's glands) open on the lateral walls of the vestibule, about 2.5 cm. caudal to the urethral orifice. The gland itself may be seen on the outside of the wall, cranial to the constrictor vestibuli and the perineal membrane (Fig 25–8). The gland sometimes becomes cystic. Only the cow, the cat, and sometimes the sheep have a gross compound major vestibular gland.

The glans clitoridis is rudimentary and barely visible in the vestibule. The body of the clitoris, however, is long and sinuous.

The vagina is relatively longer than in the mare. The rectogenital peritoneal pouch extends caudally about half the length of the vagina.

Most of the fibers of the external anal sphincter cross in the ventral decussation and pass into the opposite labium as the constrictor vulvae. The latter is dispersed in the connective tissue (see Fig. 25–4).

The constrictor vestibuli is thick at its origin from the ventral border of the levator. It passes around the vestibule and ends in a flat tendon that meets its mate under the floor of the cranial end of the vestibule. This muscle is reefed in the operation for prolapse of the vagina. It lies caudal to the perineal membrane and the major vestibular gland (Fig. 25–8).The levator ani terminates by fibers that interpenetrate, or are continuous with, the fibers of the external anal sphincter.

The vaginal artery is continued caudally by the dorsal perineal artery, which emerges lateral to the decussation of the anal sphincter and divides into the caudal rectal artery and the dorsal labial branch (see Fig. 25–5). The latter gives off a branch to the region of the tuber ischiadicum and turns ventrally in the labium. It is cut in episiotomy—a dorsolateral incision in the dorsal third of the labium. Episiotomy is performed to prevent rupture of the perineal body in parturition.

The internal pudendal artery runs back across the lateral face of the coccygeus and levator inside the lesser sciatic foramen (see Fig. 25–6). Branches are given off to the vagina, vestibule, and major vestibular gland as the artery inclines ventrally to the caudal end of the pelvic symphysis. It is accompanied by a vein and the pudendal nerve. After emerging through a foramen in the perineal membrane, it supplies the deep and dorsal arteries of the clitoris. In the majority of cows it supplies the ventral perineal arteries and a branch to the mammary gland. In some cows, these ventral perineal and mammary vessels are supplied by the dorsal labial branch of the dorsal perineal from the vaginal artery (see Fig. 25–5).

25d. DISSECTION, VAGINA, VESTIBULE, AND VULVA, BITCH

The vulva, vestibule, and vagina should be opened by a lateral incision for this demonstration. Episiotomy in the bitch is done in the median plane from the dorsal commissure.[3] The urethral tubercle is about 5 cm. from the ventral commissure of the vulva at the level of the ischial arch. On the tubercle is the urethral orifice. The urethra is relatively long, about 7 cm. The urethral tubercle marks the division between the vagina and vestibule. The vulva is the labia and commissures. The fossa clitoridis, containing the glans clitoridis, is on the floor of the vestibule just inside the labia and should not be mistaken for the urethral orifice. The vagina contributes about 9 cm. to the total of 14 cm. from the labia to the cervix. It is difficult to visualize or cannulate the external orifice of the uterus because it faces ventrally and is concealed by the dorsal median fold, which extends 2 to 3 cm. caudally from the cervix.[11]

25e. LIVE BITCH

Examine the vestibule with a speculum or a laryngoscope.[14] It is necessary to direct the speculum dorsally at first, in order to pass over the ischial arch. Find the urethral tubercle. The external orifice of the uterus cannot be seen. It is not necessary to use a speculum to pass a urethral catheter; the urethral tubercle can be palpated to guide the catheter into the urethral orifice. Vaginal fluid for a smear to determine the stage of the estrous cycle may be aspirated with a blunt pipette passed in the same manner as the speculum.

References

1. Aanes, W. A.: Surgical repair of third degree perineal laceration and rectovaginal fistula in the mare. JAVMA *144* (1964):485–491.

2. Ansari, M. M. and L. E. Matros: Surgical repair of rectovestibular lacerations in mares. Comp. Cont. Ed. *5* (1983):S129–S134.

3. Archibald, J. (ed.): Canine Surgery. Wheaton, Ill.: Am. Vet. Public., 1965.

4. Baier, W.: Die operative Behandlung des Prolapsus vaginae der Kuh. Proc. Int. Vet. Cong. Stockholm, *5* (1953):175.

5. Delahanty, D. D.: Surgical correction of contributory causes of uterine disease in the mare. JAVMA *153* (1968):1563–1566.

6. Farquharson, J.: Surgical treatment of third degree perineal lacerations. North Am. Vet. *24* (1943):220–225.

7. Freiermuth, G. J.: Episiotomy in veterinary obstetrics. JAVMA *113* (1948):231–232.

8. Habel, R. E.: A source of error in the bovine pudendal nerve block. JAVMA *128* (1956):16–17.

9. Habel, R. E.: The topographic anatomy of the muscles, nerves, and arteries of the bovine female perineum. Am. J. Anat. *119* (1966):79–96.

10. Habel, R. E.: Guide to the Dissection of Domestic Ruminants. 3rd ed., Ithaca, N. Y.: Habel, 1983.

11. Pineda, M. H., R. A. Kainer, and L. C. Faulkner: Dorsal median post cervical fold in the canine vagina. Am J. Vet. Res. *34* (1973):1487–1491.

12. Powell, D. G., J. S. E. David, and C. J. Frank: Contagious equine metritis: the present situation reviewed and a revised code of practice for its control. Vet. Rec. *103* (1978):399–402.

13. Sack, W. O. and R. E. Habel: Rooney's Guide to the Dissection of the Horse. Ithaca, N. Y.: Veterinary Textbooks, 1982.

14. Stogdale, L. and C. J. Roos: The use of the laryngoscope for bladder catheterization in the female dog. J. Am. Anim. Hosp. Assoc. *14* (1978):616–617.

CHAPTER 26

OVARY AND UTERUS

OBJECTIVES

1. To be able to recognize normal and cystic follicles and corpora lutea in the mare and cow by rectal palpation. This requires a basic understanding of the peculiar histological organization of the equine ovary.
2. To be able to palpate the ovarian bursa per rectum in the cow and mare to detect salpingitis and adhesions resulting from it. Such inflammations and adhesions indicate a bad prognosis for fertility. This examination requires a knowledge of the orientation of the bursa, the ovarian ligaments, and the course of the uterine tube.
3. To be able to find the ovaries in the abdominal cavity by palpation per rectum or in surgery.
4. To be able to palpate the horns, body, and cervix of the uterus in the mare and cow and to know the normal species difference in the size, shape, and attachment of these parts.
5. To know that the four circular folds of the bovine cervix block the lumen, except in estrus and parturition.
6. To be able to gain access to the gravid uterus for cesarean section in the cow and to make the uterine incision where it can be sutured after contraction.
7. To be able to recognize harmless cystic vestiges in the mesosalpinx and broad ligament.
8. To know where to palpate the uterus through the abdominal wall of the dog and cat.
9. To be able to palpate the cervix in ovariohysterectomy of the dog to remove as much of the body of the uterus as possible. The cervix is very short in carnivores.
10. To be able to ligate correctly the ovarian and uterine arteries in ovariohysterectomy.

26a. DISSECTION, OVARY AND UTERUS, MARE

The ovary is kidney-shaped, about 7 cm. × 3 cm., but may be much larger if it contains a mature follicle. Normal follicles may reach a diameter of 7 cm. in the mare. Follicles continue to develop for the first 70 days of pregnancy. They may reach the size of a hen's egg before regressing. Corpora lutea of the equine ovary are deeply embedded and are not palpable longer than 48 hours after ovulation. The equine ovary has a peculiar histological organization. It has a peripheral vascular zone instead of a vascular medulla, and the follicles are distributed throughout the ovary rather than concentrated in a cortex. The vessels and nerves enter the convex, attached surface. The ovarian fossa is on the free border. Ovulation always takes place in the ovarian fossa. Although ripe follicles can often be palpated per rectum on other surfaces of the ovary, post-mortem examination shows that all ripe follicles, corpora hemorrhagica, and corpora lutea have an apex directed into the ovarian fossa.[4]

The mesosalpinx, containing the uterine tube, is lateral to the caudal part of the ovary and forms the lateral wall of the ovarian bursa. The fimbriae overlap the ovarian fossa. The medial wall of the ovarian bursa is formed by the ovary and by a part of the broad ligament, the thickened free edge of which is the proper ovarian ligament, connecting the uterine end of the ovary to the uterine horn. The ovarian bursa is mostly caudal to the ovary and opens ventrally. The mesovarium is the part of the broad ligament that suspends the ovary.

The ovaries are in contact with the lumbar abdominal wall at the fourth or fifth lumbar vertebra in the non-pregnant animal. They are about 50 cm. from the vulva and 5 to 10 cm. cranial to the shaft of the ilium. With pregnancy they move ventrally.

The uterine horns are about 25 cm. long and blunt at the cranial ends. The caudal parts of the horns diverge at right angles from the body of the uterus, making transverse bicornual pregnancies possible in the mare.

The body of the uterus is 18 to 20 cm. long. The cervix is 5 to 7 cm. long and has longitudinal folds.

The gravid uterus usually lies on the ventral abdominal wall on the left of the midline.

The uterus has three arteries: (1) the uterine branch of the ovarian, (2) the uterine artery, from the origin of the external iliac, and (3) the uterine branch of the vaginal.

26b. DISSECTION, OVARY, UTERUS, COW

The ovaries are located at the ventrolateral margin of the pelvic inlet, cranial to the external iliac artery. The distance from the vulva is about 40 cm., but this is increased as the ovaries are drawn forward in pregnancy. The ovary is about the size of the distal segment of the human thumb. Normal mature follicles reach a diameter of about 15 mm.; follicles larger than 25 mm. are regarded as cystic. The corpus luteum is partly embedded in the ovary but forms a protrusion that is easily palpated 3 to 5 days after ovulation. The corpus luteum reaches its maximum size in about 7 days, when it is about 25 mm. in greatest diameter.

The orientation of the ovarian bursa and uterine tube is different from that of the bitch and the mare because the parietal attachment of the broad ligament and the ovary undergo a descent toward the pelvis in the cow. This results in the spiral of the uterine horn and gives the long axis of the ovary an obliquely transverse direction, which varies with the position of the end of the uterine horn. The tubal end of the ovary is dorsolateral, and the uterine end is ventromedial. The bursa lies lateral and cranial to the ovary. The proper ligament is medial to the orifice of the bursa and runs ventromedially toward the uterus. The mesosalpinx forms the craniolateral wall of the bursa. The uterine tube begins at the fimbriae on the free border of the mesosalpinx, near the tubal end of the ovary, turns around the dorsolateral pouch of the mesosalpinx, and runs ventromedially in the mesosalpinx to the uterus.

In a rectal examination for the presence of adhesions of the mesosalpinx to the ovary, the fingers pass over the ovary and the proper ligament and into the bursa if it is normal. Adhesions indicate salpingitis or ovaritis. Cysts may occur in the mesosalpinx or broad ligament. They are vestiges of embryonic mesonephric and paramesonephric ducts (epoöphoron, paroöphoron, hydatids).

The body of the uterus is 3 to 4 cm. long internally but appears longer on the surface because of the fusion of the caudal part of the horns. Palpate the intercornual ligaments. The ventral one is larger and is grasped per rectum to retract the uterus to palpate the horns. The latter are 35 to 40 cm. in length. The normal number of caruncles in the uterus is about 100. The cervix is 10 cm. long and has distinct external and internal orifices. The canal is occluded by circular folds, of which there are usually four, including those at the orifices.

The uterus has three arteries: (1) the uterine branch of the ovarian, (2) the uterine artery, from the internal iliac, and (3) the uterine branch of the vaginal.

The gravid uterus may lie directly upon the right abdominal floor, or it may lie within the supraomental recess with the intestines. In the latter case, it is concealed on the right by superficial and deep walls of the greater omentum. Because the supraomental recess is open caudally, the uterus may be exposed for cesarian section by drawing the greater omentum forward. The incision in the uterus should be near the ovarian end of the horn, so that the contraction of the uterus after delivery will not draw the uterine incision too far caudally to be sutured through the laparotomy incision.

Torsion of the uterus may be corrected by laying the cow down on the side toward which the torsion is directed, as determined by rectal examination.[10] The abdomen is compressed by laying a plank on the abdomen and having a person stand on the plank. This will help hold the uterus in place. The cow is then slowly rolled over to the opposite side. The cow's body moves around the uterus, correcting the torsion.

26c. DISSECTION, OVARY AND UTERUS, BITCH

Note the position and relations of the ovaries. They lie close to the caudal end of the corresponding kidney, ventral to the fourth lumbar vertebra, and half-way between the last rib and the crest of the ilium. Find the umbilicus on the abdominal wall and note that the ovary lies about 2.5 cm. caudal to the plane of the umbilicus. The right ovary is dorsal or lateral to the descending duodenum. The left ovary is dorsolateral to the descending colon and dorsomedial to the dorsal end of the spleen. In the bitch and cat, the right ovary is exposed by drawing the descending duodenum ventromedially and using the mesoduodenum to retract the other intestines. A similar maneuver with the descending colon and mesocolon exposes the left ovary.

The ovary has a mesovarian border and a free border, and the surfaces are designated medial and lateral, assuming that the mesovarian border is dorsal. Because of the mobility of the mesovarium, the ovary can swing 90 degrees medially or laterally from the sagittal plane. The ovary is completely enclosed by the bursa, except when the ovary is enlarged by ripe follicles at estrus. The ovary is in the dorsal part of the bursa—not in the pendulous part, which contains fat. The slit-like opening of the bursa is on the medial side, dorsal to the suspensory ligament. The fimbriae of the uterine tube are attached here, and the tube runs ventrally in the medial wall of the bursa, around the ventral border, and back to the uterus in the lateral wall.

Examine the ovarian arteries and veins. The arteries leave the aorta at the fourth lumbar vertebra, cross the caudal end of the kidney, and enter the mesovarian border of the ovary. The ovarian or testicular veins, especially the left one, may join the renal vein instead of the caudal vena cava. Therefore, in nephrectomy, the renal veins should be examined and ligated distal to a gonadal vein. The ovarian vein drains the cranial end of the horn of the uterus, and the artery anastomoses with the uterine artery. The uterus in carnivores has only two arteries: the uterine branch of the ovarian artery and the uterine artery, from the vaginal.

The ovary is attached to the cranial end of the uterine horn by the proper ovarian ligament. Continuous with the proper ligament is the suspensory ligament of the ovary, which is attached to the transverse fascia near the vertebral end of the last rib. These ligaments stand out if the horn of the uterus is drawn caudally. The suspensory ligament offers the main resistance to withdrawal of the ovary from the abdomen. Because of the cranial attachment of the ligament, flexion of the trunk facilitates delivery of the ovary to the incision. The suspensory ligament may be ruptured by stretching without hemostasis.

Note the relation of the uterus to the bladder and rectum. Palpate the body of the uterus. Examine the very short cervix. It is oblique so that the external orifice faces ventrally. Spread the broad ligament (often loaded with fat) and find the uterine artery as it runs cranially from the pelvis. It enters the caudal part of the broad ligament at the plane of the cervix and lies close to the caudal part of the body of the uterus, then diverges from the horn as it passes cranially, giving off 8 to 10 branches to the uterus in its course. Near the ovary, it approaches the horn again and anastomoses with the uterine branch of the ovarian artery.

26d. PALPATION AND RADIOGRAPHY OF THE UTERUS, DOG AND CAT

The following list gives the approximate size and shape of the uterine enlargements that can be palpated through the abdominal wall of an average-sized sedated bitch at various stages of gestation: 18 to 21 days—12 mm. × 8 mm.; 24 days—spherical, 15 mm.; 38 to 42 days—uterine constrictions between fetuses obliterated, abdomen distended; 42 to 50 days—rapid increase in size, fetuses palpable through the uterus and membranes.

Gestation lengths based on time of mating are less accurate than those based on ovulation as determined by the preovulatory peak in serum luteinizing hormone.[6] This is 1 to 2 days before ovulation. The normal interval from the day of peak luteinizing hormone level to parturition is 65 days. The following radiographic features of canine pregnancy are based on the period of time following the day of luteinizing hormone peak.[6, 8, 9] Uterine enlargement is first detectable at 30 days (35 days before parturition) by the presence of pear-shaped enlargements. By 35 days of gestation these are spherical, and by 41 days they are tubular or ovoid. Fetal mineralization is not detectable until 45 days in a lateral radiograph. Up until then it is difficult to tell if the uterine enlargement is due to pregnancy or a disease process. The presence of spherical shapes is highly suggestive of pregnancy. In pyometra, the distended uterus has a smooth outline with no evidence of segmentation and often a larger diameter than the coils of small intestine that it displaces. The time when these enlargements of the pregnant uterus are first detectable is variable. It will be the earliest when a high-detailed radiographic technique is used in a thin, quiet animal after evacuation of the bowel and bladder. Applying pressure to the caudal abdomen with a radiolucent paddle or injecting air into the peritoneal cavity will contribute to earlier visualization of these enlargements.

Fetal mineralization is first seen at 45 days of gestation in the vertebrae, skull, and ribs. Radiographic evidence of skeletal mineralization proceeds as follows: 48 days—scapula, humerus, femur; 52 days—radius, ulna, tibia; 54 days—pelvis and 13 countable ribs; 61 days—caudal vertebrae, fibula, calcaneus, paws, and deciduous teeth. In late pregnancy, the fetuses lie in the cranioventral part of the abdomen crowding the intestines dorsally.

Fetal death between 30 and 45 days of gestation may be suggested by the failure of the uterus to enlarge and the presence of gas in the uterus. After fetal mineralization the most reliable radiographic features of intrauterine fetal death are: overriding of the skull bones or extreme deformity of the skull, abnormal fetal posture with increased flexion of the trunk or pelvic limb extension, and intrafetal or perifetal gas accumulation.[1, 8]

The data on the radiographic features of pregnancy in the cat are less precise.[5] For the following features the stage of gestation was based on crown to rump length measurements of the fetuses performed at autopsy at the time of radiography: 25 to 35 days—uterine enlargement with a more cranial position in the abdomen; 38 days—mineralization of the skull, scapula, humerus, and femur; 41 days—mineralization of the radius and ulna; 43 days—mineralization of the tibia, fibula, and pelvis; 49 days—mineralization of the metatarsal and metacarpal bones; 52 days—mineralization of the digits, sternum, and calcaneus; 58 days—mineralization of deciduous teeth.

References

1. Ackerman, N.: Radiographic evaluation of the uterus: a review. Vet. Radiol. 22 (1981):252–257.
2. Amoroso, E. C., J. L. Hancock, and J. W. Rowlands: Ovarian activity in the pregnant mare. Nature 161 (1948):355.
3. Andrews, F. N. and F. F. McKenzie: Estrus, ovulation,

and related phenomena in the mare. Mo. Agr. Exp. Sta. Res. Bull. 329 (1941): 1–114.
4. Bergin, W. C. and W. D. Shipley: Genital health in the mare. I: Observations concerning the ovulation fossa. Vet. Med.—Small Anim. Clin. 63 (1968):362–365.
5. Boyd, J. S.: The radiographic identification of the vari-

ous stages of pregnancy in the domestic cat. J. Small Anim. Pract. *12* (1971):501–506.

6. Concannon, P. and V. Rendano: Radiographic diagnosis of canine pregnancy: onset of fetal skeletal radiopacity in relation to times of breeding, preovulatory luteinizing hormone release and parturition. Am. J. Vet. Res. *44* (1983):1506–1511.

7. Kirk, H.: Index of Diagnoses, 3rd. ed. Baltimore: Williams & Wilkins, 1947.

8. Rendano, V. T.: Radiographic evaluation of fetal development in the bitch and fetal death in the bitch and queen. *In* Kirk R. W. (ed.): Current Veterinary Therapy VIII. Philadelphia: W. B. Saunders, 1983, pp.947–952.

9. Rendano, V. T., D. H. Lein, and P. W. Concannon: Radiographic evaluation of prenatal development in the beagle. Correlation with time of breeding, LH release, and parturition. Vet. Radiol. *25* (1984):132–141.

10. Roberts, S. J. and R. B. Hillman: An improved technique for the relief of bovine uterine torsion. Cornell Vet. *63* (1973):111–116.

11. Schnelle, G. B.: Radiology in Canine Practice. Evanston, Ill.: North Am. Vet. Public., 1950.

12. Scott, E. A. and D. J. Kunze: Ovariectomy in the mare: presurgical, surgical, and postsurgical considerations. J. Eq. Med. Surg. *1* (1977):5–12.

CHAPTER 27

MAMMARY GLAND

OBJECTIVES

1. To understand the definition of a mammary gland and to know how many glands and how many duct systems are present in each species.
2. To understand the comparative nomenclature.
3. To know the surgical anatomy of the bovine teat: the layers of the wall, the vascular pattern, the distribution of smooth muscle, and the annular fold and venous ring at the base.
4. To appreciate the protective function of the lining of the teat canal.
5. To understand the suspensory apparatus of the bovine udder, especially the relation of the lateral laminae to the superficial inguinal ring and the external pudendal vessels.
6. To be able to trace the blood vessels of the mammary glands in the bitch and the cow and to know the direction of flow of the blood in the veins.
7. To be able to palpate the superficial inguinal (mammary) lymph nodes in the cow and to palpate the next lymph node in the chain draining the bovine udder (see Chapter 24).
8. To be able to anesthetize the whole udder or one teat.
9. To be able to palpate swollen superficial inguinal and axillary lymph nodes resulting from metastasis of mammary neoplasms in the bitch.
10. To know which mammary glands are drained by these lymph nodes in the bitch. Given a malignant neoplasm in a certain mammary gland, what other glands and which lymph node should be removed with it?

Table 27–1. MAMMARY GLANDS AND DUCT SYSTEMS

Species	Glands	Duct Systems per gland
Cat	8	5–7
Bitch	10	8–14
Sow	14	2
Cow	4	1
Ewe	2	1
Mare	2	2

A mammary gland is the glandular complex associated with one teat (papilla mammae). It is a modified skin gland developed from a linear epidermal thickening, the mammary ridge, visible on the lateral surface of the trunk in the 14 mm. pig embryo. The length of the ridge varies with the species. In carnivores and swine, it reaches from the axilla to the inguinal region, but in ruminants and the horse, it is limited to the groin. As the dorsal part of the trunk grows, the mammary ridges undergo a relative ventral displacement. Cellular proliferation at intervals along the mammary ridge produces a series of round thickenings, which grow deeper into the mesenchyme, become more spherical, and are called mammary buds. There are usually more buds than the normal number of mammary glands, and some of them degenerate along with the intervening segments of the ridge. In cattle, mammary buds persisting caudal to the normal mammary glands or between them give rise to accessory mammary glands. These are usually called supernumerary teats, but they also have glandular tissue. In sheep, the accessory glands occur cranial to the normal ones.[17]

The number of duct systems in one mammary gland varies with the species of domestic animal from 1 to 14, depending on the number of primary epithelial sprouts that grow from the mammary bud into the mesenchyme (Table 27–1). A collective term, udder, is applied to all of the mammary glands in the ruminant and horse.

The secretory unit is the alveolus, about 200 of which are grouped in a lobule measuring 1.5 × 1 × 0.5 mm.[18, 19] The alveolar ducts are drained by lactiferous ducts to the lactiferous sinus. This has two parts in the cow: the gland sinus and the teat sinus. In carnivores, the lactiferous sinus is a simple fusiform enlargement of the lactiferous duct. The papillary duct, or teat canal, is a narrow passage from the lactiferous sinus to the exterior.

27a. UDDER, MARE

There are two mammary glands: right and left. Each has a teat, which is flattened sagittally and bears two orifices. Each orifice leads to a separate teat canal, lactiferous sinus, and duct system. The skin of the udder and teats bears fine hairs and many sebaceous and sweat glands. The sebaceous glands are especially large near the teat orifices.

27b. DISSECTION IN SITU, UDDER, COW

To observe the suspensory apparatus of the udder, one pelvic limb must be removed distal to the mid-thigh region. Each half of the udder is supported by a medial elastic lamina and several lateral, mostly collagenous, laminae. The connective tissue of both medial and lateral laminae is continuous with the stroma, integrating the gland with its supporting tissue. The udder is not a bag. The most superficial lateral lamina is attached to the skin at the line of reflection from udder to thigh. It is cut near the cutaneous attachment when the skin is reflected ventrally from the lateral side of the udder.

Observe the dorsocaudal course of the lymphatics in the superficial laminae of the suspensory apparatus. The lymphatics drain to the superficial inguinal (mammary) lymph nodes, which lie deep to the caudal border of the lateral lamina. The efferent lymphatics from these nodes pass through the abdominal wall to the deep inguinal nodes (see Section 24b) at the origin of the deep circumflex iliac artery from the external iliac.

The lateral laminae can be separated and traced to their insertions into the gland. The superficial lateral laminae pass under the udder and join the medial lamina. Deeper laminae enter the gland at successively higher levels on the lateral surface. The fibers run mainly cranioventrally. The lateral laminae originate from the symphysial tendon caudally and the lateral crus of the superficial inguinal ring (aponeurosis of the external oblique) cranially.

The halves of the udder can be separated between their medial laminae, which are composed mostly of elastic tissue derived from the yellow abdominal tunic. The caudal borders, however, originate from the symphysial tendon and are collagenous. The entire suspensory apparatus can now be visualized. Relaxation or overloading of the medial laminae lets the udder down in the midline and causes the teats to project laterally. The fact that the median septum is composed of two separate sheets facilitates amputation of one half of the udder.

An incision through the lateral laminae at the base of the udder will expose the external pudendal artery near its division into cranial and caudal mammary arteries. The cranial mammary artery is the same as the caudal superficial epigastric. The caudal artery is the same as the ventral labial artery of other species, but in the cow it becomes very small caudal to the udder, where it is continuous with the mammary branch of the internal pudendal. There is usually a sigmoid flexure in the external pudendal artery. Note the large external pudendal vein and the genitofemoral nerve (from L 2, 3, 4). The external pudendal artery and vein are the primary mammary vessels. A cow with gangrenous mastitis may be salvaged by cutting these vessels between ligatures. The affected glands slough out, and the wound heals more rapidly than it does when the circulation is intact.[4] Note the course of the cranial and caudal mammary arteries and the artery to the superficial inguinal lymph node.

The small mammary branch of the internal pudendal artery courses superficially from the vulva toward the udder. The large accompanying vein and the mammary branch of the pudendal nerve are deeper (see Fig. 25–4). Anesthesia of the udder is obtained by paravertebral injection of lumbar nerves 1, 2, 3, and 4 and injection of the nerves below the vulva (see Sections 20f, p.214 and 25b, p.272). Lumbar nerves 1 and 2 reach the cranial part of the udder by passing around the abdomen in the flank. Lumbar nerves 3 and 4 and part of 2 form the genitofemoral nerve and reach the udder through the inguinal canal.[16]

The large vein that extends from the vulva to the udder (see Fig. 25–4) is the result of the end-to-end anastomosis of the mammary vein from the internal pudendal and the ventral labial (caudal mammary) vein from the external pudendal. Formerly called the perineal vein, it may be single or bilateral and it often is convoluted. Right and left caudal mammary veins anastomose near the superficial inguinal lymph nodes.

A study of the valves in the ventral labial vein indicated that the blood flows toward the external pudendal vein as in the bitch and mare.[3] Ventral lymphatics of the vulva also drain toward the udder to the superficial inguinal lymph nodes.

At the cranial extremity of the udder examine the large caudal superficial epigastric vein and the small artery. These are the same as the cranial mammary vessels. The vein is directly continuous with the cranial superficial epigastric vein (subcutaneous abdominal or milk vein). Trace it caudally through the gland to the external pudendal. Trace the subcutaneous abdominal vein cranially to the "milk well," where it perforates to the internal thoracic vein. Rarely, there is an anastomosis with the superficial thoracic, resulting in a "milk vein" all the way to the axillary vein in the axilla.

Most of the superficial veins of the udder drain cranially toward the subcutaneous abdominal. The veins and lymphatics can be distinguished through the skin of the udder of the live cow because the course of the lymphatics is predominantly perpendicular to that of the veins.

A venous ring is formed around the base of the udder by the cranial and caudal mammary veins on each side and by anastomotic branches between right and left mammary veins cranial and caudal to the udder. In the lactating cow, the large veins are dilated so much that the valves are incompetent and blood can flow in either direction: toward the external pudendal or toward the subcutaneous abdominal. Many of the large veins of the udder have no valves.

It has been shown that the subcutaneous abdominal veins can be ligated without ill effect.[8] The direction of blood flow in the caudal superficial epigastric vein in sheep and goats has been determined.[11] In the virgin, the flow was toward the external pudendal. In lactation, the vessel was dilated; the valves did not occlude it, and the flow was toward the cranial superficial epigastric vein.

To summarize: For each half of the udder, there is one large artery, the external pudendal. There are two large veins: the external pudendal and the subcutaneous abdominal. The ventral labial vein carries blood from the vulva toward the external pudendal vein, with the possible exception of conditions causing dilatation of the vein and incompetence of the valves.

27c. DISSECTION, DETACHED UDDER AND TEATS

Unlike the mare, cat, and bitch, the cow and sow do not have hair or glands in the skin of the teats. Examine a skinned teat to see the superficial arterial network, fed by two or three longitudinal arteries.

The main papillary artery can be seen best in corrosion casts. It enters the teat on the medial, lateral, or caudal side and runs straight distally near the inside of the teat wall, covered by the larger veins. Examine cross sections of a teat in which the venous plexus is engorged. The veins are large and thick-walled. The middle layer of the teat wall, between the skin and the mucosa, contains longitudinal and circular smooth muscle fibers in addition to the vessels. The middle layer has been described as an erectile tissue that reduces the lumen of the teat sinus, stiffens the teat, and increases its volume before milking.[14] After the milk is "let down," the erectile tissue is collapsed, and the teat sinus is distended with milk. This venous plexus is of surgical importance.

Examine a teat opened by an incision from the teat orifice to the glandular tissue. Note the papillary duct or teat canal at the apex of the teat. The duct is 8 to 12 mm. long from the teat orifice to the teat sinus. It is lined by a special stratified squamous epithelium, which is thrown into longitudinal folds. The cells of this epithelium undergo a sebaceous transformation that produces a plug of fatty desquamated cells in the canal. This is an important factor in resistance to infection.[1] The teat canal is surrounded by the teat sphincter of smooth muscle. The cavity of the teat is the teat sinus. This is lined with two-layered columnar epithelium. The sharp line of demarcation between the stratified epithelium of the teat canal and the columnar epithelium of the teat sinus is easily seen. The folds of mucosa of the teat canal are continued a short distance into the teat sinus, forming a radial structure (Fuerstenberg's rosette). Although no mechanical function has been found for this mucosal rosette at the teat canal, subepithelial inflammatory cells accumulate beneath the columnar epithelium at its junction with the stratified squamous epithelium of the teat canal. These may offer protection against invading pathogens.[13]

Observe the folds and pockets of mucosa lining the teat sinus. The folds may proliferate and occlude the lumen. The gland sinus is in the body of the gland above the base of the teat. It may or may not be partially separated from the teat sinus by an annular fold of mucosa. The prominence of the annular fold is subject to individual variation. Pathologically, it may occlude the lumen. A venous circle surrounds the base of the teat at this level and receives the blood from the papillary veins. In operating through the teat canal to relieve a stenosis near the annular fold ("high spider"), the instrument should be guided to the center of the lumen by palpation to avoid cutting the venous circle. This same venous circle should be avoided when local anesthetic is injected around the base of the teat and when the teat is incised longitudinally to correct the fibrotic occlusion of the teat sinus.

The diverticula of the gland sinus receive the large lactiferous ducts. Attempt to trace some of these. It is difficult because the lactiferous ducts, unlike the ducts of other glands, have many dilations and constrictions. Many of them are superficial, and when they become distended, the resulting "milk knots" are palpable.

27d. LIVE COW

Palpate the superficial inguinal (mammary) lymph nodes. There are usually two on each side, and the caudal node is larger. These are located dorsal to the gland between the medial and lateral laminae of the suspensory apparatus of the udder and cranial to the thick, fat-filled connective tissue in the perineum below the ischial arch. Push your fingers firmly into the fold of skin between the attachment of the udder and the pelvic limb and palpate medially. The borders of the nodes can be felt through the lateral laminae.

These nodes enlarge in cows with mastitis. They are drained to the deep inguinal nodes at the origin of the deep circumflex iliac artery from the external iliac. When enlarged deep inguinal nodes are palpated per rectum, be sure to examine for enlarged superficial inguinal nodes and mastitis before considering lymphosarcoma.

Identify the subcutaneous abdominal vein and trace it cranially from the venous circle at the base of the udder to the palpable aperture where it penetrates the rectus abdominis to join the internal thoracic vein. From the latter, blood returns to the heart via the brachiocephalic vein and the cranial vena cava. Changes occur in the subcutaneous abdominal vein as an early sign of congestive heart failure from such conditions as pericarditis, pericardial lymphosarcoma, or endocarditis. The vein will be abnormally distended and will feel more firm, like a rope, and a pulse will be evident associated with ventricular systole. This vein should not be used for venipuncture because of the danger of a hematoma causing udder edema and subsequent mastitis or a local infection leading to endocarditis.

27e. DISSECTION, MAMMARY GLANDS, BITCH

There are usually five pairs of mammary glands in the bitch. If the number is reduced, the missing gland is No. 1, the cranial thoracic. Gland No. 2 is the caudal thoracic, Nos. 3 and 4 are the cranial and caudal abdominal, and No. 5 is the inguinal gland. The frequency of all mammary tumors in the dog increases from cranial to caudal, and a majority originate in glands 4 and 5.[6] Mammary gland neoplasia comprises about 50 percent of all canine neoplasms, with 50 percent of the mammary gland neoplasms being malignant.[9, 12] In cats, the incidence of mammary gland neoplasia is 17 percent of all feline neoplasms, and 84 percent of the former are malignant.[9]

In the dog, each gland has 8 to 14 lactiferous duct systems that open on the teat. The lactiferous duct systems of the glands do not communicate. The arterial supply and the venous and lymphatic drainage are roughly divided into cranial and caudal zones. The line of division may pass between glands 3 and 4 or through gland 3. The lymphatics of the cranial three glands anastomose, and those of the caudal two glands anastomose. Sometimes the lymphatics of glands 3 and 4 anastomose. Metastasis to lymph nodes and to adjacent glands is common.[12] Lymph node metastasis from mammary neoplasms originating in glands 1 and 2 is seen in the axillary and sternal lymph nodes; from glands 4 and 5 it goes to the superficial inguinal node. Actual lymph node metastasis from gland 3 is usually to the axillary lymph node, but in a few dogs the metastatic lesion is in the superficial inguinal lymph node.[6] In these dogs, a neoplasm of gland 4 could not be ruled out.

The small ventral labial branch from the external pudendal artery may be seen at the caudal end of the inguinal gland. It is quite superficial and is accompanied by a vein.

On the deep surface of the inguinal gland, the external pudendal artery and vein may be seen emerging from the superficial inguinal ring. These vessels are continued cranially on the deep surface of the glands as the caudal superficial epigastric vessels. The artery supplies gland 5, perforates gland 4, becomes superficial, and anastomoses with the cranial superficial epigastric artery between glands 3 and 4.

Just superficial and medial to the origin of the caudal superficial epigastric artery is the superficial inguinal lymph node. This node normally receives lymphatic drainage from glands 4 and 5, and sometimes part of 3.[2]

The cranial superficial epigastric artery perforates the abdominal wall in the xiphoid region. It supplies the cranial abdominal mammary gland (No. 3) and anastomoses with the caudal superficial epigastric. The thoracic mammary glands are supplied by the perforating branches of the internal thoracic vessels. These branches emerge through the interchondral spaces and between the xiphoid and ninth costal cartilages close to the midline. The lateral part of the thoracic mammary glands is supplied by the lateral thoracic vessels from the axilla.

The axillary lymph node of the dog and cat lies on the second rib deep (dorsal) to the pectoral muscles, caudal to the axillary vein, and medial to the insertion of the latissimus dorsi and teres major. This node drains mammary glands 1, 2, and all or part of 3. It is difficult to palpate. The inconstant accessory axillary node can be palpated in the dog and cat if present. It is between the fifth and sixth ribs in the angle between the latissimus dorsi and deep pectoral and covered by the cutaneous trunci. Lay the hand flat on the thorax caudal to the arm and stroke caudally. Glands 1, 2, and 3 also have lymphatics that penetrate the ventral thoracic wall to the sternal node.[2]

Because of the high incidence of malignancy in cats, the usual surgical procedure is a radical mastectomy with removal of all the glands on the affected side and the axillary and superficial inguinal lymph nodes. In dogs, there is no evidence that the postoperative survival time is improved by the method of surgery: removal of only the neoplastic gland, removal of the neoplastic and adjacent glands, or removal of all the glands on one side and lymphadenectomy.[10]

27f. LIVE DOG

Palpate the axilla for the presence of an accessory axillary lymph node. Palpate the external pudendal vessels emerging from the superficial inguinal ring and the superficial inguinal lymph node subcutaneously just cranial and ventral to the ring.

References

1. Adams, E. W. and C. G. Rickard: The antistreptococcic activity of bovine teat canal keratin. Am. J. Vet. Res. *24* (1963):122–135.
2. Baum, H.: Das Lymphgefässsytem des Hundes. Hirschwald: Berlin, 1918, pp. 118–119.
3. Becker, R. B. and P. T. Dix: Circulatory system of the cow's udder. Fla. Agric. Exp. Sta. Bull. *379* (1942) 1–18.
4. Brewer, R. L.: Mammary vessel ligation for gangrenous mastitis. JAVMA *143* (1963):44–45.
5. Emmerson, M. A.: Anatomy of the udder. *In* Little R. B., and W. N. Plastridge (eds.) Bovine Mastitis. McGraw-Hill, New York, 1946.
6. Fidler, I. J. and R. S. Brodey: A necropsy study of canine malignant neoplasms. JAVMA *151* (1967):710–715.
7. Foust, H. L.: The surgical anatomy of the teat of the cow. JAVMA *98* (1941):143–150.
8. Graves, R. R.: An experiment with milk veins. Hoard's Dairyman *52* (1916):687 and 717.
9. Harvey, H. J.: General priniciples of veterinary oncologic surgery. J. Am. Anim. Hosp. Assoc. *12* (1976):335–339.
10. Harvey, H. J.: Department of Clinical Sciences, New York State College of Veterinary Medicine, Cornell University, Ithaca, N. Y., 1985. Personal communication.
11. Linzell, J. L. and L. E. Mount: Variations in the direction of venous blood-flow in the mammary region of the sheep and goat. Nature (Lond.) *176* (1955):37–38.
12. Moulton, J. E., D. O. N. Taylor, C. R. Dorn, and A. C. Anderson: Canine mammary tumors. Path. Vet. *7* (1970):289–320.
13. Nickerson, S. C. and J. W. Pankey: Cytologic observations of the bovine teat end. Am. J. Vet. Res. *44* (1983):1433–1441.
14. Peeters, G., L. Massart, W. Oyaert, et al.: Volumewijzigingen der Rundertepels. Vlaams Diergeneeskundig Tijdschrift, *17*(1948):59–68.
15. Riederer, T.: Ueber den Bau der Papilla mammae des Rindes. Arch. Tierhlk. *29* (1903):593–623.
16. St. Clair, L. E.: The nerve supply to the bovine mammary gland. Am. J. Vet. Res. *3* (1942):10–16.
17. Turner, C. W.: The Mammary Gland. Columbia, Mo.: Lucas Brothers, 1952.
18. Weber, A. F., R. L. Kitchell, and J. H. Sautter: Mammary gland studies I. The identity and characterization of the smallest lobule unit in the udder of the dairy cow. Am. J. Vet. Res. *16* (1955):255–263.
19. Weber, A. F.: The bovine mammary gland: structure and function. JAVMA *170* (1977):1133–1136.
20. Zietzschmann, O.: Bau und Funktion der Milchdrüse. *In* Grimmer, W. (ed.): Chemie und Physiologie der Milch. Berlin; Paul Parey, 1910.

CHAPTER 28

PENIS, ACCESSORY GLANDS, AND ISCHIORECTAL FOSSA

OBJECTIVES

1. In connection with surgery of the penis, to understand the blood supply and the marked difference between the horse and other species.
2. To be able to anesthetize the field for urethrotomy in the horse by blocking the perineal nerves.
3. To be able to block the pudendal nerve in the horse or bull to anesthetize the penis.
4. To understand the layers of the prepuce in the horse and their relation to the prepuce of other species.
5. To understand the structure and relationships of the three erectile tissues of the penis: the corpus cavernosum penis, corpus spongiosum penis, and the glans penis in all species.
6. In connection with breeding injuries and semen collection, to understand the mechanism of erection.
7. To be able to palpate the corpus cavernosum and bulbospongiosus muscle along the body of the horse penis.
8. To be able to palpate the major structures of the dog penis: long part of glans, bulb of glans, os penis, corpora cavernosa penis, and ischiocavernosus and bulbospongiosus muscles.
9. To understand the position of the canine os penis in relation to the glans and urethra and to be able to palpate the caudal end where calculi often accumulate.
10. To understand the peculiar orientation of the feline penis and the anatomy of urethrostomy in the cat.
11. To be able to identify the accessory genital glands by palpation per rectum. To know which glands are present in each species.
12. To know the surgical anatomy of the prostate in the dog and the changes in its position due to hyperplasia with increasing age.
13. To appreciate the effect of the long preprostatic urethra in the cat on the position of the bladder.
14. To be able to find the openings of the anal sacs in the dog and to be able to remove the sacs without damage to the external anal sphincter.
15. To understand the surgical anatomy involved in the repair of perineal hernia.
16. To be able to identify the major urogenital structures on radiographs of the dog.

28a. DISSECTION, VESSELS OF PENIS, PERINEAL AND PUDENDAL NERVES, HORSE

1. The internal pudendal artery of most male animals terminates as the artery of the penis, and this immediately divides into three branches: the artery of the bulb of the penis, the deep artery of the penis, and the dorsal artery of the penis. In the horse, the internal pudendal appears to terminate as the artery of the bulb because the deep artery of the penis originates elsewhere, and the dorsal artery is very small or absent. The field of the dorsal artery is supplied in the horse by anastomosing branches of the middle and cranial arteries of the penis. The artery of the bulb enters the corpus spongiosum just before the latter turns around the ischial arch.

2. The obturator vessels can be seen on the ventral surface of the tuber ischiadicum. The obturator artery of the horse, unlike that of other species, supplies a middle artery of the penis, which divides into cranial and caudal branches. The caudal branch anastomoses with the dorsal artery of the penis, if present, and gives off the deep arteries of the penis, which enter the deep surface of the crus penis and run forward to the corpus cavernosum. The cranial branch supplies the penis and anastomoses with the cranial artery of the penis.

3. The external pudendal artery of most animals gives a branch to the scrotum and continues as the caudal superficial epigastric, which gives branches to the prepuce. In the horse, the external pudendal also supplies the cranial artery of the penis, a major source of blood for the corpus cavernosum and glans. The branches of the cranial vein form a dense plexus on the sides and dorsum of the penis.

Anesthesia of the area from the anus to the scrotum may be obtained by blocking the superficial perineal nerves. The nerves emerge on both sides of the anus and run ventrally around the ischial arch to the scrotum. One branch is subcutaneous and the other is under the deep fascia. The point of injection is 2 cm. dorsal to the ischial arch and an equal distance lateral to the anus. Anesthetic is deposited subcutaneously and subfascially (0.5 cm. deeper). Anesthesia and protrusion of the penis may be obtained by blocking the pudendal nerves. This is accomplished from one of the perineal nerve injection points. The needle is advanced until it strikes the ischial arch on the midline, where the pudendal nerves turn around the arch to become the dorsal nerves of the penis.[28]

28b. DISSECTIONS, PENIS AND PREPUCE, HORSE

The prepuce of most animals consists of an external lamina of haired skin, which is continuous at the preputial orifice with the internal lamina. The latter is attached to the penis at the caudal end of the preputial cavity and is drawn out and applied to the surface of the penis in erection. Hair and skin glands extend only a short distance inside the preputial orifice, where the sebaceous glands are especially well developed. The remainder of the internal lamina, as well as the skin on the free part of the penis, lacks hair and glands, but the cells of the stratified squamous epithelium undergo a fatty transformation and are desquamated to form a large part of the smegma.

The prepuce of the horse is complicated by the preputial fold, a cylindrical fold of the internal lamina, which is doubled on itself at the preputial ring. In erection, the whole prepuce is drawn out and applied to the body of the penis. The preputial ring can be recognized as a thickened band on the extended penis and serves as a surgical landmark. In the horse, the rudimentary hairs and large skin glands extend to the preputial ring, so that a much larger area of the internal lamina than in other species is furnished with glands.

Study a cross section of the penis. The corpus cavernosum penis is dorsal. (This term is used in the singular in ungulates because right and left corpora cavernosa are not divided by a median septum as they are in the dog.) It is surrounded by a thick tunica albuginea. White fibrous trabeculae from the tunic traverse the cavernous tissue, which is composed of venous spaces and muscular trabeculae. The deep arteries of the penis and branches of the other arteries of the penis ramify in the erectile tissue.

In the ventral groove of the corpus cavernosum penis lies the urethra, surrounded by the corpus spongiosum penis. The bulbospongiosus muscle covers the corpus spongiosum ventrally. Outside the bulbospongiosus is the paired, longitudinal retractor penis.

The glans penis is continuous with the corpus spongiosum. It covers the end of the penis, and its dorsal process extends 10 cm. caudally on the dorsum. The horse has a urethral process surrounded by the fossa glandis. A dorsal diverticulum of the fossa, the urethral sinus, is often filled with smegma.

The equine penis is subject to paralysis; it hangs out of the prepuce and may become edematous. The muscular disorder is not in the retractor penis muscles, because these can be cut in the horse without causing elongation of the penis. The paralysis is in the smooth muscle of the trabeculae of the corpus cavernosum. The tonic contraction of this muscle is maintained in the contracted penis by sympathetic impulses. This is illustrated by the paralysis of the penis caused by propiopromazine, a tranquilizer that blocks adrenergic effects.[32, 42] Erection is a parasympathetic reaction requiring a release of sympathetic tonus of the smooth muscle of the trabeculae and of the helicine arteries. The latter are closed by their circular muscle and a longitudinal bundle of muscle fibers on one side of the lumen. When this eccentric muscle relaxes, the arteries uncoil and deliver arterial blood directly to the venous spaces of the corpus cavernosum. The drainage of the venous spaces is retarded by compression of the outflow veins against the inside of the tunica albuginea. This passive sympathetic release mechanism does not produce full erection. The pumping action of the ischiocavernosi on the crura generates venous pressure in the corpus cavernosum many times greater than systolic arterial pressure (see Section 28d). After ejaculation the sympathetic tonus is restored, the helicine arteries are closed, and the trabeculae contract, gradually expelling the blood from the corpus cavernosum.

28c. MALE URETHRA AND ACCESSORY GENITAL GLANDS, HORSE

The genital fold containing the ureters and deferent ducts is on the dorsal surface of the bladder. The most cranial glands are the paired seminal vesicles. Their cranial surfaces are covered with peritoneum. The next gland caudally, composed of two lateral lobes and an isthmus, is the prostate.

Two or three centimeters caudal to the prostate is another pair of glands, the bulbourethrals. These are located just cranial to the point where the urethra turns ventrally around the ischial arch. The arteries of the bulb penetrate the bulbospongiosus to enter the corpus spongiosum.

The right and left retractor penis muscles pass around the rectum, decussate, and become adherent to each other on the penis. The large fusiform bodies lateral to the urethra at the ischial arch are the crura of the penis, enclosed in the ischiocavernosus muscles. The crura unite to form one corpus cavernosum penis in the horse.

28d. GENITALIA, BULL

The vesicular glands are lobulated. The prostate has only a small body palpable on the dorsal surface, but a large pars disseminata is distributed in the wall of the pelvic urethra. The bulbourethral glands are present at the ischial arch. Palpation of the bulbourethral glands is a useful method of differentiating castrated from cryptorchid lambs. Although cryptorchidism is rare in the bull and goat, the incidence is 5 to 15 percent of ram lambs. The bulbourethral glands in the uncastrated or cryptorchid lamb are about the size of a hazelnut (1.25 cm.) at 4 to 6 months. In lambs that were castrated early, the glands are about the size of a pea and almost impossible to palpate per rectum.[15]

The retractor penis is large and functional. It originates from caudal vertebrae 2–3 or 3–4 and is inserted on the penis distal to the sigmoid flexure, maintaining the flexure and retraction of the penis by its tonus. (The fibrous architecture of the corpus cavernosum penis and tunica albuginea also tends to maintain the flexure of the penis.) The tonic contraction of the retractor, which is all smooth muscle, is stimulated by a continuous discharge of adrenergic impulses and is released during erection by cholinergic inhibitory impulses from the pelvic nerves.[24] Larson's pudendal and caudal rectal nerve block not only anesthetizes the penis but also interrupts the sympathetic impulses, permitting relaxation of the retractor and protrusion of the penis.[26] An antiadrenergic tranquilizer has the same relaxing effect but produces no anesthesia. Epidural anesthesia does not block the sympathetic impulses unless the dose is large enough to extend cranially to the origins of the preganglionic sympathetic fibers from the lumbar cord. This "high epidural" will cause a paresis or paralysis of the hind limbs that is dangerous in a large bull. An antiadrenergic tranquilizer combined with a "low epidural" that blocks only the sacral nerves will provide penile relaxation and anesthesia.

It is important that the penis of the bull receives almost all of its blood supply from the caudal end. The dorsal and deep arteries (from the internal pudendal) are therefore large. The dorsal arteries, paired at the beginning, form a single artery at a variable distance from the ischial arch. In bovine urethrotomy, considerable hemorrhage may be avoided by separating the dorsal arteries from the deep surface of the penis before sectioning the latter.

The dorsal nerves of the penis accompany the artery. They may be blocked at the ischial arch, as described in section 28a. An easier and more accurate method is that used by Larson in which the pudendal and caudal rectal nerves are blocked on the medial surface of the sacrosciatic ligament (see Fig 25–7).[26] The pudendal nerve is located by rectal palpation. It runs downward and backward from the third sacral nerve to the lesser sciatic foramen, the cranial border of which is palpable. The nerve is dorsal to the internal iliac artery, identified by its pulse near the ischiatic spine. A 12.5 cm. needle is inserted medial to the sacrotuberous ligament (caudal border of the sacrosciatic ligament) and guided to the nerve by the hand in the rectum. After blocking the pudendal nerve, the injection is continued as the needle is withdrawn to infiltrate the caudal rectal nerves. The importance of blocking the pudendal nerve again at D (see Fig. 25–7) in the bull is disputed.

The preputial cavity is about 40 cm. long when the penis is retracted. There is a short urethral process on the side of the glans. In the sheep and goat, this process is long, composed of erectile tissue, and extends beyond the glans. It is a site of obstruction by calculi and causes difficulty in passing a catheter. When a urethral catheter is passed through the penis of a buck, it often enters a dorsal diverticulum of the urethra at the ischial arch.[23] This prevents advancement into the pelvic urethra. In bulls and rams, it may lodge in mucosal folds around the excretory ducts of the bulbourethral glands.

There are three types of penis, differing in the proportion of musculocavernous to fibrous tissue and in the presence or absence of an os penis:

1. The musculocavernous type has a large expansible corpus cavernosum penis and a large glans, as in man and the horse.

2. The fibrous type has a dense, thick tunica albuginea that does not expand very much in erection, the protrusion of the penis being largely due to the rapid straightening of the sigmoid flexure caused by a great increase in pressure in the narrow corpus cavernosum. The glans is very small. This type occurs in the ruminants and the pig (Fig. 28–1).

3. The type with an os penis is a further development in the stiffening of the corpora cavernosa penis, in that the part enclosed by the large glans is converted to bone. This type is seen in the dog and cat and in many wild species.

The mechanism of rapid erection in the bull and ram has been described.[41] The venous spaces of each crus are drained by a large, thick-walled vein that begins in the distal part of the crus. These

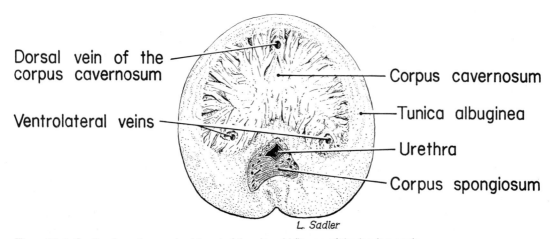

L. Sadler

Figure 28–1. Section from the proximal bend of the sigmoid flexure of the bovine penis.

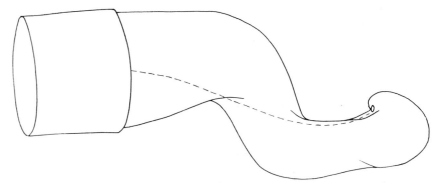

Figure 28–2. Spiral resulting from protrusion of the penis of an adult bull. Dorsal view. The axis of the spiral is the raphe of the penis, shown by a broken line. (Reprinted by permission from Ashdown, et al.: J. Anat. *103* (1968): 567–572 Cambridge University Press.)

two veins unite to form a single vessel that courses distally in the dorsal part of the corpus cavernosum penis to the sigmoid flexure, where it is connected by anastomoses with two ventrolateral veins, one on each side of the urethral groove (Fig. 28–1). These vessels extend from one end of the corpus cavernosum to the other and have their largest diameter in the sigmoid flexure. Their side branches lead to the cavernous spaces. Both the ventral vessels and their branches have thick walls of elastic and muscular tissue. The cavernous spaces of the crura are filled with blood from branches of the deep artery of the penis, as in other species. Then repeated contractions of the ischiocavernosus muscles pump blood rapidly from the venous spaces of the crura through the dorsal and ventrolateral veins of the corpus cavernosum to the venous spaces of the sigmoid flexure, causing it to straighten out rapidly. The blood pressure in the corpus cavernosum penis of the bull during coitus is 60 times as high as the systolic carotid pressure.[9] Similar results (27 times arterial pressure) were obtained in the horse.[8] Electromyographic records indicated that the ischiocavernosus muscles acted as a booster pump.

Angiographic studies in the ram and buck show that at peak erection, contraction of the ischiocavernosus muscles occludes both the arterial inflow and venous outflow from the corpus cavernosum penis producing a closed system.[10] Impotence due to inability to obtain or maintain erection has been associated with acquired or congenital vascular shunts from the corpus cavernosum penis to adjacent vessels.

Hematomata of the bovine penis usually occur in the region of the second bend of the sigmoid flexure. This is at the preputial orifice in erection. If they are not treated, they lead to scar formation with deviation of the penis. The rupture may be of the tunica albuginea or of the dorsal vessels on the surface. The prognosis is better in the latter case, and a careful diagnosis should be made before condemning the animal.[31, 44]

Hemorrhage from rupture of the tunica albuginea of the corpus cavernosum also occurs proximally in the first 12 cm. of the body of the penis at a site proximal to a fibrous occlusion of the large dorsal vein in the corpus cavernosum penis.[7] This obstruction may cause abnormally high pressures associated with the pumping action of the ischiocavernosus muscles during erection and result in rupture of the vein and of the tunica albuginea. This may produce a visible or palpable swelling caudal and dorsal to the scrotum. Ruptures distal to the sigmoid flexure usually cause swelling cranial to the scrotum.

Urinary calculi in cattle often lodge in the urethra of the distal portion of the sigmoid flexure of the penis. In palpation, these should not be confused with the retractor penis at this level.

A spiral deviation of the end of the penis was observed in more than half of the ejaculations of normal bulls.[36] After intromission into a transparent artificial vagina, the distal end of the penis twisted in a left hand spiral around the axis of the raphe of the penis. The anatomical structures that cause the spiral include (see Figs. 28–2 to 28–5):[4, 5]

1. The subcutaneous tissue of the free end of the penis is more densely fibrous than the dermis of the skin and is composed of spiral fibers running around the penis from the raphe. The raphe runs from the ventral surface of the penis to the right side of the glans. The subcutaneous spiral

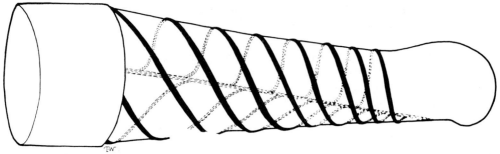

Figure 28–3. Arrangement of collagen fibers in the subcutaneous tissue of the bovine penis. Dorsal view. The longitudinal fibers of the raphe are shown by broken lines. The course of the fibers around the penis is shown by solid (dorsal) and broken (ventral) lines. (Reprinted by permission from Ashdown et al.: J. Anat. *103* (1968): 567–572 Cambridge University Press.)

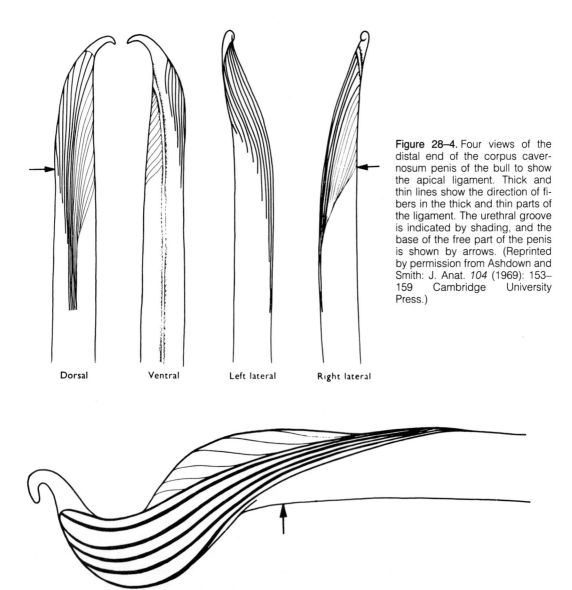

Dorsal   Ventral   Left lateral   Right lateral

Figure 28–4. Four views of the distal end of the corpus cavernosum penis of the bull to show the apical ligament. Thick and thin lines show the direction of fibers in the thick and thin parts of the ligament. The urethral groove is indicated by shading, and the base of the free part of the penis is shown by arrows. (Reprinted by permission from Ashdown and Smith: J. Anat. *104* (1969): 153–159 Cambridge University Press.)

Figure 28–5. Cranial and left lateral view of the distal end of the corpus cavernosum penis of the bull to show the normal displacement of the thick part of the apical ligament to the left in spiral deviation. The base of the free part of the penis is indicated by the arrow. (Reprinted by permission from Ashdown and Smith: J. Anat. *104* (1969): 153–159 Cambridge University Press.)

fibers run from the raphe dorsally and to the right, to join the raphe again more distally. The fibers are loosely attached to adjacent turns on the side opposite the raphe, causing the erect penis to bend toward the nonextensile raphe.

2. The fibers of the tunica albuginea have a similar architecture to that of the subcutaneous tissue, permitting the end of the penis to bend ventrally and to the right.

3. The apical ligament of the penis originates dorsally from the longitudinal fibers of the tunica albuginea along a 7-cm. strip beginning distal to the sigmoid flexure. The fibers on the left side are much thicker than those on the right. They are attached to the distal end of the tunica albuginea. When the free end of the penis deviates ventrally and to the right under the pressure of erection, the apical ligament slips over to the left side and retains the tip of the penis, forming a spiral. If the ligament is cut, a smooth bend ventrally and to the right persists. Premature spiraling prevents intromission and can be corrected by shortening the apical ligament and suturing it to the tunica albuginea, but the latter must not be perforated lest erection be impaired.[40]

The epithelial surfaces of the skin of the penis and internal lamina of the prepuce are fused at birth and separate as the calf matures sexually. The frenulum is a band of connective tissue that attaches the ventral surface of the penis to the prepuce. This normally degenerates as the epithelia separate, and the process is usually completed by 8 to 11 months. The penile raphe represents the site of attachment of the frenulum. A strand of the frenulum near the glans may persist. It is composed of connective tissue covered by epithelium, and it usually contains a vein and sometimes an artery. It is strong enough to cause a marked deviation of the penis during erection.[3, 44] This can be corrected surgically, but these bulls should not be used for breeding because of the suspected inheritance of the condition.

28e. GENITALIA, BOAR

The vesicular glands are large. The body of the prostate is exposed on the dorsal surface of the urethra, and the rest of the gland is disseminated in the wall of the urethra. The bulbourethral glands are large and elongated. These glands are all markedly reduced in size in pigs castrated early in life.

The boar penis is a fibrous type with a sigmoid flexure similar to that of ruminants, except that it is prescrotal. The free end is pointed and curved in a spiral and surrounded by a thin glans.

The prepuce has a small orifice. The cranial part is dilated and opens into a dorsal diverticulum. The latter is lined by skin with sebaceous and tubular glands, the secretion of which is mixed with decomposing urine to produce a foul-smelling liquid. For this reason the diverticulum must be avoided in evisceration of slaughtered swine.

28f. DISSECTION, GLANS PENIS, DOG

At the caudal end of the preputial cavity, the internal lamina of the prepuce is continuous with the skin on the glans. The erectile tissue of the glans can be demonstrated by a longitudinal incision. The glans surrounds the os penis and consists of a bulbous part caudally and a long part cranially. In the ventral groove of the os penis, the urethra is enclosed in the corpus spongiosum. The latter is continuous over the os penis with the bulb of the glans, not to be confused with the bulb of the penis at the other end of the organ between the crura.

The vascular anatomy involved in erection in the dog has been described.[13] In the dog, the right and left corpora cavernosa penis are divided by a median septum. The first stage of erection results from release of arterial blood from helicine arteries in the corpora cavernosa and in the corpus spongiosum, especially its enlargement, the bulb of the penis. Contractions of the ischiocavernosus muscles are correlated with pressure peaks in the corpora cavernosa that reach about 40 times arterial systolic pressure at intromission.[34] These findings have greatly increased our estimate of the importance of the corpora cavernosa in canine erection. The stiffening of this structure facilitates intromission.

In the second stage, the penis is gripped behind the glans by the female vestibular bulbs and constrictor vestibuli. This pressure reflexly stimulates tonic contraction of the ischiourethralis and rhythmic contractions of the bulbospongiosus.[22] The ischiourethralis muscles throttle the common dorsal vein of the penis inside the ischial arch, where it passes through a slit between their conjoined tendons and the transverse perineal ligament.[30] This slows outflow from the bulb of the glans while the bulbospongiosus pumps blood distally through the corpus spongiosum to the glans. The result is rapid enlargement, first of the bulb and then of the long part of the glans. The flow in the dorsal artery of the penis is increased, and this contributes to the erection of the long part of the glans. During this stage the male pelvic thrust is repeated rapidly, and sperm-rich ejaculation occurs. The rhythmic contractions of the bulbospongiosus also pump the semen distally.

In the third stage, usually called the tie, and lasting 5 to 45 minutes, the male steps over the female with one hind limb and faces the opposite direction. The penis turns laterally 180°, bending in its body at the level of the neck of the scrotum. The bulb of the glans is firmly attached to the os penis and is locked in the vagina by the vestibular bulbs and the constrictor vestibuli. The penile muscles exhibit only intermittent contraction during the tie. They are not necessary to maintain erection because the veins draining the glans—the superficial veins to the caudal superficial epigastrics through the prepuce and the dorsal veins of the penis—are compressed by the reversed, stretched, and twisted prepuce and preputial muscle. During this stage voluminous sperm-free ejaculation occurs.[19]

The corona glandis is the rim around the distal end of the glans. Touching it before intromission causes a reflex detumescence, which could benefit the species; if premature erection of the glans prevents intromission, detumescence provides another chance. The reflex also has practical importance in collecting semen for artificial insemination: the corona should not be touched. The most sensitive area for stimulation of ejaculation is not the glans but the body of the penis caudal to the glans.[21]

Section of the ischiourethralis muscles prevents the tie, demonstrating the importance of dorsal vein compression in erection of the bulb of the glans. Dogs that have these muscles cut will remate several times in 10 minutes after failure of the tie. Normal dogs will not attempt coitus for several hours after a tie has occurred.[22]

The os penis is the ossified cranial portion of the corpora cavernosa penis. The caudal end of the os penis is just cranial to the scrotum. It can be felt in the live dog. Calculi passing down the urethra are often caught at the caudal end of the os penis where the expansion of the urethra is prevented by the bony walls of the urethral groove. One side of the groove may be removed surgically if necessary.[2] Surgical incision into the urethra to remove calculi should be directly on the ventral median plane, where the retractor muscles can be displaced and only the corpus spongiosum covers the urethra.[38] Incision to either side will cause extensive bleeding from the corpus cavernosum.

28g. PELVIS AND MALE GENITAL ORGANS, DOG

The large prostate gland surrounds the urethra caudal to the bladder. There are no seminal vesicles or bulbourethral glands. At 8 months of age, the prostate is in the pelvis. With sexual maturity it gradually increases in size and extends into the abdominal cavity. In most dogs 4 years old, two-thirds of the prostate is abdominal, i. e., in front of the pubis. After 10 years, the whole gland is abdominal.[18] If the prostate cannot be palpated through the abdominal wall it should be palpated per rectum, pushing the bladder back into the pelvis with the other hand.[12]

The blood supply, which must be ligated in prostatectomy,[1] consists of two branches of the prostatic artery on each side. The pelvic nerves accompany the prostatic artery and are joined by the hypogastric nerve to form the pelvic plexus. These nerves should be spared as well as the branches of the plexus that go to the bladder and urethra.[17] In many dogs, a large amount of fat accumulates in the lateral ligaments of the bladder and is found cranial and ventral to the prostate. This fat is supplied by a branch of the caudal epigastric artery or pudendoepigastric trunk. Removal of this fat will expose the blood and nerve supply to the prostate covered dorsally by a single layer of peritoneum of the wall of the rectogenital pouch. The latter is continuous cranially with the lateral ligament of the bladder.

As the urethra turns around the ischial arch, it is surrounded by an enlargement of the corpus spongiosum, the bulb of the penis (not to be confused with the bulb of the glans). The bulb of the penis is covered by the bulbospongiosus muscle. The retractor penis is a thin median band of muscle. The fusiform muscles on both sides of the bulbospongiosus are the ischiocavernosus muscles, which cover the crura of the penis. The latter unite ventrally and continue forward under the pelvis as the corpora cavernosa penis. Examine the dorsal arteries and veins of the penis.

28h. DISSECTION, ISCHIORECTAL FOSSA, MALE DOG

The ischiorectal fossa contains fat and fascia, which must be removed to see the boundaries.

The muscle forming the lateral boundary of the ischiorectal fossa is the superficial gluteal. Medial to the muscle is the sacrotuberous ligament. Originating from the ischial end of the ligament and the tuber ischiadicum is the biceps femoris. The medial wall of the ischiorectal fossa is formed by two muscles: the lateral one is the coccygeus, and the muscle lying on the rectum cranial to the external sphincter is the levator ani. The floor of the fossa is formed by the ischium and the obturator internus.

On the lateral wall of the pelvis, the sciatic nerve and the large caudal gluteal vessels are cranial to the sacrotuberous ligament. The caudal cutaneous femoral nerve passes across the medial surface of the ligament and runs down over the tuber ischiadicum. It has a large area of distribution to the skin on the caudal surface and caudal half of the lateral surface of the thigh. It overlaps with the lateral cutaneous femoral nerve laterally and the superficial perineal nerve medially. The internal pudendal vessels and the pudendal nerve course into the floor of the fossa from lateral to the coccygeus muscle and toward the midline of the ischial arch. The caudal rectal vessels and nerve, originating from the pudendal trunks, are short. They pass dorsally, caudal to the levator ani, and are distributed to the external anal sphincter and adjacent perineum. The superficial perineal nerve is usually a branch of the pudendal nerve near the coccygeus muscle.[37] It emerges from the fossa and passes over the ischial arch, where it is superficial just lateral to the midline. It supplies the skin of the perineum and scrotum. Deep perineal nerve(s) branch from the pudendal within the fossa and supply the muscles of the penis and urethra. The genitofemoral nerve (L 3, L 4) emerges from the inguinal canal to supply the skin of the prepuce and medial thigh but not the scrotum.[37]

In perineal hernia, the levator and coccygeus muscles are often atrophied, and the hernial contents usually pass between the levator and the external sphincter or through the levator.[11] The caudal rectal vessels and nerve may be stretched across the hernial sac and should be spared to avoid paralysis of the sphincter ani in bilateral operations. After removal of the herniated tissues (fat, tumors) or replacement of organs (bladder, prostate, gut), the pelvic diaphragm is reconstructed by suturing the cranial border of the external anal sphincter to the coccygeus dorsolaterally, to the sacrotuberous ligament laterally, and to the internal obturator ventrally. A flap of fascia from the lateral margin of the hernia is then sutured to the caudal border of the external anal sphincter.[33] A modification of this procedure utilizes transposition of the internal obturator muscle into the fossa to help close the ventral aspect of the hernia.[20] The tendon is incised at the lesser sciatic notch, and the muscle is elevated from the ischium but left attached to the pubis. The freed portion is reflected dorsally and sutured to the external anal sphincter medially and the sacrotuberous ligament and superficial gluteal laterally.

Perineal hernias occur almost exclusively in males. One study has shown that the levator ani of the female is longer, larger, and heavier and has a larger termination in the external anal sphincter than in the male.[14] In this study, alterations of the levels of testosterone did not influence the anatomy of the levator ani in the male.

The orifice of the anal sac (sinus paranalis) opens on the lateral wall of the cutaneous zone of the anal canal. The sac is covered by the external anal sphincter. Microscopic glands in the wall of the sac are the source of the secretions that fill it.

28i. RADIOGRAPHS, DOG AND CAT

Compare the normal position of the bladder in the abdomen of the dog and cat. Note the long preprostatic urethra in the cat, which accounts for the more cranial position of its bladder. In normal young dogs, the bladder neck should be at the level of the pelvis. It will be displaced cranially when the bladder is full and as the prostate enlarges. Note the relationship of the prostate to the bladder in older dogs. Contrast studies may show a distortion of the lumen of the urethra and the neck of the bladder if the prostate is enlarged.[29] As a rule, hyperplasia and prostatitis tend to cause more symmetrical prostatic enlargement than cysts, neoplasms, or prostatic abscesses.[39]

Observe the canine os penis. Normal variations in its shape are common. Note its caudal extent with relation to the scrotum. In looking for calculi, the pelvic limbs should be pulled caudally to avoid confusion with the gastrocnemius sesamoids at the stifle joint.

28j. LIVE MALE DOG

Palpate the following structures:
1. Bulbospongiosus and ischiocavernosus muscles at the root of the penis.
2. The part of the shaft of the penis composed of the cavernous bodies. Appreciate its flexibility. Note the groove for the urethra ventrally.
3. Os penis. Find its junction caudally with the cavernous bodies where calculi sometimes lodge. Note the ventral groove for the urethra.
4. The long and bulbar parts of the glans.

28k. MALE GENITALIA, CAT

The urethra lies on the pelvic floor. The bulbourethral glands are at the ischial arch. The prostate lies at the pelvic inlet. There are no vesicular glands. Note the long preprostatic urethra. This places the bladder farther ahead of the pubis than it is in other species. The more cranial location must be taken into account when the bladder is punctured through the abdominal wall to relieve distention.

Knowledge of the anatomy of the feline penis is important in the surgical treatment of urethral calculi: The relaxed penis is directed ventrally and caudally. The tip of the penis is covered by a glans that is continuous with the corpus spongiosum around the urethra. The skin of the glans bears cornified spines directed proximally. These are most developed in the intact male. There is a small os penis in the glans in the adult that is continuous with the corpora cavernosa penis, which form most of the shaft of the penis. The crura are attached proximally to the ischiatic tubers and are covered by the ischiocavernosus muscles. The pelvic urethra passes caudally between the bulbourethral glands at the ischial arch and narrows as it enters the penis. It is surrounded by a thin layer of corpus spongiosum and lies in the groove on the urethral surface of the penis. This surface faces dorsocaudally because the penis is directed caudoventrally. This groove is formed by the cavernous bodies and the os penis. The bulbospongiosus muscle covers the urethra at the ischial arch and the paired retractor penis muscle passes caudally over the bulbospongiosus muscle and penis to the glans. During erection the penis increases 50 percent in length, doubles its diameter, and curves downward and forward to assume a position more like that of the canine penis. The change in form during erection is related to the structure of the tunica albuginea and trabeculae, but most important is the presence of a median dorsal apical ligament.[35]

In perineal urethrostomy an incision is made over the penis, and it is dissected free from the adjacent connective tissue.[43] Proximally on the deep surface, the ischiocavernosus muscles with the enclosed crura are cut at their attachment on the ischiatic tubers. The suspensory ligament between the caudal symphysis pelvis and the penis is severed. The pelvic urethra is freed from the floor of the pelvis. The penis is then drawn caudoventrally, and the urethral surface is exposed by removing the retractor penis and incising the bulbospongiosus muscle. The urethra is slit open up to the pelvic urethra between the bulbourethral glands. The purpose of this is to open the pelvic urethra, because it has a larger diameter (4 mm.) than the penile urethra. The edges of the opened urethra are sutured to the skin around the incision that freed the penis, to include the proximal two-thirds of the penile urethra. The body of the penis is ligated with a mattress suture at this point, and the rest of the penis is amputated.

References

1. Archibald, J. and A. J. Cawley: Canine prostatectomy. JAVMA *128* (1956):173–177.

2. Arnold, R. A.: A technic for partial ostectomy of the canine penis. Small Anim. Clin. *1* (1961):366–372.

3. Ashdown, R. R.: Persistence of the penile frenulum in young bulls. Vet. Rec. *74* (1962):1464–1468.

4. Ashdown, R. R., S. W. Ricketts, and R. C. Wardley: The fibrous architecture of the integumentary coverings of the bovine penis. J. Anat. *103* (1968):567–572.

5. Ashdown, R. R. and J. A. Smith: The anatomy of the corpus cavernosum penis of the bull and its relationship to spiral deviation of the penis. J. Anat. *104* (1969):153–159.

6. Ashdown, R. R. and H. Pearson: Studies on "corkscrew" penis in the bull. Vet. Rec. *93* (1973):30–35.

7. Ashdown, R. R. and C. E. Glossop: Impotence in the bull: 3. Rupture of the corpus cavernosum penis proximal to the sigmoid flexure. Vet. Rec. *113* (1983):30–37.

8. Beckett, S. D., R. S. Hudson, D. F. Walker, et al.: Blood pressures and penile muscle activity in the stallion during coitus. Am. J. Physiol. *225* (1973):1072–1075.

9. Beckett, S. D., D. F. Walker, R. S. Hudson, et al.: Corpus cavernosum penis pressure and penile muscle activity in the bull during coitus. Am. J. Vet. Res. *35* (1974): 761–764.

10. Beckett, S. D., T. M. Reynolds, and J. E. Bartels: Angiography of the crus penis in the ram and buck during erection. Am. J. Vet. Res. *39* (1978):1950–1954.

11. Bojrab, M. J.: Perineal herniorrhaphy. Comp. Cont. Ed. *3* (1981):8–15.

12. Bovee, K. C.: Physical examination of the urinary system. Vet. Clin. North Am. *1* (1971):119–128.

13. Christensen, G. C.: The urogenital system. *In* Evans, H. E., and G. C. Christensen, Miller's Anatomy of the Dog. 2nd ed. Philadelphia: W. B. Saunders, 1979.

14. Desai, R.: An anatomical study of the canine male and female pelvic diaphragm and the effect of testosterone on the status of the levator ani of male dogs. J. Am. Anim. Hosp. Assoc. *18* (1982):195–202.

15. Dietz, O. and G. K. Dorn: Diagnose und Operation des Kryptorchismus beim Schaf. Monatsch. Vet. Med. *14* (1959):205–208.

16. Dorr, L. D. and M. J. Brody: Hemodynamic mechanisms of erection in the canine penis. Am. J. Physiol. *213* (1967):1526–1531.

17. Gordon, N.: Surgical anatomy of the bladder, prostate gland, and urethra. JAVMA *136* (1960):215–221.

18. Gordon, N.: The position of the canine prostate gland. Am. J. Vet. Res. *22* (1961):142–146.

19. Grandage, J.: The erect dog penis: a paradox of flexible rigidity. Vet. Rec. *91* (1972):141–147.

20. Hardie, E. M., R. J. Kolata, T. D. Earley, et al.: Evaluation of internal obturator muscle transposition in treatment of perineal hernia in dogs. Vet. Surg. *12* (1983):69–72.

21. Hart, B. L. and R. L. Kitchell: Penile erection and contraction of penile muscles in the spinal and intact dog. Am. J. Physiol. *210* (1966):257–262.

22. Hart, B. L.: The action of extrinsic penile muscles during copulation in the male dog. Anat. Rec. *173* (1972):1–6.

23. Hinkle, R. F., J. L. Howard, and J. L. Stowater: An anatomic barrier to urethral catheterization in the male goat. JAVMA *173* (1978):1584–1586.

24. Klinge, E.: The effect of some substances on the isolated bull retractor penis muscle. Acta Physiol. Scand. *78* (1970):280–288.

25. Klinge, E., P. Pohto, and E. Solatunturi: Adrenergic innervation and structure of bull retractor penis muscle. Acta Physiol. Scand. *78* (1970):110–116.

26. Larson, L. L.: The pudendal nerve block for anesthesia of the penis and relaxation of the retractor penis muscle. JAVMA *123* (1953):18–27.

27. Larson, L. L., and R. L. Kitchell: Neural mechanisms in sexual behavior II. Gross neuroanatomical and correlative neurophysiological studies of the external genitalia of the bull and the ram. Am. J. Vet. Res. *19* (1958):853–865.

28. Magda, I. I.: Local anesthesia in operations on the male perineum in horses. (Abstr.) JAVMA *113* (1948):559.

29. Matera, E. A. and J. Archibald: Prostate gland. *In* Archibald, J. (ed.) Canine Surgery. Wheaton, Ill.: Am. Vet. Public., 1965.

30. Nitschke, T.: Der M. compressor venae dorsalis penis s. clitoridis des Hundes. Anat. Anz. *118* (1966):193–208.

31. Noordsy, J. L., D. M. Trotter, D. L. Carnahan, and J. G. Vestweber: Etiology of hematoma of the penis in beef bulls—A clinical survey. *In* McFeely, R. A. and E. I. Williams (eds.) VIth Intern Congr. on Cattle Dis. 1970, Am. Ass. Bovine Pract. pp. 333–338.

32. Pearson, H. and B. M. Q. Weaver: Priapism after sedation, neuroleptanalgesia and anesthesia in the horse. Eq. Vet. J. *10* (1978):85–90.

33. Pettit, G. D.: Perineal hernia in the dog. Cornell Vet. *52* (1962):261–279.

34. Purohit, R. C. and S. D. Beckett: Penile pressures and muscle activity associated with erection and ejaculation in the dog. Am. J. Physiol. *231* (1976):1343–1348.

35. Redlich, G.: Das Corpus penis des Katers und seine Erektionsveränderung, eine funktionell-anatomische Studie. Gegenbaur's Morph. Jahrb. *104* (1963):561–584.

36. Seidel, G. E. and R. H. Foote: Motion picture analysis of bovine ejaculation. J. Dairy Sci. *50* (1967):970–971.

37. Spurgeon, T. L. and R. L. Kitchell: Electrophysiological studies of the cutaneous innervation of the external genitalia of the male dog. Zentralbl. Veternärmed. C. *11* (1982):289–306.

38. Stone, E. A.: Surgical management of urolithiasis. Comp. Cont. Ed. *3* (1981):627–635.

39. Thrall, D. E.: Radiographic aspects of prostatic disease in the dog. Comp. Cont. Ed. *3* (1981):718–724.

40. Walker, D. F.: Deviations of bovine penis. JAVMA *145* (1964):677–682.

41. Watson, J. W.: Mechanism of erection and ejaculation in the bull and ram. Nature *204* (1964):95–96.

42. Wheat, J. D.: Penile paralysis in stallions given Propiopromazine. JAVMA *198* (1966):405–406.

43. Wilson, G. P. and J. W. Harrison: Perineal urethrostomy in cats. JAVMA *159* (1971):1789–1793.

44. Wolfe, D. F., R. S. Hudson, and D. F. Walker: Common penile and preputial problems in bulls. Comp. Cont. Ed. *5* (1983):S447–S455.

45. Young, S. L., R. S. Hudson, and D. F. Walker: Impotence in bulls due to vascular shunts from the corpus cavernosum penis. JAVMA *171* (1977):643–648.

CHAPTER 29

TESTIS, SCROTUM, AND CORD

OBJECTIVES

1. To be able to palpate the epididymis and differentiate it from the testis. This is necessary for the diagnosis of epididymitis and disease of the testis. It requires a knowledge of the orientation of the testis in the scrotum in each species.
2. To be able to crush or ligate the artery of the testis in castration. To know the origin and course of the testicular vessels and the lymph nodes that receive the testicular lymphatics.
3. To know that the nerves of the testis, like the vessels, are separate from those of the scrotum. Anesthesia of the testis requires an injection into the spermatic cord and will not affect the site of incision in the scrotum.
4. To know the components of the spermatic cord and be able to palpate it from the superficial inguinal ring to the testis.
5. In connection with vasectomy of teaser animals, one should be able to find the ductus deferens. It is on the medial side of the cord except in ruminants, where it is on the cranial side.
6. To know the layers of the tunica vaginalis and which layer is incised in open castration.
7. To know the layers of the scrotum and its blood and nerve supply.

29a. TESTIS AND SCROTUM, STALLION

The wall of the scrotum is composed of skin and the tunica dartos—a layer of connective tissue and smooth muscle. The dartos is very closely adherent to the skin and is cut with the skin in castration. It also forms the scrotal septum.

The external pudendal blood vessels supply the scrotum. The nerves are derived from the iliohypogastric (L 1), ilioinguinal (L 2), genitofemoral (mostly L 3, partly L 2 and L 4), and superficial perineal (S 2 to S 5). These vessels and nerves descend into the scrotum, outside the tunica vaginalis. The lymphatics of the scrotum go to the superficial inguinal lymph nodes. The cremasteric artery from the external iliac supplies the cremaster muscle.

The testis of the horse lies in the scrotum with its long axis almost parallel with the vertebral column. The capsule of the testis, the tunica albuginea, is covered by a serous coat, the visceral layer of the vaginal tunic. When the testis is removed in open castration, it is still covered by the visceral layer of the tunic; only the parietal layer has been opened. (If the knife goes into the parenchyma of the testis, the visceral layer and the tunica albuginea to which it is fused are cut at the same time, but they are not peeled off the testis.) In a closed castration, the vaginal tunic is not incised but is stripped out of the spermatic fascia intact and ligated or crushed with the enclosed cord. The distinction between open and closed castration is whether or not the vaginal cavity, a diverticulum of the peritoneal cavity, is opened before the testis is removed.

The epididymis is attached to the dorsal border of the testis and overlaps the lateral surface slightly, forming a testicular bursa between the epididymis and the testis. The epididymis is enlarged at both ends. The head is attached to the cranial end of the testis where it is continuous with the rete testis. The tail is attached to the caudal end by the proper ligament and is continuous with the ductus deferens (see Fig. 29–1). Like the testis, the epididymis is covered by a serous coat, the visceral layer of the vaginal tunic. The fold between the testis and the tail of the epididymis is the proper ligament of the testis. The ligament of the tail of the epididymis is the thickened distal free border of the mesorchium. It connects the tail of the epididymis to the parietal layer of the tunic. The mesorchium is the homologue of the mesovarium, the fold of serous membrane containing the testicular vessels and nerves. It extends from the origin of the testicular vessels from the aorta and caudal vena cava or renal vein to the testis. In the spermatic cord proximal to the epididymis, the mesoductus deferens is attached to the medial side of the mesorchium. The thin part of the mesorchium between the mesoductus deferens and the parietal layer of the tunic may be called the mesofuniculus.

In open castration, many operators incise the parietal layer of the vaginal tunic over the cranial end of the testis and evert the tunic, exposing the testis. They perforate the mesofuniculus and grasp the ligament of the tail of the epididymis with one finger. This provides a grip on the testis and vaginal tunic as the spermatic fascia is stripped off the tunic to the level of the superficial inguinal ring. In young horses, the emasculator is placed around the outside of the entire parietal tunic. In older horses, the parietal layer is incised up to the superficial inguinal ring, and the mesorchium is separated from the mesoductus deferens. One emasculator is placed around the testicular vessels and the other is placed around the ductus deferens, cremaster, and vaginal tunic. Thus, the entire tunic is severed and removed with the testis in either the open or closed method. Various methods of castration have been well described, including an aseptic technique with primary closure.[1, 3]

The proper ligament of the testis and the ligament of the tail of the epididymis are remnants of the gubernaculum testis. The descent of the testis and cryptorchidism are discussed in Chapter 21.

The spermatic cord comprises the following elements:

1. Testicular artery. It has a flexuous course in the mesorchium, runs caudally on the epididymal border of the testis, turns ventrally around the caudal end, and runs cranially on the free border, giving off branches to the lateral and medial surfaces.

2. Testicular vein. In the horse, dog, and cat, it may be a branch of the renal vein. Its branches form the pampiniform plexus around the artery.

3. Lymphatics of the testis and epididymis ascend directly to the medial iliac and lumbar lymph nodes.

4. The testicular plexus of autonomic and visceral sensory nerves accompanies the vessels.

5. The ductus deferens ascends from the tail of the epididymis. It is attached by the meso-ductus to the medial side of the mesorchium in all domestic mammals, except ruminants, where it is attached to the cranial side of the mesorchium because of the rotated position of the testis (Fig. 29–1). The ductus deferens is supplied by a special deferential artery from the umbilical artery.

6. Visceral layer of the tunica vaginalis. This is the serous covering of structures 1 to 5.

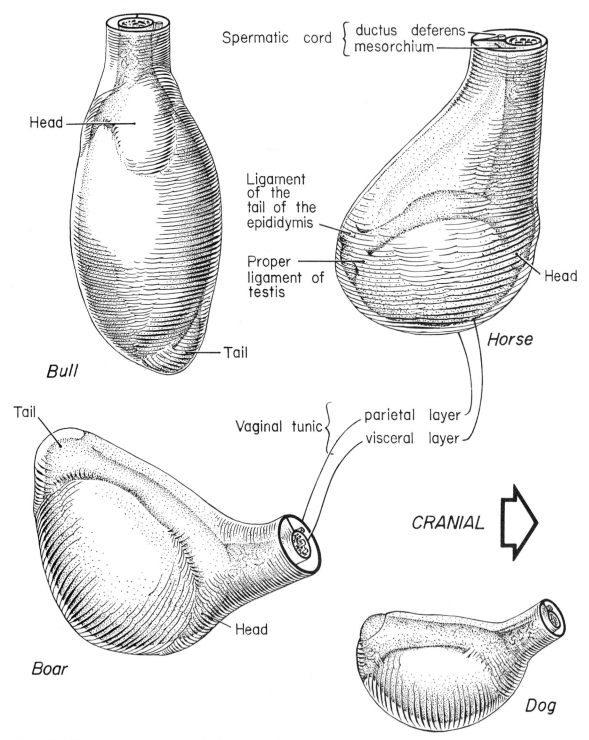

Figure 29–1. Right testis and vaginal tunic, lateral view. The head and tail of the epididymis are labeled. The cremaster is not shown.

Covering the spermatic cord, but technically not included in it, are the parietal layer of the tunic, the cremaster muscle and cremasteric fascia, and the internal and external spermatic fasciae. The latter are separated by the cremaster, but the distinction between the layers of fascia has no practical importance. Most of the spermatic fascia is stripped off of the vaginal tunic in castration.

Torsion of the spermatic cord has been associated with an elongate epididymis, mesoepididymis, proper ligament of the testis, and ligament of the tail of the epididymis.[4] These elongated structures resemble the normal anatomical relationships that occur during the descent of the testis.

29b. TESTIS AND SCROTUM, BULL

The tunica dartos of the bovine scrotum is thick. The cremaster is large, and the spermatic fascia is thick.

The testis is elongated and the long axis is vertical, so that the head of the epididymis is dorsal and the tail is ventral. The epididymal border of the testis of ruminants is medial and the free border is lateral (Fig. 29–1). Compared with the horse, the ruminant testis is rotated first on its short axis through 90° and then on its long axis through 90°.

Examine a cast of the testicular artery. After a convoluted course in the spermatic cord, the artery passes along the caudolateral border of the epididymis and around the ventral end of the testis to the free border, where, unlike that of the carnivores, swine, and horse, it immediately divides into several sinuous branches. Straight branches may be seen passing into the gland. The small arteries in the cord are the convoluted accessory artery of the testis and the long epididymal artery.

The head of the epididymis covers the dorsal end of the testis. The body lies on the caudal side of the medial border of the testis, and the tail is attached to the ventral end. The ligament of the tail of the epididymis is attached to the parietal layer of the vaginal tunic. There is only one duct in the epididymis of any species, and its convolutions do not anastomose. Excision of any part of the body or tail of the epididymis will interrupt the flow of sperm. This may be done intentionally, as in the sterilization of teaser bulls by cutting off the tail of the epididymis, or accidentally when biopsy of the testis is intended.

The spermatic cord has the same components as that of the horse. The ductus deferens, originating from the tail of the epididymis in the fundus of the scrotum, must run dorsally the full length of the testis on the cranial side of the epididymis before reaching the spermatic cord. It is accessible here for vasectomy, which can be performed bilaterally through a single cranial midscrotal incision.[2]

Local anesthesia for humane castration should include injection into the spermatic cord as well as subcutaneous infiltration at the site of the scrotal incision.

29c. TESTIS AND SCROTUM, BOAR

The scrotum of the boar is close to the ischial arch. The long axis of the testis is directed dorsocaudally. The epididymis lies on the dorsocranial border of the testis, head down. The tail of the epididymis is attached by its ligament and fascia to the dorsocaudal extremity of the scrotum.

29d. TESTIS AND SCROTUM, DOG.

The long axis of the canine testis is slightly inclined dorsocaudally. The epididymis lies on the dorsal border of the testis. The tail of the epididymis is prominent and palpable on the caudal end of the testis in the live animal. In the dog and cat, the tip of the tail of the epididymis is not covered by the vaginal tunic but is weakly adherent to the spermatic fascia. The ligament of the tail of the epididymis is represented by the tough annular reflection of the visceral to the parietal tunic around this area of adhesion. The ductus deferens runs cranially on the medial side of the epididymis.

A specific type of male pseudohermaphrodism occurs in Miniature Schnauzers in which these cytogenetically male (XY) dogs have testes that are usually retained but are attached to the ends of uterine horns. If a testis is in the scrotum, the uterine horn may be palpated in the spermatic cord.[6]

29e. MALE GENITALIA, CAT

The scrotum is close to the anus and dorsal to the prepuce. The long axis of the testis is directed dorsocaudally. The spermatic cord is very long, as in the boar.

29f. LIVE CAT

Locate the spermatic cord ventral to the pelvis, where the ductus deferens can be exposed for vasectomy. Palpate the tail of the epididymis on the caudal pole of the testis, where intraepididymal injection of a sclerosing agent will produce sterilization.[5]

References

1. Heinze, C. D.: Methods of equine castration. JAVMA *148* (1966):428–432.
2. Lofstedt, R. M.: Vasectomy in ruminants: a cranial midscrotal approach. JAVMA *181* (1982):373–375.
3. Lowe, J. E. and R. Dougherty: Castration of horses and ponies by a primary closure method. JAVMA *160* (1972):183–185.
4. Pascoe, J. R., T. V. Ellenburg, M. R. Culbertson, et al.: Torsion of the spermatic cord in the horse. JAVMA *178* (1981):242–245.
5. Pineda, M. H. and M. P. Dooley: Surgical and chemical vasectomy in the cat. Am. J. Vet. Res. *45* (1984):291–300.
6. Marshall, L. S., M. L. Oehlert, M. E. Haskins, et al.: Persistent Müllerian duct syndrome in Miniature Schnauzers. JAVMA *181* (1982):798–801.

APPENDIX

The following tables of skeletal development list the ossification centers for the horse and the dog and cat along with the approximate age at which growth plate closure is observed on radiographs.

Table 1. SKELETAL DEVELOPMENT, HORSE

Ossification Centers at (or After) Birth	Approximate Age at Growth Plate Closure Observed on Radiographs
Vertebrae, except C 1, C 2	
Cranial epiphysis _ _ _ _ _ _ _ _ _	2–3 Y[5, 6]
Body	
Caudal epiphysis _ _ _ _ _ _ _ _ _	4.5–6 Y[2, 6] (some incomplete ventrally)
Two sides of arch	
Epiphysis of spinous process _ _ _ _ _ _	7–15 Y[4]
Constant on T 2–T 5,	
Occasional on T 6–T 9 (6–12 M)	
Atlas	
Ventral arch _ _ _ _ _ _ _ _ _ _	6 M[3]
Two sides of dorsal arch _ _ _ _ _ _ _	6 M[3]
Axis	
Dens and cranial articular surface_ _ _ _ _	7–9 M[5]
Intercentrum _ _ _ _ _ _ _ _ _ _	2–4 Y[3, 5]
Body	
Caudal epiphysis _ _ _ _ _ _ _ _ _	5 Y[5]
Two sides of arch	
Thoracic Limb	
Scapula	
Dorsal border (9–12 M) _ _ _ _ _ _	after 3 Y[3]
Body	
Supraglenoid tubercle and coracoid _ _ _	10–12 M[2]
process	
Cranial part of ventral angle _ _ _ _ _	12 M[3]
Humerus	
Major tubercle _ _ _ _ _ _ _ _ _ _ _	2–3 Y[1]
Proximal epiphysis (head and minor tubercle)_ _	18–30 M[1]
Diaphysis	
Distal epiphysis _ _ _ _ _ _ _ _ _ _	14–21 M[1, 3]
Medial epicondyle _ _ _ _ _ _ _ _ _	6–12 M[1]
Radius	
Proximal epiphysis_ _ _ _ _ _ _ _ _ _	14–21 M[1, 3]
Diaphysis	
Distal epiphysis _ _ _ _ _ _ _ _ _ _	22–32 M[1, 3]
Styloid process (distal ulna) _ _ _ _ _ _	2–9 M[1, 3] (usually incomplete, may never close)
Ulna	
Olecranon tubercle (12 M)_ _ _ _ _ _ _	23–37 M[1]
Diaphysis	
Carpus	
One center for each bone	
Metacarpal III	
Proximal epiphysis_ _ _ _ _ _ _ _ _ _	before birth
Diaphysis	
Distal epiphysis _ _ _ _ _ _ _ _ _ _	6–12 M[1, 3]
Digit	
Phalanx I	
Proximal epiphysis _ _ _ _ _ _ _	6–9 M[1, 3]
Diaphysis	
Distal epiphysis _ _ _ _ _ _ _ _	before birth to 1 M[3]

Table 1. SKELETAL DEVELOPMENT, HORSE *(continued)*

Ossification Centers at (or After) Birth	Approximate Age at Growth Plate Closure Observed on Radiographs
Phalanx II	
Proximal epiphysis — — — — — — —	6–9 M[1,3]
Diaphysis	
Distal epiphysis — — — — — — — —	by birth[3]
Phalanx III	
One center	
Pelvic Limb	
Os coxae	
Ilium ⎫	
Ischium ⎬ — — — — — — — — —	10–12 M[2,3] (18–24 M[1])
Pubis ⎭	
Iliac crest ⎫	
Tuber coxae ⎪	
Ischiatic tuberosity ⎬ — — — — —	4–5 Y[2,3]
Caudal border ischium ⎪	
Acetabular bone ⎭	
Pelvic symphysis	inconstant closure
Femur	
Third trochanter	
Major trochanter — — — — — — — —	18–30 M[1]
Head — — — — — — — — — — —	24–36 M[1]
Diaphysis	
Distal epiphysis — — — — — — — —	21–30 M[1,3]
Tibia	
Tibial tuberosity ⎫ — — — — 8–14 M[1] ⎫	
Proximal epiphysis ⎭	⎬ 23–38 M[1,3]
Diaphysis — — — — — — — — — — ⎭	
Distal epiphysis — — — — — — — —	16–25 M[1]
Lateral malleolus (distal fibula) — — — — —	3–6 M[1,3]
Fibula	
Proximal epiphysis (after birth) — — — — —	may never close
Body (after birth)	
Tarsus	
Calcaneus	
Tuber calcanei — — — — — — —	19–30 M[1,3]
Diaphysis	
Tarsals I and II — — — — — — — —	before birth
Other tarsal bones	
One center for each	

1. Adams, O. R.: Lameness in Horses. 3rd Ed. Philadelphia: Lea & Febiger, 1974.
2. Barone, R.: Anatomie comparée des mammifères domestiques. Volume 1. Osteology. 2nd. ed. Paris: Vigot, 1976.
3. Getty, R.: Sisson and Grossman's The Anatomy of the Domestic Animals. 5th Ed. Philadelphia: W. B. Saunders, 1975.
4. Hertsch, B. and E. Grimmelmann: Röntgenologische Untersuchungen der Ossifikations-vorgänge am Widerrist beim Pferd. Zentralbl. Veterinärmed. (A) *26* (1979):191–200.
5. Hertsch, B. and A. El S. Ragab: Röntgenologische Untersuchungen der Epiphysen-fugenschliessung an den Halswirbeln beim Pferd. Berl. Münch. Tierärztl. Wochenschr. *90* (1977):172–176.
6. Rendano, V. T. and C. B. Quick: Equine radiology, the cervical spine. Mod. Vet. Pract. *59* (1978):921–927.

Table 2. SKELETAL DEVELOPMENT, DOG AND CAT

Ossification Centers at (or After) Birth	Approximate Age at Growth Plate Closure Observed on Radiographs	
	Dog	Cat[6]
Vertebrae, except C 1, C 2		
Cranial epiphysis (2–8 W) — — — — — — —	7–14 M[2]	
Body		
Caudal epiphysis (2–8 W) — — — — — — —	7–14 M[2]	
Two sides of arch		
Atlas		
Ventral arch		
Two sides of dorsal arch — — — — — — —	4 M[3]	
Axis		
Apex of dens (3–4 M) — — — — — — — —	3–4 M[3]	
Dens and cranial articular surface — — — — —	7–9 M[3]	
Intercentrum (3 W) — — — — — — — — —	4 M[3]	
Body		
Caudal epiphysis (3 W) — — — — — — —	7–9 M[3]	
Two sides of arch — — — — — — — —	3 M[3]	
Thoracic Limb		
Scapula		
Body		
Supraglenoid tubercle (7 W) — — — — —	3–7 M[4, 8] — — — — — — — — —	3.5–4 M
Humerus		
Proximal epiphysis (1–2 W) (head and tubercles) —	10–15 M[4, 8] — — — — — — — —	18–24 M
Diaphysis		
Distal epiphysis — — — — — — — — — —	5–8 M[4, 8] — — — — — — — —	4 M
Lateral part of condyle (2–3 W) } — — — —	5 M[7] — — — — — — — —	3.5 M
Medial part of condyle (2–3 W)		
Medial epicondyle (6–8 W) — — — — — —	5–6 M[7, 9] — — — — — — —	4 M
Lateral epicondyle — — — — — — —	at birth — — — — — — — —	3.5 M
Radius		
Proximal epiphysis (3–5 W) — — — — — —	5–11 M[4, 8] — — — — — — —	5–7 M
Diaphysis		
Distal epiphysis (2–4 W) — — — — — —	6–12 M[4, 8] — — — — — — —	14–22 M
Ulna		
Olecranon tubercle (6–8 W) — — — — — —	5–10 M[4, 7, 8, 9] — — — — — —	9–13 M
Diaphysis		
Anconeal process (12 W)* — — — — —	3–5 M[10]	
Distal epiphysis (6–8 W) — — — — — —	6–12 M[4, 8, 9] — — — — —	14–25 M
Carpus		
Radial carpal (3–4 W)		
Three centers — — — — — — — —	3–4 M[1, 4, 5]	
Accessory Carpal		
Diaphysis (3 W)		
Epiphysis (7 W) — — — — — — —	3–6 M[1, 4, 7, 8] — — — — — — —	4 M
Other carpal bones		
One center each		
Metacarpus		
Metacarpal I		
Proximal epiphysis (5 W) — — — — — —	6–7 M[4]	
Diaphysis		
Metacarpal II–V		
Diaphysis		
Distal epiphysis (4 W) — — — — — — —	5–7 M[4, 7, 8] — — — — — — — —	7–10 M
Digit		
Phalanx I and II		
Proximal epiphysis (4–5 W) — — — — — —	5–7 M[1, 4, 8, 9] — — — — — — —	4–5.5 M
Diaphysis		
Phalanx III		
One center		

Table 2. SKELETAL DEVELOPMENT, DOG AND CAT *(continued)*

Ossification Centers at (or After) Birth	Approximate Age at Growth Plate Closure Observed on Radiographs	
	Dog	**Cat** [6]
Pelvic Limb *(continued)*		
Os coxae		
Ilium		
Ischium	4–6 M [1, 4, 9]	
Pubis		
Acetabular bone (7 W)		
Iliac crest (4 M)	15 M–5.5 Y [4]	
Ischiatic tuberosity, caudal border of ischium (3 M)	8–14 M [4, 9]	
Caudal pelvic symphysis (7 M) (interischiatic bone)	15 M–5 Y [4, 9]	
Pelvic symphysis closure (cranial to caudal)	2.5–6 Y [4]	
Femur		
Minor trochanter (8 W)	8–13 M [1, 4, 9]	8–11 M
Major trochanter (8 W) } 6–9 M [4, 8]		
Head (2 W)	6–12 M [4, 8]	7–10 M
Diaphysis		
Distal epiphysis (3 W)	6–12 M [4, 8]	13–19 M
Trochlea (3 W)	3M [9]	
Patella (9 W) [9]		
Tibia		
Tibial tuberosity (8 W)	8–10 M	
Proximal epiphysis (3 W) } 6–9 M [4, 9]		
Diaphysis	6–15 M [4, 7, 8]	12–18 M
Distal epiphysis (3 W)	5–11 M [4, 8]	10–13 M
Medial malleolus (3 M)	4–5 M [4, 9]	
Fibula		
Proximal epiphysis (9 W)	6–12 M [4, 9]	13–18 M
Diaphysis		
Distal epiphysis (2–7 W)	5–13 M [4, 8]	10–14 M
Sesamoids		
Gastrocnemius m. (3 M dog [9], 2.5–4 M cat [1])		
Popliteus m. (3 M dog [9], 4–5 M cat [1])		
Tarsus		
Calcaneus		
Tuber calcanei (6 W)	3–8 M [4, 7, 8, 9]	7–13 M
Diaphysis		
Other tarsal bones (2–4 W)		
One center each		
Metatarsus		
Diaphysis		
Distal epiphysis (4 W)	5–7 M [4, 8]	8–11 M
Digit similar to thoracic limb		

*Not a separate ossification center in all dogs. Growth plate closes at 14 to 15 weeks in Greyhounds, 16 to 20 weeks in German Shepherds.

1. Chapman, W. L.: Appearance of ossification centers and epiphyseal closures as determined by radiographic techniques. JAVMA *147* (1965):138–141.
2. Hare, W. C. D.: Zur Ossifikation und Vereinigung der Wirbelepiphysen beim Hund. Wien. Tierärztl. Monat. *48* (1961):210–215.
3. Hare, W. C. D.: Radiographic anatomy of the cervical region of the canine vertebral column. JAVMA *139* (1961):209–220.
4. Hare, W. C. D.: The age at which epiphyseal union takes place in the limb bones of the dog. Wien. Tierärztl. Monat. *9* (1972):224–245.
5. Pomriaskynski-Kobozieff, N. and N. Kobozieff: Etude radiologique de l'aspect du squelette normal de la main du chien aux divers Stades de son évolution de la naissance à l'âge adult. Rec. Méd. Vét. *130* (1954): 617–646.
6. Smith, R. N.: Fusion of ossification centers in the cat. J. Small Anim. Pract. *10* (1969):523–530.
7. Smith, R. N. and J. Allcock: Epiphyseal fusion in the Greyhound. Vet. Rec. *72* (1960):75–79.
8. Sumner-Smith, G.: Observations on the epiphyseal fusion of the canine appendicular skeleton. J. Small Anim. Pract. *7* (1966):303–311.
9. Ticer, J. W.: Radiographic Technique in Small Animal Practice. Philadelphia: W. B. Saunders, 1975, p. 101.
10. Van Sickle, D. The relationship of ossification to elbow dysplasia. Anim. Hosp. *2* (1966):24–31.

INDEX

Page numbers in *italics* refer to illustrations; a t following a page number indicates a table.